Problems in Anesthesia: Cardiothoracic Surgery

In loving memory of
Derek Sydney Hardy (1938–2000)

Problems in Anesthesia: Cardiothoracic Surgery

Edited by

Joseph E Arrowsmith, MD, MRCP (UK), FRCA

Consultant Anaesthetist
Papworth Hospital
Cambridge, UK

John Simpson, MB, FRCA

Honorary Consultant Anaesthetist
Royal Brompton Hospital
London, UK

informa
healthcare

New York London

CONTENTS

LIST OF CONTRIBUTORS

Joseph E Arrowsmith
Anaesthesia
Papworth Hospital
Papworth Everard
Cambridge CB3 8RE, UK

Matthew J Barnard
Anaesthesia
The Heart Hospital
University College London Hospitals
London W1N 8AA, UK

David J Bihari
Intensive Care Unit
Prince of Wales Hospital
Randwick, NSW 2031, Australia

Christopher J Broomhead
Department of Anaesthesia
The London Chest Hospital
Bonner Road
London E2 9JX, UK

Michelle J Capdeville
Cardiothoracic Anesthesia
Case Western Reserve University School of
Medicine
11100 Euclid Avenue
Lakeside 2531
Cleveland, OH 44106-5007, USA

Alan M Cohen
Department of Anaesthesia
Bristol Royal Infirmary
Marlborough Street
Bristol BS2 8HW, UK

M Peter Colvin
Department of Anaesthesia
The London Chest Hospital
Bonner Road
London E2 9JX, UK

Heather P Duncan
Paediatric Intensive Care Unit
Bristol Royal Hospital for Children
Upper Maudlin Street
Bristol BS2 8BJ, UK

John Dunning
Cardiothoracic Surgery
Papworth Hospital
Papworth Everard
Cambridge CB3 8RE, UK

David JR Duthie
Department of Anaesthesia
Leeds General Infirmary
Great George Street
Leeds LS1 3EX, UK

Andrew I Gardner
Anaesthesia
Sir Charles Gairdner Hospital
Hospital Street
Nedlands, Western Australia 6009, Australia

Shane George
Department of Anaesthesiology
Royal Brompton and Harefield NHS Trust
Sydney Street
London, SW3 6NP, UK

Neville M Gibbs
Department of Anaesthesia
Sir Charles Gairdner Hospital
Hospital Street
Nedlands, Western Australia 6009, Australia

Fiona M Gibson
Anaesthesia
Royal Hospital Trust
Belfast BT12 6BA, Northern Ireland, UK

Stuart J Gold
Department of Anaesthesia
Leicester Royal Infirmary
Leicester LE1 5WW, UK

Andrew A Grace
Cardiology
Papworth Hospital
Papworth Everard
Cambridge CB3 8RE, UK

Catherine R Grebenik
Oxford Heart Centre
John Radcliffe Hospital
Headley Way
Oxford OX3 9DU, UK

Katherine P Grichnik
Cardiothoracic Anesthesia
Duke Heart Center
Box 3094, Duke University Medical Center
Durham, NC 27710, USA

Alina M Grigore
Texas Heart Institute
Room O-250
6720 Bertner Street
Houston, TX 77030, USA

Hilary P Grocott
Cardiothoracic Anesthesia and Critical Care
Medicine
Box 3094, Duke University Medical Center
Durham, NC 27710, USA

Ian Hardy
Department of Anaesthesia
Papworth Hospital
Papworth Everard
Cambridge CB3 8RE, UK

Elaine L Hill
Oxford Heart Centre
John Radcliffe Hospital
Headley Way
Oxford OX3 9DU, UK

Cindy Horst
University Department of Anaesthesia
Glenfield Hospital
Groby Road
Leicester LE3 9PG, UK

Eric Jacobsohn
Department of Anaesthesology and Critical Care
Washington University School of Medicine
Campus Box 8054
660 South Euclid Avenue
St Louis, MO 63110–1093, USA

John D Kneeshaw
Department of Anaesthesia
Papworth Hospital
Papworth Everard
Cambridge CB3 8RE, UK

Colleen Gorman Koch
Department of Cardiothoracic Anesthesia G-3
The Cleveland Clinic Foundation
9500 Euclid Avenue
Cleveland, OH 44195, USA

Marc de Kock
Anesthesiology
Cliniques Universitaires St Luc
Avenue Hippocrates 0.1821
1200 Brussels, Belgium

Raymond D Latimer
Department of Anaesthesia
Papworth Hospital
Papworth Everard
Cambridge CB3 8RE, UK

Trevor WR Lee
Department of Anaesthesology and Critical Care
Medicine
University of Manitoba Health Sciences Center
GE 706-820 Sherbrooke Street
Winnipeg, Manitoba R3A 1R9, Canada

A Timothy Lovell
University Department of Anaesthesia
Bristol Royal Infirmary
Marlborough Street
Bristol BS2 8HW, UK

Gregory R McAnulty
Anaesthesia and Cardiothoracic Intensive Care
St George's Hospital
Blackshaw Road
London SW17 0QT, UK

William T McBride
Cardiothoracic Anaesthesia
Royal Victoria Hospital
Belfast BT12 6BN, Northern Ireland, UK

Helena M McKeague
Cardiothoracic Anaesthesia and Intensive Care
General Infirmary at Leeds
Great George Street
Leeds LS1 3EX, UK

Mark Messent
Department of Anaesthesia
The London Chest Hospital
Bonner Road
London E2 9JX, UK

Berend Mets
Department of Anaesthesiology
PH5 Stem
Columbia University
CPMC 630 West 168 Street
New York, NY 10032, USA

Sheena A Millar
Department of Anaesthesia
Papworth Hospital
Papworth Everard
Cambridge CB3 8RE, UK

Rosalind J Mills
Department of Anaesthesia
Yorkshire Heart Centre
Leeds General Infirmary
Great George Street
Leeds LS1 3EX, UK

Peter J Murphy
Paediatric Intensive Care Unit
Bristol Royal Hospital for Children
Paul O'Gorman Building
Upper Maudlin Street
Bristol BS2 8BJ, UK

Vilas U Navapurkar
Department of Anaesthesia and Intensive Care
Addenbrooke's Hospital
Hills Road
Cambridge CB2 2QQ, UK

Roddy O'Donnell
Paediatric Intensive Care Unit
Box 7
Adenbrooke's Hospital
Hills Road
Cambridge CB2 2QQ, UK

Michael J O'Leary
Intensive Care Unit
St George Hospital
Gray Street
Kogarah, NSW 2217, Australia

Martin J Platt
Department of Anaesthesia
The London Chest Hospital
Bonner Road
London E2 9JX, UK

M Krishna Prasad
Department of Anaesthesia
Papworth Hospital
Papworth Everard
Cambridge CB3 8RE, UK

Stephen J Pryn
Department of Anaesthesia and Critical Care
Bristol Royal Infirmary
Bristol BS2 8HW, UK

Bernhard JCJ Riedel
Department of Anesthesiology
University of Texas MD Anderson Cancer Center
1515 Holcombe Boulevard, Box 42
Houston, TX 77030, USA

Andrew J Ritchie
Cardiothoracic Surgery
Papworth Hospital
Papworth Everard
Cambridge CB3 8RE, UK

Gary W Roach
Kaiser Permanente Medical Center
2425 Geary Boulevard
San Francisco, CA 94705, USA

Christopher J Rozario
Department of Anaesthesia
Papworth Hospital
Papworth Everard
Cambridge CB3 8RE, UK

Rana A Sayeed
Cardiothoracic Surgery
Papworth Hospital
Papworth Everard
Cambridge CB3 8RE, UK

Ajeet D Sharma
Anesthesiology
Prince George Regional Hospital
2000 15th Avenue
Prince George, BC V2M 2S2, Canada

Andrew D Shaw
Division of Anesthesiology and Critical Care
University of Texas MD Anderson Cancer Center
1515 Holcombe Boulevard, Box 42
Houston, TX 77030, USA

Avinash C Shukla
Department of Anaesthesia
The London Chest Hospital
Bonner Road
London E2 9JX, UK

Virinder S Sidhu
Anaesthesia
St Mary's Hospital
Praed Street
Paddington
London W2 1NY, UK

John C Simpson
Anaesthesia
Royal Brompton Hospital
Sydney Street
London SW3 6NP, UK

Thomas F Slaughter
Anesthesiology
Box 3094
Duke University Medical Center
Durham, NC 27710, USA

Gautam Sreeram
Anesthesiology
Box 3094, Duke University Medical Center
Durham, NC 27710, USA

Mark Stafford-Smith
Anesthesiology
Box 3094, Duke University Medical Center
Durham, NC 27710, USA

David P Stansfield
University of Michigan Health System
CS Mott Children's Hospital
Section of Pediatric Anesthesiology
1500 East Medical Center Drive
Ann Arbor, MI 48109-2011, USA

Justiaan LC Swanevelder
University Department of Anaesthesia
Glenfield Hospital
Groby Road
Leicester LE3 9PG, UK

Sally Tomkins
Department of Anaesthesia
Bristol Royal Infirmary
Marlborough Street
Bristol BS2 8HW, UK

Alain Vuylsteke
Anaesthesia and Intensive Care
Papworth Hospital
Papworth Everard
Cambridge CB3 8RE, UK

Andrew R Wolf
Paediatric Intensive Care Unit
Bristol Royal Hospital for Children
Upper Maudlin Street
Bristol BS2 8BJ, UK

Susan J Wright
Department of Anaesthesia
University College Hospitals
London W1N 8AA, UK

FOREWORD

Cardiothoracic surgery anesthesia has become more complex as a more diverse set of conditions are now treated surgically, and as technology has changed so that very different approaches to even common problems can be used. This book brings to the reader a better understanding of the breadth and depth of modern-day cardiothoracic anesthesiology.

This essayist believes that the best way to learn is from experience. The experience need not be first-hand, but can be learned from others. The format of this book is to present a case and then an approach to the case. Some of the cases and topics are the result of things that did not go well. One always learns more from complications and problem cases because there is generally a lesson on what not to do. When things go completely well there is no lesson and one is left wondering what, out of the many things done, was the difference between success and failure. Many of the topics covered in the book are here because the authors have learned from their experiences what to do and, more importantly, what not to do!

The format of the chapters makes for an organized and helpful presentation. The case-based teaching relates the material to the clinic and the discussion explains the options in approach. The conclusion of each chapter highlights the essential tips in dealing with the various cases. The cases themselves range from the common (for example, off-pump coronary artery bypass) to the rather rare (for example, anesthetic management of the patient with carcinoid heart disease). There are many topics, all important to the current-day practitioner.

A final point about this book is that, unlike many textbooks, it has a generous representation of anesthesiologists (anesthetists) from both sides of the Atlantic. This is a vitally important aspect of the book because it shows that, despite our global knowledge and the information age in which we live, we still have variable practices. It is reassuring to know that medicine has still not advanced to the point where there is only one way to do things, particularly in difficult cases as most of these are. This leaves room for more investigation and continued advancement of the field.

JG Reves
Professor of Anesthesiology
Dean School of Medicine
Vice President for Medical Affairs
Medical University of South Carolina
Charleston, SC, USA

INTRODUCTION

'Up from the ashes, grow the roses of success' (R & R Sherman in *Chitty Chitty, Bang Bang*, MGM, 1968)

Cynics have described anesthesiology as '99% boredom and 1% sheer terror'. It is perhaps fortunate that few patients share this perception. Experience has taught the anesthesiologist to expect, and prepare for, the worst-case scenario. With luck he will learn, not from his own misfortune, but from the successes and failures of others. 'It's hard to learn ...', Reves and Hall remind us in *Common Problems in Cardiac Anesthesia*, '... when all goes well.

In this volume an international panel of authors have used illustrative case histories to describe a wide variety of problems encountered in the practice of modern cardiothoracic anesthesia. The brief was simple – present a case history, describe how you dealt with the problem, reveal the outcome and justify your course of action. Other than seeking expansion and clarification in some areas, and influencing the manner in which information has been presented, editorial 'interference' has been kept to a minimum. Although the reader, and indeed the editors, may not agree with every course of action taken, we have encouraged our contributors to support their decisions with reasoned scientific and evidence-based argument. It is the reader who must decide whether this has been achieved!

The editors come from two generations of anesthesiologists: one has used pen, paper and a wheezing fax machine; the other the full range of tools available to the 'paperless' generation. It is fortunate that most of our contributors fall into the second category and we are indebted to them for their hard work. We thank our families for their great forbearance during the preparation of this volume. Lastly we thank Annick Ireland of Martin Dunitz Ltd, and Maire Collins and Rowena Milan of Harwood Academic Publishers for their patience and encouragement.

Having digested the cases presented, we suspect that you the reader will have in mind an interesting case or clinical scenario of your own. If you would like to share your experience with others, we would encourage you to send brief details either to the publisher or by email to JArrowsmith@doctors.org.uk.

Joe Arrowsmith, Cambridge, UK
John Simpson, London, UK

1

Anesthesia for cardiac surgery during pregnancy

Elaine L Hill and Catherine R Grebenik

Introduction

In the developed world, heart disease is the leading indirect cause of maternal mortality, accounting for 39 of 134 (29%) deaths in the most recent confidential enquiry into maternal deaths (1994–1996).[1] The prevalence of heart disease during pregnancy is quoted at between 1 and 4%. The spectrum varies in different parts of the world, but the majority of cases are due to rheumatic heart disease, although the proportion due to congenital problems is increasing as survival to adult life with treated or palliated disease becomes common.[2] Bacterial endocarditis, aortic dissection and ischemic heart disease also occur in pregnant patients.

Ideally, women with known heart disease should be fully evaluated and counselled before pregnancy is considered. For example, pregnancy in women with Eisenmenger's complex is said to carry approximately 35% mortality, and is thus absolutely contraindicated. Where possible, necessary cardiac surgery should be performed either prior to pregnancy or, if the patient has sufficient cardiac reserve, delayed until after delivery. Occasionally women will require cardiac surgery during pregnancy, and there may be a conflict between maternal and fetal interests with regard to the timing of surgery and delivery. The management of these patients requires a coordinated team approach with good communication between obstetricians, cardiologists, neonatologists, anesthetists and surgeons, and a contingency plan for obstetric emergencies. Advances in neonatology, with greatly improved infant survival after premature delivery, have signifi-

cantly changed management. This should be borne in mind when counselling patients and their partners about the timing of surgery. The literature relating to cardiac surgery in pregnancy consists of case reports and series from the past 50 years, and suggests that definitive cardiac surgery during pregnancy is remarkably safe for the mother, with reasonable levels of fetal survival. Mortality rates are said to be little different from procedures performed in non-pregnant patients. This may, however, be a function of the selective reporting of successful cases. It is a brave team that reports two or more deaths from one operation.

Case History

A 28-year-old mother of three had an aortic valve replacement for congenital aortic stenosis. A porcine xenograft was used as she wished to have more children. Three years later she became pregnant, and was seen at 15 weeks gestation when the aortic prosthesis was found to be working normally. At 26 weeks gestation she was admitted to hospital with a 2-week history of malaise, tiredness, and night sweats. *Streptococcus sanguis*, sensitive to gentamicin sulphate and benzyl penicillin, was grown from blood cultures and a diagnosis of bacterial endocarditis was made. The cause of her endocarditis was unclear, but she admitted to having had a mouth abscess in early pregnancy, which she had 'lanced' with a pin.

There was no evidence of heart failure and she was managed initially with high-dose intra-

Past medical history	Aortic valve replacement 18 months earlier. Three uncomplicated pregnancies – all spontaneous vaginal deliveries.
Regular medications	Gentamicin 60 mg IV TDS, benzyl penicillin 2.4 g IV 4 hourly.
Examination	Weight 59 kg. Height 1.6 m. Pulse 106 bpm – slow upstroke. BP 98/78 mmHg. Respiratory rate 24 bpm. Persistent pyrexia $\geq$ 37.4 °C. A few scattered splinter hemorrhages and a single conjunctival hemorrhage. Gallop rhythm with high-pitched systolic murmur radiating to the carotids. Lung fields clear. Liver/spleen not palpable.
Investigations	Hb 8.4 g dl^{-1}, WBC 7.2 $\times$ 10^9 l^{-1}, platelets 267 $\times$ 10^9 l^{-1}, INR 1.1, ESR 92 mm hr^{-1}, [Na$^+$] 138 mmol l^{-1}, [K$^+$] 3.3 mmol l^{-1}, urea 16 mg dl^{-1} (5.7 mmol l^{-1}), creatinine 0.7 mg dl^{-1} (60 μmol l^{-1}). C-reactive protein 4.0 mg dl^{-1}. **ECG:** Sinus tachycardia. LV hypertrophy. PR interval 280 ms. **TTE:** Sizeable vegetations on ventricular surface of prosthetic valve cusps. Mobile vegetation seen to move into and partially obstruct valve orifice during systole. Peak systolic velocity 6 ms^{-1} equating to an outflow gradient of 144 mmHg. LV function – 'vigorous'. No aortic regurgitation.

venous antibiotics. Transthoracic echocardiography demonstrated prolific vegetations on the aortic valve, one of which prolapsed and partially obstructed the valve ring during systole. There was no aortic regurgitation, but a systolic outflow gradient of 144 mmHg was recorded. The other major concern was a progressive increase in PR interval on her electrocardiogram (ECG) suggestive of the development of abscess formation within the aortic root. Obstetric ultrasound showed satisfactory fetal growth.

A multidisciplinary approach was clearly necessary for optimal management of this difficult case. Consideration of the timing of fetal delivery had to be weighed against the risk to the mother in view of her deteriorating clinical condition, the increasing cardiovascular stress imposed by the growing fetus and consequent operative risk, and the risk of coronary or cerebral embolism from the infected prosthesis. Clearly, maternal health was the principle consideration.

There was no doubt that aortic valve re-replacement was required, but it was decided to continue antimicrobial treatment for another 2 weeks to allow the fetus to reach 28 weeks gestation, at which point the prospects of survival would be quite high. It was agreed, however, that any form of embolic event would be an indication for immediate surgery. The patient and her partner accepted this plan. Medical management and serial monitoring therefore continued for a further 2 weeks. A combined Cesarean section with tubal ligation and redo aortic valve replacement was scheduled.

On the day of surgery the patient was premedicated with ranitidine 150 mg and metoclopramide 10 mg by mouth 90 minutes preoperatively. In the anesthetic room a wedge was placed under the right flank to produce left lateral displacement of the uterus and avoid aortocaval compression. Sodium citrate 0.3M 30 ml was administered orally before induction, and intravenous access and intra-arterial blood pressure monitoring were established under local anesthesia. A pulmonary artery flotation catheter was inserted via the right internal jugular vein. Additional monitoring consisted of a five-lead ECG and a pulse oximeter. The fetal heart rate was monitored externally using ultrasonic cardiography. After preoxygenation a modified rapid sequence induction with cricoid pressure was performed, utilizing fentanyl citrate 1 mg, thiopental 125 mg and suxamethonium 100 mg. The trachea was intubated and the lungs ventilated to normocapnia with 50% oxygen in nitrous oxide and 0.5% halothane. Pancuronium 6 mg was given after intubation. A further 1 mg fentanyl was given at sternotomy, followed by another 1 mg at the start of cardiopulmonary bypass (CPB). Hemodynamic stability was adequate, with systolic pressures of between 90 and 110 mmHg before CPB. The fetal heart tracing showed no ill effects from anesthesia.

As this was a reoperative procedure, it was felt prudent to prepare for CPB before delivery of the fetus, in case there was an acute deterioration in the condition of the mother during the Cesarean section. The chest was therefore opened first and pericardial adhesions from previous surgery dissected. Purse string sutures were placed into the ascending aorta and right atrium in preparation for cannulation. At this stage, almost 2 hours after the induction of anesthesia, a routine lower segment Cesarean section was performed and a live male infant weighing 1.3 kg was delivered. The infant was intubated immediately after birth and given intramuscular naloxone. Intravenous ergometrine 0.25 mg was administered immediately after delivery. The uterus was closed in two layers with special attention being paid to hemostasis. Tubal ligation was performed and the abdominal wound left open to allow inspection of the uterus during the cardiac procedure. After full heparinization, CPB was established and the patient was cooled to 32°C. The aortic xenograft with its vegetations was removed and replaced with a Starr–Edwards mechanical prosthesis. The patient was weaned easily from CPB without inotropic support in sinus rhythm. Total CPB time was 65 minutes. Protamine was given as usual, followed by closure of the abdominal and sternotomy wounds. There was no evidence of major hemorrhage from the uterine incision. A total of 1000 ml modified gelatin solution and 5 units of blood were transfused during the procedure.

At the end of the 4-hour operation, the patient was transferred to the postoperative recovery unit where she was extubated after 1 hour. She had an uneventful postoperative course and remained in hospital for a 4-week course of intravenous antibiotic treatment. The infant was admitted to the special care baby unit, where he made satisfactory progress, and was discharged to the district general hospital at 6 weeks of age. Both mother and baby were well at 1-year follow-up.

Discussion

Physiological changes in pregnancy

The anesthetic management of the pregnant patient undergoing cardiac surgery must take account of the physiological changes of pregnancy, which will exacerbate the problems of pre-existing cardiovascular disease. Other factors to be considered include the risks of aortocaval compression in the supine position – a potential problem from about 20 weeks gestation – and acid aspiration. The possible effects of drugs on the fetus and alterations in uteroplacental blood flow must also be taken into account. Cardiothoracic anesthetists will be familiar with the important physiological changes that occur during pregnancy, but a brief summary is provided here.

There is a gradual and progressive rise in cardiac output with an increase of 40% by the third trimester; accounted for by a 30% rise in stroke volume and a 15% rise in heart rate. This increase starts early; by 8 weeks gestation cardiac output has already risen by 1 l min^{-1}. Increases in myocardial wall tension and contractility result in a further increase in myocardial oxygen demand. Total body oxygen consumption rises by 15–18%. Blood volume increases by about one-third, with plasma volume increasing more (45%) than red blood cell volume (20%) resulting in the 'physiological anemia of pregnancy'. There is a decrease in both systemic and pulmonary vascular resistance resulting in virtually unchanged pulmonary capillary wedge pressure and central venous pressure, despite the increased volume load. Systolic arterial pressure is unaltered in pregnancy, unless pre-eclampsia supervenes; diastolic blood pressure tends to fall in the first two trimesters and returns to non-pregnant levels by term. A significant fall in colloid osmotic pressure increases the likelihood of developing pulmonary edema.

Increased minute ventilation is achieved by a rise in respiratory rate associated with a fall in $PaCO_2$ and a decreased buffering capacity. Functional residual capacity falls. These changes together with splinting of the diaphragm may induce a sensation of breathlessness.

An increase in the concentrations of plasma clotting factors, fibrinogen and fibrin degradation products leads to a hypercoagulable state, so that women with mechanical heart valves are at high risk of valve thrombosis if anticoagulation is inadequate.[3,4] Coumadin and its derivatives cross the placenta and are associated with fetal teratogenicity; heparin given subcutaneously has no fetal effects but is unpleasant for the patient and liable to be associated with variable levels of anticoagulation.[5]

The pregnant patient with cardiac disease may be intolerant of these physiological changes. Stenotic valvular lesions, in particular, are poorly tolerated because of the limitation they impose on increasing cardiac output. Early onset of congestive symptoms is an ominous sign. The cardiovascular stress of pregnancy is considerable by 12 weeks gestation, is maximal by 28–32 weeks gestation, but peaks with labor, delivery and the immediate postpartum period. In labor, cardiac output increases by another 15–40% with a further 10–25% increase during uterine contractions. Autotransfusion from the contracted uterus increases cardiac output still further in the immediate postpartum period. Recovery of the cardiovascular system to preconception levels may take up to 12 weeks.[6] The likely effects on the maternal cardiovascular system influence the choice of management, in terms of medical versus surgical treatment, timing of surgery (i.e. pre- or post-delivery) and the mode and timing of delivery.

Case discussion

The case presented illustrates a successful approach to the problem of a pregnant woman who required urgent replacement of a prosthetic aortic valve. Medical management enabled cardiac surgery and operative delivery of the fetus to be delayed until week 28 of gestation. The likelihood of survival after pre-term delivery is related to both birth weight and gestational age, but is around 80–90% at 28 weeks for all but the smallest infants.[7,8] Interestingly female infants have better survival rates than males of the same weight and gestational age. Delaying surgical intervention was possible in this case, because there was no acute maternal hemodynamic decompensation, although there was an ever-present risk of systemic embolization. The major concern was the possibility of uterine hemorrhage during or after CPB – a concern that ultimately proved unfounded. Although Cesarean section has been performed on CPB,[9] in most reports of combined procedures, delivery has been performed immediately prior to

cardiac surgery and CPB.[10–13] Bleeding from the uterus does not appear to be a major problem although in one case prophylactic hysterectomy was performed before cardiac surgery.[14] The use of aprotinin has been suggested when CPB is needed in the early puerperium.[11]

Had this woman presented much earlier in pregnancy, there would have been no option other than to replace her aortic valve while hoping to preserve the fetus. The optimal gestational age for good fetal outcome after cardiac surgery is uncertain. Surgery during the first trimester of pregnancy carries a risk of spontaneous miscarriage and congenital fetal abnormality; the effects on organogenesis are unclear, although no anesthetic agent has been proven to be teratogenic.[15] Surgery in the second trimester is complicated by the risks of intrauterine fetal death and premature labor. When delivery occurs before 26 weeks gestation, fetal morbidity and mortality is substantial with a high risk of long-term neurological sequelae in survivors.

Closed mitral valvotomy during pregnancy was first reported in 1952 by two of the great pioneers in cardiac surgery.[16,17] Since then a large number of closed mitral valvotomies have been performed in pregnancy with maternal death rates of 3% or less, and fetal mortality of 10% or less.[18,19] The first report of CPB during pregnancy, published in 1959, described a patient undergoing repair of septal defect and pulmonary valve commissurotomy at 6 weeks gestation.[20] The mother survived, but the fetus spontaneously aborted 3 months later. Since then many further cases have been published.

Various authors have reviewed the collected reported outcomes of cardiac surgery with CPB during pregnancy.[21–27] The majority of these reports concern patients with valvular heart disease. The maternal death rate varies markedly according to surgical procedure, with the highest rate being 22% for aortic-arterial dissection. Pomini et al reported a 3% maternal and 20% fetal mortality rate for 69 cases performed between 1958 and 1992.[22] Weiss et al, analysing cases between 1984 and 1996, reported mortality rates of 6 and 30% respectively.[21] Extreme emergency significantly affects maternal outcome, as might be expected. Whilst many authors have observed that maternal mortality is not, or only marginally increased – compared with procedures in the non-pregnant patient –

Weiss *et al* question this and note that there may be an inherent bias in the reporting of such cases, with under-reporting of cases with poor outcomes.[21] Other authors have also remarked on this bias.[28] Even if CPB during pregnancy does not appear to cause excessive maternal risk, fetal survival is severely compromised by surgery. Nevertheless, healthy babies have been born following operations using CPB although there is little or no data on their long-term developmental outcome. Indeed, there is a report of the birth of a healthy infant even after an operation involving hypothermic total circulatory arrest.[29]

Weiss *et al* examined the effect of the timing of surgery relative to delivery with respect to maternal morbidity and mortality, and noted that the maternal mortality was not significantly different between patients operated on during pregnancy, immediately after delivery or with a delay until the postpartum period.[21] However maternal morbidity was significantly greater in patients operated on immediately after delivery or delayed until the postpartum period. In contrast, fetal outcome was improved if surgery was performed at or after delivery. Such observations reflect the difficulties and complexities of deciding on a management plan for both mother and fetus.

If pregnancy has reached 28 weeks or more, there seems to be little to gain and much to lose in attempting surgery without delivery of the fetus. A recent case report documents acute hemodynamic deterioration following a mitral valve replacement performed at 31 weeks gestation. Emergency Cesarean section, performed 12 hours postoperatively resulted in dramatic hemodynamic improvement with maternal survival, but sadly, the infant perished.[30] Thus, in these circumstances we would recommend Cesarean section immediately followed by cardiac surgery. However, where the maternal condition mandates cardiac surgery before 28 weeks gestation, all efforts should be made to minimize the adverse effects of CPB on the fetus. One team avoided the use of CPB by performing off-pump coronary artery bypass grafting on a pregnant woman with intractable angina.[31]

Laboratory studies have examined the effects of CPB on fetal lambs,[32] but the findings cannot be directly extrapolated to humans. For obvious reasons there are no experimental studies of the effects of CPB on the human fetus, and the only data comes from case reports. Clearly the use of CPB represents a major risk to the fetus, with particular areas of concern being the effects of hypotension, non-pulsatile perfusion, hypothermia, heparinization, hemodilution, complement activation and release of vasoactive substances, particulate and air embolism, and alterations in maternal acid–base balance. From published work the following recommendations can be made.

Management of CPB in the pregnant patient

Maintenance of uteroplacental flow

Uteroplacental blood flow is not subject to autoregulation – flow through the intervillous space being pressure dependent and inversely proportional to uterine vascular resistance. A fall in maternal blood pressure is therefore likely to reduce placental perfusion. Alpha-adrenoceptor agonists will increase uterine vascular tone and reduce uteroplacental blood flow, although when maternal blood pressure is very low, the overall effect of vasoconstriction is beneficial. Ephedrine, with its combination of direct and indirect alpha and beta adrenergic effects, is recommended as the safest vasopressor agent. Fetal heart monitoring with external cardiotocography (CTG) has been used as an indirect monitor of placental flow since the mid-1970s. Fetal bradycardia and loss of heart variability have been reported in response to both maternal hypotension and the onset of CPB at 'normal' flow rates. Increasing maternal arterial pressure and increasing pump flows have resulted in improved CTG traces in some cases, although not in others. Compensatory fetal tachycardia may occur once normal maternal circulation is restored. Most authors advocate higher than normal perfusion pressures during CPB; a minimum of 70 mmHg is frequently advocated. A slow transition to CPB may help to minimize hypotension at the start of CPB. Allowance should also be made for the increased cardiac output of the pregnant woman, with flow rates of at least $2.4 \ l \ min^{-1} \ m^{-2}$ recommended. Poor fetal outcome has been documented despite the use of high flows and normal arterial pressure.[33] The effect of pulsatile versus non-pulsatile flow remains uncertain. Although it has been suggested that pulsatile flow may be more efficient in preserving uterine perfusion,[34] there is currently insufficient data to confirm or refute this. Few of the operations reported have been performed with pulsatile flow.[35] It seems probable that, as always in cardiac surgery, expeditious surgery with a short pump run will achieve the best outcome.

Temperature during CPB

The optimum temperature for CPB during pregnancy is another matter for debate – balancing risks to the woman against those to the fetus. Cooling and rewarming have been suggested to have adverse effects on the fetus;[36] Pomini et al noted that embryo-fetal mortality was 24% when hypothermia was used, against a zero fetal mortality with normothermia, suggesting that the use of hypothermia is a serious risk factor for fetal death.[22] Fetal bradycardia is a common response to cooling, and rewarming is associated with arrhythmias. In a recently reported case, serious fetal bradycardia of 50 beats min^{-1} with loss of beat-to-beat variability persisted for 50 min during hypothermic CPB at 28°C, with recovery only when rewarming occurred.[37] In addition to fetal dysrhythmia, cooling may also provoke uterine contractions. Thus, when possible, cardiac surgery should be performed with normothermic or tepid (32–35°C) CPB. If difficult and prolonged surgery is anticipated, however, then moderate hypothermia (28–32°C) may be necessary to reduce systemic oxygen requirements and provide cardiac and cerebral protection to the mother.

Monitoring of uterine activity

Uterine contractions appear to be an important problem during and after CPB and should be monitored continuously peroperatively and for several days postoperatively. Uterine instability during CPB may be due to dilution of circulating progesterone or a result of increased prostaglandin production. Sick cardiac patients may tolerate tocolytic drugs poorly and their prophylactic use is not advised. If premature labor or uterine irritability is detected then treatment can be started to reduce the risk of fetal demise. Currently used tocolytics include magnesium sulfate, calcium-channel blockers, nitrates and β_2 agonists (e.g. salbutamol and ritodrine). These agents, however, may have deleterious effects on the pregnant patient with decompensated heart disease.

Acid–base balance

Alpha-stat management of acid–base balance is advocated; care is needed to avoid maternal alkalemia, which, by shifting the oxyhemoglobin dissociation curve to the left, reduces oxygen transfer to the fetus. It is suggested that maternal PaO_2 should be maintained in the range 188–300 mmHg (25–40 kPa) during CPB, although there is no objective evidence to support this practice.

Heparinization

Surprisingly, no morbidity or mortality appears to be directly attributable to anticoagulation. Heparin, a large molecule, does not cross the placental barrier and thus has no effect on the fetus.

Hemodilution

There is no available information on the effects of hemodilution during bypass on the fetus. It seems likely that moderate hemodilution is well tolerated although it may be prudent to avoid excessive falls in hematocrit.

Fetal monitoring

The normal baseline fetal heart rate is 120–150 beats min^{-1} and a normal range of variability is a sign of fetal well-being. Fetal heart variability is reduced by maternal anesthesia. Fetal tachycardia may occur secondary to maternal administration of sympathomimetic drugs or atropine. Fetal bradycardia is usually a response to hypoxia and acidosis, and may presage death in utero. The fetal heart can be monitored reliably transabdominally from as early as 12 weeks gestation.

Anesthetic management

The outcome of surgery is likely to be related to the maternal condition requiring surgery, rather than to the use or avoidance of any particular anesthetic technique or drug. All care should be taken to optimize maternal and fetal conditions. As previously mentioned, attention must be paid to the risks of acid aspiration at induction of anesthesia, and of aortocaval compression. The commonly used chronotropic and inotropic agents are safe when used appropriately.

Ethical issues

A discussion of this case would be incomplete without some mention of the ethical issues involved. In the first trimester of pregnancy, the fetus, essentially an extension of the mother is normally of secondary concern. If the mother requires urgent surgical intervention the fetus is non-viable in an extrauterine environment and survival is dependent on the survival of the mother. Cardiac surgery may result in death of the fetus, despite the best attempts to maintain the pregnancy. On the other hand, later in pregnancy when independent fetal viability is possible, there may be a conflict between maternal and fetal well-being, and the issue of 'fetal rights' may be raised.[38] Morally responsible motherhood may require the mother to consider the best interests of her unborn child, but few would argue that she should do this at the risk of her own life. The mother is entitled to autonomy – that is to determine what may or may not be done with her body. Recent cases have clarified the situation to the extent that to force treatment on to a pregnant woman to protect her fetus is almost never justifiable.[39]

Conclusions and key learning points

- Pregnancy imposes ever-increasing cardiovascular stress up to the third trimester; this may precipitate the need for cardiac surgery and necessitate premature delivery of the fetus.
- Cardiac surgery with CPB can be performed during pregnancy although fetal mortality rates are 20–30%. In many published series maternal mortality rates are comparable to those for non-pregnant patients, but selective reporting of successful cases may have biased this.
- If CPB is attempted during pregnancy specific allowance must be made for the changes in maternal physiology; a high-flow, high-pressure, normothermic technique is advocated, with expeditious surgery.
- The anesthetic technique should take account of the pregnancy, with maneuvers to reduce the risk of aspiration and aortocaval compression, and consideration of drug effects on the uterus and fetus.
- Where the pregnancy has reached 28 weeks or more, Cesarean section followed immediately by cardiac operation may offer the best chance of saving both mother and child.
- A multidisciplinary approach is essential for the successful management of pregnant women with life threatening cardiovascular disease.

References

1. Department of Health. *Why mothers die – report on confidential enquiries into maternal deaths in the United Kingdom 1994-6.* The Stationery Office, 1998.

2. Oakley CM. Pregnancy and congenital heart disease. *Heart* 1997;**78**:12–4 (erratum in *Heart* 1997;**78**:322).

3. Iturbe-Alessio I, Fonseca MC, Mutchinik O *et al.* Risks of anticoagulant therapy in pregnant women with artificial heart valves. *N Engl J Med* 1986;**315**:1390–3.

4. Salazar E, Zajarias A, Gutierrez N, Iturbe I. The problem of cardiac valve prostheses, anticoagulants, and pregnancy. *Circulation* 1984;**70**:I169–77.

5. Chan WS. What is the optimal management of pregnant women with valvular heart disease in pregnancy? *Haemostasis* 1999;**29 (Suppl S1)**:105–6.

6. Capeless EL, Clapp JF. When do cardiovascular parameters return to their preconception values? *Am J Obstet Gynecol* 1991;**165**:883–6.

7. Draper ES, Manktelow B, Field DJ, James D. Prediction of survival for preterm births by weight and gestational age: retrospective population based study. *BMJ* 1999;**319**:1093-7.

8. Koh TH, Harrison H, Casey A. Prediction of survival for preterm births. Survival table was not easy to understand. *BMJ* 2000;**320**:647.

9. Martin MC, Pernoll ML, Boruszak AN, Jones JW, LoCicero Jd. Cesarean section while on cardiac bypass: report of a case. *Obstet Gynecol* 1981;**57(6 Suppl)**:41S-5S.

10. Tzankis G, Morse DS. Cesarean section and reoperative aortic valve replacement in a 38-week parturient. *J Cardiothorac Vasc Anesth* 1996;**10**:516-8.

11. Lamarra M, Azzu AA, Kulatilake EN. Cardiopulmonary bypass in the early puerperium: possible new role for aprotinin. *Ann Thorac Surg* 1992;**54**:361-3.

12. Shemin RJ, Phillippe M, Dzau V. Acute thrombosis of a composite ascending aortic conduit containing a Bjork-Shiley valve during pregnancy: successful emergency cesarean section and operative repair. *Clin Cardiol* 1986;**9**:299-301.

13. Pinosky ML, Hopkins RA, Pinckert TL, Suyderhoud JP. Anesthesia for simultaneous cesarean section and acute aortic dissection repair in a patient with Marfan's syndrome. *J Cardiothorac Vasc Anesth* 1994;**8**:451-4.

14. Gonzalez-Santos JM, Vallejo JL, Rico MJ *et al.* Thrombosis of a mechanical valve prosthesis late in pregnancy. Case report and review of the literature. *Thorac Cardiovasc Surg* 1986;**34**:335-7.

15. Duncan PG, Pope WD, Cohen MM, Greer N. Fetal risk of anesthesia and surgery during pregnancy. *Anesthesiology* 1986;**64**:790-4.

16. Brock RC. Valvulotomy in pregnancy. *Proc Roy Soc Med* 1952;**45**:538-42.

17. Cooley DA. Mitral commisurotomy during pregnancy. *JAMA* 1952;**150**:1113-6.

18. Becker RM. Intracardiac surgery in pregnant women. *Ann Thorac Surg* 1983;**36**:453-8.

19. Harken DE, Taylor WJ. Cardiac surgery during pregnancy. *Clin Obstet Gynecol* 1961;**4**:697-709.

20. Dubourg G, Broustet H, Bricaud H. Correction d'une triade de Fallot, en circulation extra-corporelle, chez une femme enceinte. *Arch Mal Coeur Vais* 1959;**52**:1389-93.

21. Weiss BM, von Segesser LK, Alon E *et al.* Outcome of cardiovascular surgery and pregnancy: a systematic review of the period 1984-1996. *Am J Obstet Gynecol* 1998;**179**:1643-53.

22. Pomini F, Mercogliano D, Cavalletti C *et al.* Cardiopulmonary bypass in pregnancy. *Ann Thorac Surg* 1996;**61**:259-68.

23. Parry AJ, Westaby S. Cardiopulmonary bypass during pregnancy. *Ann Thorac Surg* 1996;**61**:1865-9.

24. Chambers CE, Clark SL. Cardiac surgery during pregnancy. *Clin Obstet Gynecol* 1994;**37**:316-23.

25. Bernal JM, Miralles PJ. Cardiac surgery with cardiopulmonary bypass during pregnancy. *Obstet Gynecol Surv* 1986;**41**:1-6.

26. Strickland RA, Oliver WC Jr, Chantigian RC *et al.* Anesthesia, cardiopulmonary bypass, and the pregnant patient. *Mayo Clin Proc* 1991;**66**:411-29.

27. Becker RM. Intracardiac surgery in pregnant women. *Ann Thorac Surg* 1983;**36**:453-8.

28. Westaby S, Parry AJ, Forfar JC. Reoperation for prosthetic valve endocarditis in the third trimester of pregnancy. *Ann Thorac Surg* 1992;**53**:263-5.

29. Buffolo E, Palma JH, Gomes WJ *et al.* Successful use of deep hypothermic circulatory arrest in pregnancy. *Ann Thorac Surg* 1994;**58**:1532-4.

30. Baraka A, Kawkabani N, Haroun-Bizri S. Hemodynamic deterioration after cardiopulmonary bypass during pregnancy: resuscitation by postoperative emergency Cesarean section. *J Cardiothorac Vasc Anesth* 2000;**14**:314-5.

31. Silberman S, Fink D, Berko RS *et al.* Coronary artery bypass surgery during pregnancy. *Eur J Cardiothorac Surg* 1996;**10**:925-6.

32. Hawkins JA, Paape KL, Adkins TP *et al.* Extracorporeal circulation in the fetal lamb. Effects of hypothermia and perfusion rate. *J Cardiovasc Surg (Torino)* 1991;**32**:295-300.

33. Khandelwal M, Rasanen J, Ludormirski A *et al.* Evaluation of fetal and uterine hemodynamics during maternal cardiopulmonary bypass. *Obstet Gynecol* 1996;**88**:667-71.

34. Tripp HF, Stiegel RM, Coyle JP. The use of pulsatile perfusion during aortic valve replacement in pregnancy. *Ann Thorac Surg* 1999;**67**:1169–71.

35. Golden LP. Aortic valve repair and arch replacement during pregnancy: a case report. *AANA J* 1996;**64**:243–54.

36. Goldstein I, Jakobi P, Gutterman E, Milo S. Umbilical artery flow velocity during maternal cardiopulmonary bypass. *Ann Thorac Surg* 1995;**60**:1116–8.

37. Kawkabani N, Kawas N, Baraka A *et al*. Case 3—1999. Severe fetal bradycardia in a pregnant woman undergoing hypothermic cardiopulmonary bypass. *J Cardiothorac Vasc Anesth* 1999;**13**:346–9.

38. Draper H. Women, forced cesareans and antenatal responsibilities. *J Med Ethics* 1996;**22**:327–33.

39. Committee on Ethics, American College of Obstetricians and Gynecologists: Patient choice: maternal-fetal conflict. Washington, D.C.: American College of Obstetricians and Gynecologists, 1987.

2

Tumor extraction from the inferior vena cava and right atrium requiring cardiopulmonary bypass

Ajeet D Sharma, Gautam Sreeram and Thomas F Slaughter

Introduction

Renal cell carcinoma is one of the few malignancies that directly invades the inferior vena cava (IVC) and the right side of the heart in the absence of distant metastases. Current treatment involves radical nephrectomy with extraction of tumor/thrombus from the IVC and right heart. Depending on the extent of IVC and right heart involvement, tumor extraction may necessitate cardiopulmonary bypass (CPB) and, in rare cases, deep hypothermic circulatory arrest (DHCA) may be required.

Case report

A 56-year-old female presented to the emergency room with a 14-hour history of right flank pain accompanied by painless hematuria and a weight loss of 5 kg over 4 months. Physical examination revealed a fullness in the right upper quadrant of the abdomen. Subsequent investigation revealed a right renal mass extending into the IVC and right atrium. A percutaneous biopsy of the renal mass confirmed the diagnosis of renal cell carcinoma.

Since there was no evidence of metastatic spread, a decision was made to perform a radical nephrectomy with extraction of tumor/thrombus from the IVC and right atrium under CPB. The night before surgery the patient was sedated with diazepam 5 mg by mouth. One hour before surgery the patient was premedicated with methadone 5 mg by mouth.

In the anesthesia induction room a right forearm vein was cannulated with a 14-G cannula and an infusion of 0.9 % saline commenced. After administration of intravenous midazolam 2 mg, a right radial artery catheter was placed. Following the administration of 0.9 % saline 500 ml the patient was tipped 'head down' and the right internal jugular vein cannulated. Because the tumor within the IVC was known to be 'free floating' and not adherent to the vessel wall, it was considered prudent not to insert a cannula for pressure monitoring in either the IVC or femoral vein.

After adequate preoxygenation, anesthesia was induced with thiopental 250 mg and fentanyl 300 µg. Pancuronium 8 mg was administered after positive pressure mask ventilation had been established. Following endotracheal intubation, the lungs were ventilated with oxygen in air (FiO$_2$ 0.5) and anesthesia was maintained with isoflurane 0.5–1.5% and incremental doses of fentanyl.

Multiplane transesophageal echocardiography (TEE) revealed a dilated IVC with a large mobile complex mass (4 cm diameter) extending into the right atrium. The right internal jugular vein cannula was visualized above the mass. Color-flow Doppler imaging demonstrated blood flow around the tumor in the IVC. The mass was seen to prolapse into the right ventricle during diastole but there was no right ventricular outflow tract obstruction. The tricuspid valve

Past medical history	Hypertension. Hypercholesterolemia. Frequent urinary tract infections. No history of gastroesophageal reflux or peptic ulcer disease.
Regular medications	Furosemide 20 mg BD, simvastatin 10 mg OD, famotidine 20 mg PRN. No known drug allergies.
Examination	Obese. Weight 80. 5 kg. Height 1. 64 m. [BMI 30 kg m^{-2}]Pulse 78 min^{-1} BP 140/90. Fullness in right upper quadrant of abdomen – no masses palpable. No facial or cervical fullness. Upper chest wall veins not dilated.
Investigations	Hb 13 g dl^{-1}, WBC 11. 5 × 10^9 l^{-1}, platelets 250 × 10^9 l^{-1} [Na$^+$] 134 mmol l^{-1}, [K$^+$] 4. 0 mmol l^{-1}, [Ca^{2+}] 2. 25 mmol l^{-1}, urea 28 mg. dl^{-1} (10 mmol. l^{-1}), creatinine 1. 5 mg. dl^{-1} (130 μmol l^{-1}). **CXR:** Heart size normal, lungs clear. **ECG:** Sinus rhythm. **CT Abdomen and pelvis:** 10.5-cm diameter heterogeneous, complex cystic, right renal mass extending into the right renal vein, IVC, and right atrium. The adrenal glands, left kidney, pancreas, liver, and spleen appeared normal. **CT chest:** No evidence of metastatic disease. **Radionucleotide bone scan:** No evidence of metastatic disease.

was competent, and the pulmonary arteries free of tumor. There was no pericardial involvement or effusion, and left ventricular function was normal.

With the patient in the supine position, a midline abdominal surgical incision was made from the xiphisternum to the pubis. Radical right nephrectomy and regional lymphadenectomy were then performed without incident. Following anticoagulation with heparin 300 u kg^{-1}, CPB was established between the superior vena cava (SVC) and the ascending aorta. The right atrial appendage was then opened and the tumor/thrombus extracted. At the same time a cardiotomy suction cannula was placed in the right atrium to drain any remaining blood. Venous drainage was thus achieved by cannulae in both the SVC and the right atrium. After tumor extraction the right atrial cannula was removed, the atriotomy closed and the SVC cannula manipulated into the right atrium. The total duration of CPB was 30 minutes. The anticoagulant effect of heparin was reversed with protamine and, having achieving hemostasis, the abdominal and thoracic wounds were closed. The patient remained hemodynamically stable throughout surgery. There were no intraoperative complications and the estimated blood loss was 750 ml.

A repeat TEE examination after surgical resection revealed no residual tumor in either the right atrium or the IVC. Histological examination of the resected kidney confirmed renal cell carcinoma with no extracapsular extension or pelvic lymph node involvement. The IVC wall was free of tumor infiltration. No malignant cells were demonstrated in the thrombus removed from the right atrium. The remainder of the patient's postoperative course was unremarkable, and she was discharged home on the fifth postoperative day.

Discussion

Renal cell carcinoma accounts for the majority of all primary renal cell neoplasms.[1] The peak age incidence occurs between 55 and 60 years, with a 2:1 male preponderance.[1] Renal cell carcinoma invades the IVC in up to 10% of cases and can extend to the right atrium in as many as 1% of patients.[2,3] An aggressive surgical approach, which involves extraction of the tumor/thrombus from the IVC and right atrium, provides the only hope for cure in these patients.

Patients with renal cell carcinoma present with the triad of hematuria, flank pain, and a palpable mass.[1] Intermittent fever, in the absence of infection, may be the only presenting sign. The disease may be associated with several paraneoplastic syndromes that have implications for anesthetic management.[4] These include hyperglycemia, hypercalcemia, renin secretion, and insulin production. Cytokines and hormones produced by renal cell carcinoma can promote gluconeogenesis and glycogenolysis leading to hyperglycemia. Tumor renin secretion may cause severe hypertension and hypokalemia. Hepatosplenomegaly and abnormal liver function tests are not uncommon. The vascularity of renal cell carcinoma may result in arteriovenous fistulae, cardiomegaly, and ultimately congestive cardiac failure. The tumor may obstruct the SVC producing a syndrome characterized by distension of cervical and upper thoracic veins, conjunctival edema, edema and cyanosis of the face, neck, and upper chest, and, on occasion, symptoms of raised intracranial pressure.

The operative approach is determined by the extent of cephalic extension of the tumor/thrombus.[5,6] Therefore, accurate imaging of the IVC is critical. Common preoperative imaging modalities include inferior venacavography, transabdominal ultrasonography, magnetic resonance imaging (MRI), computerized tomography (CT), and TEE. Inferior venacavography is recognized as the 'gold standard' for evaluation of the IVC. Superior venacavography, in addition to inferior venacavography, is necessary to define the extent of cephalic spread of the tumor in cases of complete IVC obstruction. Due to overlying bowel gas or obesity, abdominal ultrasonography is unable to visualize the IVC in up to 30% of cases.[7] Glazer and colleagues compared preoperative TEE with contrast venacavography and MRI for evaluation of caval tumor/thrombus.[8] Their findings revealed diagnostic accuracies of 90, 85, and 75% for MRI, TEE, and contrast venacavography, respectively. The authors concluded that MRI was the preferred investigative modality for caval tumor/thrombus evaluation because it is non-invasive and can be performed without the administration of contrast media.

With the availability of newer technologies, IVC pressure monitoring is rarely performed. In the case described, the renal tumor was free-floating and had not infiltrated the wall of the IVC. Although the IVC was dilated, color-flow Doppler confirmed flow around the tumor mass indicating minimal obstruction. In some cases renal cell carcinoma infiltrates the IVC walls necessitating resection and reconstruction of the IVC. In these cases renal venous pressure measurements can influence decisions regarding IVC reconstruction. Normal renal venous pressure can be up to 22 cmH$_2$O. If the tumor is on the right side and the collateral veins between the left renal vein and systemic venous circulation are abundant, IVC reconstruction may not be required. In order to determine the need for caval reconstruction, left renal pressure can be measured before and after clamping the IVC.[9] Nishiyama and colleagues performed IVC reconstruction only in those patients with right renal cell carcinoma in whom clamping of the IVC was associated with highly elevated left renal venous pressure measurements (pressure change from 22 to 61 cmH$_2$O). If the pressure change was negligible – indicating adequate collateral venous return – IVC reconstruction was not performed. The same principles can be utilized for left-sided renal cell carcinomas with IVC wall infiltration.

The surgical approach to extraction of tumor/thrombus involving the IVC is determined by the extent of cephalic spread. For tumor/thrombus extending from the renal veins to the atriocaval junction, extraction can be performed without CPB[10] whereas tumors extending beyond the atriocaval junction into the right side of the heart invariably require CPB.[11] In cases where the tumor does not extend above the hepatic veins, a tourniquet can be placed around the IVC below the hepatic veins and a relatively easy IVC excision and extraction can be anticipated. For tumors extending to the atriocaval junction, extraction can be performed by threading a balloon catheter into the right atrium, inflating the balloon and gently pulling it back through the IVC.[12] Complete balloon occlusion of the IVC above the hepatic veins can impede hepatic venous drainage into the right atrium leading to systemic hypotension and elevated IVC pressures. The degree of hypotension produced is influenced by the extent of collateral venous flow from the infrarenal IVC to the SVC via the azygos and lumbar veins. Once the balloon is pulled below the hepatic veins, hepatic venous drainage occurs and arterial and IVC pressures are restored. Complications associated with balloon extraction include IVC laceration, incomplete tumor extraction, severe hemorrhage and pulmonary embolization from friable tumor/thrombus.[13]

For complex tumors involving the right atrium or ventricle, tumor extraction is performed utilizing CPB either with or without systemic hypothermia.[11] This approach provides a relatively 'bloodless' operative field, good visualization, and the potential for complete excision of tumor infiltrating the IVC wall. Disadvantages include bleeding associated with heparin administration and postoperative renal, pulmonary, and cerebral dysfunction. Venous cannulation can be difficult if the right atrium contains tumor/thrombus. In this situation, the SVC is first cannulated and the right atrial appendage opened. While the tumor is being extracted, a second cannula is placed in the right atrium to supplement venous drainage from the SVC. Once the tumor is extracted the venous cannula is inserted into the right atrium and the atrial appendage closed.

Central venous cannulation must be performed with great care so as to avoid dislodging or fragmenting tumor in the right atrium. Inserting the catheter to a level above the superior atriocaval junction under TEE guidance is advisable. To prevent tumor embolization, pulmonary artery flotation catheters are best avoided until after extraction of the tumor/thrombus. Right-sided heart outflow obstruction can occur if the tumor mass prolapses and obstructs the tricuspid valve. Precautionary steps to minimize the risk of this complication include increasing right-sided filling pressures with fluid administration, and placing the patient in Trendenlenburg position to direct the tumor/thrombus away from the tricuspid valve.

Transesophageal echocardiography offers several advantages for perioperative monitoring of the patient with advanced renal cell carcinoma. First, TEE provides high-quality near-field images of the atria, IVC, and SVC. Cephalic extension of renal cell tumor/thrombus is frequently found to be greater than predicted by conventional imaging techniques of MRI, CT, or inferior venacavography.[14] TEE is superior to transthoracic echocardiography for imaging the right atrial chamber, and this information is critical to determine the optimal surgical approach and the need for CPB. Second, tumor embolism

is a potentially fatal intraoperative complication.[14] Acute changes in the superior extension of the tumor/thrombus, or the presence of new echogenic material in the pulmonary arteries may be demonstrated by TEE. Third, information provided by TEE may lead to an alteration in surgical approach. Tumors confined to the hepatic veins portend relatively straightforward extraction by clamp application, incision, and extraction of the tumor from the infrahepatic IVC. For tumor/thrombus extending above the hepatic veins, surgical approaches include (a) balloon catheter 'pull-through' from the IVC and/or (b) hypothermic CPB and DHCA to facilitate tumor extraction.[12]

Following successful tumor extraction, TEE provides information regarding residual tumor/thrombus, IVC obstruction, and tumor embolization,[15,16] and importantly, TEE provides real-time information about cardiac anatomy and myocardial and valvular function.

Surgical excision of renal cell carcinoma involving the IVC and right heart can be curative. Depending upon the extent of cephalad spread of these tumors, CPB may be required. Important issues for consideration in these patients include thorough preoperative evaluation to exclude paraneoplastic syndromes, careful central venous cannulation, hemodynamic instability during balloon catheter inflation and extraction, the risk of pulmonary tumor/thromboembolism, and the potential for excessive bleeding from venous collaterals and IVC laceration (40–68% after complete surgical excision).[3]

Conclusions

• Renal cell carcinoma tumor/thrombus can directly spread to the IVC and right atrium. Aggressive surgical extraction of tumor with or without CPB can improve survival.
• A thorough preoperative evaluation should be performed to exclude paraneoplastic syndromes.
• Central venous cannulation should be performed with caution. TEE guidance is advised.
• Optimization of right heart filling can reduce the risk of outflow obstruction.
• Hemodynamic compromise may occur during

balloon catheter extraction of tumor/thrombus – especially if hepatic venous drainage is obstructed.

- Severe bleeding and pulmonary embolization may occur during tumor extraction.
- TEE provides valuable information regarding the optimal surgical approach, pulmonary embolism, residual tumor/thrombus, IVC obstruction, valvular, and myocardial function.
- Rarely, in cases of IVC and/or right atrial wall infiltration, tumor extraction may be attempted under deep hypothermic circulatory arrest.

References

1. Motzer RJ, Bander NH, Nanus DM. Renal-cell carcinoma. *N Engl J Med* 1996;**335**:865–75.

2. Sigman DB, Hasnain JU, Del Pizzo JJ, Sklar GN. Real-time transesophageal echocardiography for intraoperative surveillance of patients with renal cell carcinoma and vena caval extension undergoing radical nephrectomy. *J Urol* 1999;**161**:36–8.

3. Hatcher PA, Anderson EE, Paulson DF *et al*. Surgical management and prognosis of renal cell carcinoma invading the vena cava. *J Urol* 1991;**145**:20–3.

4. Papac RJ, Poo-Hwu WJ. Renal cell carcinoma: a paradigm of lanthanic disease. *Am J Clin Oncol* 1999;**22**:223–31.

5. Pritchett TR, Lieskovsky G, Skinner DG. Extension of renal cell carcinoma into the vena cava: clinical review and surgical approach. *J Urol* 1986;**135**:460–4.

6. Hatcher PA, Paulson DF, Anderson EE. Accuracy in staging of renal cell carcinoma involving vena cava. *Urology* 1992;**39**:27–30.

7. Webb JA, Murray A, Bary PR, Hendry WF. The accuracy and limitations of ultrasound in the assessment of venous extension in renal carcinoma. *Br J Urol* 1987;**60**:14–7.

8. Glazer A, Novick AC. Preoperative transesophageal echocardiography for assessment of vena caval tumor thrombi: a comparative study with venacavography and magnetic resonance imaging. *Urology* 1997;**49**:32–4.

9. Nishiyama H, Nakamura K, Nishimura M *et al*. Inferior vena caval resection for renal cell carcinoma: usefulness of renal venous pressure measurement. *Hinyokika Kiyo* 1991;**37**:1029–34.

10. Koide Y, Mizoguchi T, Ishii K, Okumura F. Intraoperative management for removal of tumor thrombus in the inferior vena cava or the right atrium with multiplane transesophageal echocardiography. *J Cardiovasc Surg (Torino)* 1998;**39**:641–7.

11. Marshall FF, Reitz BA. Technique for removal of renal cell carcinoma with suprahepatic vena caval tumor thrombus. *Urol Clin North Am* 1986;**13**:551–7.

12. Mizoguchi T, Koide Y, Ohara M, Okumura F. Multiplane transesophageal echocardiographic guidance during resection of renal cell carcinoma extending into the inferior vena cava. *Anesth Analg* 1995;**81**:1102–5.

13. Montie JE, Pontes JE, Novick AC *et al*. Resection of inferior vena cava tumor thrombi from renal cell carcinoma. *Am Surg* 1991;**57**:56–61.

14. Katz ES, Rosenzweig BP, Rorman D, Kronzon I. Diagnosis of tumor embolus to the pulmonary artery by transesophageal echocardiography. *J Am Soc Echocardiogr* 1992;**5**:439–43.

15. Treiger BF, Humphrey LS, Peterson CV Jr *et al*. Transesophageal echocardiography in renal cell carcinoma: an accurate diagnostic technique for intracaval neoplastic extension. *J Urol* 1991;**145**:1138–40.

16. Allen G, Klingman R, Ferraris VA *et al*. Transesophageal echocardiography in the surgical management of renal cell carcinoma with intracardiac extension. *J Cardiovasc Surg (Torino)* 1991;**32**:833–6.

3
Cardiopulmonary bypass in a patient with a brain tumor

Hilary P Grocott and Alina M Grigore

Introduction

Cardiac surgery performed with cardiopulmonary bypass (CPB) is known to be associated with significant organ dysfunction. Arguably, one of the most devastating complications is cerebral injury, which may manifest as neurocognitive dysfunction and stroke.[1] Even in patients with no known pre-existing cerebral pathology, brain dysfunction has been reported, and cerebral edema has been reported in otherwise healthy patients following CPB.[2] This edema may be due to changes in blood–brain barrier (BBB) permeability.[3]

The aetiology of CPB-associated BBB alteration is likely multifactorial with microembolic events, alterations in cerebral blood flow (including global hypoperfusion), and a CPB-triggered 'whole body' inflammatory response representing possible mechanisms for increased BBB permeability.[2–4] In addition, the stress of CPB results in an increased production of antidiuretic hormone (ADH), which decreases plasma osmolarity thereby contributing to cerebral swelling.[5–7] The patient with a brain tumor who requires cardiac surgery with CPB presents a unique situation in which there is a potential to further increase injury in a brain that is already compromised.

Case history

A 79-year-old female presented to her physician with unexplained confusion and was subsequently found to be hyponatremic. Her past history was remarkable for a successful resection of a cancerous right upper lobe lung tumor 9 years previously. Three years prior to presentation she was diagnosed has having a 3-cm brain tumor near the right cavernous sinus that, due to

Past medical history	Bronchial carcinoma – operated 9 years earlier. Intracranial meningioma. Personality disorder. Hypothyroidism. Chronic airflow obstruction. Asymptomatic bilateral internal carotid artery stenosis (80%).
Regular medications	Phenytoin, furosemide, levothyroxine, metoprolol, captopril, beclomethasone, albuterol.
Examination	Weight 65 kg. BMI 27.1 kg. m^{-2}. No focal neurological signs. No signs of raised intracranial pressure.
Investigations	[Na$^+$] 135 mmol. l^{-1}. Phenytoin level – 'therapeutic'. **Coronary angiography:** 80% stenosis of left main coronary artery **TTE:** Impaired LV function (LVEF 40%), left atrial enlargement. Mild mitral regurgitation. **Cranial MRI:** Brain lesion unchanged. No mass effect.

its CT and MRI characteristics, was considered to be a benign meningioma. At the time, the tumor was indenting the medial part of the right temporal lobe and, due to the position and size of the tumor, it was felt that conservative management (including seizure prophylaxis and regular follow-up) would be most appropriate.

Following a thorough medical evaluation, the hyponatremia was thought to be consistent with psychogenic polydipsia and was successfully treated with water restriction. However, while hospitalized for treatment, she suffered a non-Q wave myocardial infarction associated with pulmonary edema. Findings at coronary angiography prompted urgent scheduling for coronary artery bypass graft surgery (CABG).

Her preCABG evaluation demonstrated no signs of increased intracranial pressure (ICP), and there was no other neurological dysfunction or localizing signs. Other laboratory results were within normal limits. A contrast-enhanced MRI showed no recent enlargement of the brain lesion, and no mass-effect was noted.

Prior to induction of anesthesia, arterial and pulmonary artery catheters were placed under local anesthesia. Anesthesia was induced with midazolam 0.05 mg kg^{-1}, fentanyl 10 µg kg^{-1}, and thiopental 4 mg kg^{-1} with neuromuscular blockade achieved using pancuronium 0.1 mg kg^{-1}. Following endotracheal intubation, anesthesia was maintained with isoflurane 0.5–1.0 % in oxygen/air (FiO$_2$ 0.3–1.0) and intermittent boluses of fentanyl and midazolam. Moderate hyperventilation was employed throughout to maintain a PaCO$_2$ of 30–35 mmHg (3.9–4.6 kPa).

The CPB prime consisted of Hetastarch 500 ml and lactated Ringer's (LR) 1000 ml to which 3.2% saline 100 ml was added — final [Na$^+$] 206 mmol. l^{-1}, ~ 450 mOsm. l^{-1}. Immediately after the initiation of CPB, dexamethasone 4 mg was administered. During CPB, the patient was cooled to a nasopharyngeal (NP) temperature of 28°C. Mean arterial pressure (MAP) was maintained between 60 and 80 mmHg using boluses of phenylephrine and/or sodium nitroprusside by infusion, as required. Alpha-stat acid–base management was utilized during hypothermia with the PCO$_2$ maintained at 30–35 mmHg (3.9–4.6 kPa). Serum sodium levels were between 132–138 mmol. l^{-1}, and serum glucose levels were controlled with intermittent administration of small boluses (2–5 units) of soluble insulin. Hematocrit was maintained at ≥17% with the administration of packed red blood cells (PRBC) as necessary. Following the institution of CPB, two coronary artery bypass grafts were fashioned during a single application of an aortic cross-clamp. Cold antegrade blood cardioplegia was used for myocardial protection. The patient was rewarmed over 20 minutes, avoiding NP temperatures >36°C, and separated from CPB without inotropic support. Prior to transfer to the ICU, an additional dose of dexamethasone 4 mg was administered.

The patient awakened approximately 4 hours after the completion of surgery, with no clinical signs of increased ICP or other neurologic deficits, and was extubated. With the exception of a transient and self-limiting episode of atrial fibrillation, she made an uneventful recovery and was discharged home in stable condition on the sixth postoperative day.

Discussion

Cardiac surgery with CPB is well known to be associated with detrimental cerebral effects.[1] The potential adverse CNS effects of the brain tumor superimposed on the effects of CPB may have an added adverse effect on cerebral homeostasis. Brain tumors pose a variety of considerations for the anesthesiologist, most of which are related to the potential for increased ICP, local alterations in CBF and disturbances in BBB permeability. The altered BBB results from an increased permeability of brain capillaries resulting from structural injury to the cerebral endothelium, opened cellular endothelial tight junctions, increased pinocytosis, and cellular disruption.[8] Metabolic impairment of the endothelial transport system can also occur, as well as neovascularization of the tumor and surrounding tissue by vessels lacking normal BBB characteristics. Meningiomas, in particular, are known to produce vascular endothelial growth factor (VEGF), a potent stimulus both for angiogenesis and peritumoral edema formation.[9,10]

CPB produces cerebral edema formation[2,3] (with the potential for associated increases in ICP) likely resulting from BBB disruption induced by inflammatory and microembolic events occurring during CPB. Elevated ICP may lead to global cerebral ischemia that may be responsible for the neurologic dysfunction that can present after cardiac surgery.[11] The cerebral edema documented following CPB appears to be primarily cortical in origin.[2] The cortical location of cerebral edema is consistent with the findings of small capillary and arteriolar dilations (SCADs) in the cortex and deep gray matter in patients and experimental animals having undergone CPB.[12] This association of edema and SCADs supports the theory of microembolic injury contributing to oedema formation as SCADS are thought to represent the 'ghosts' of lipid soluble microemboli.[12]

Preoperative preparation of a patient requiring cardiac surgery in whom a brain tumor is known to exist should include a thorough clinical examination focusing on identifying any signs of increased ICP as well as any neurologic dysfunction (including localizing signs). Computed tomography or MRI needs to be performed to evaluate tumor size and position as well as any mass effect, cerebral edema and/or obstructive hydrocephalus. The presence of these signs should alert the physician to the presence of impairment in cerebral elastance (and compliance) and as a result, plans to compensate for this impairment should be made.[13]

Careful consideration should be given to any recent history of hyponatremia. In this particular case, in the absence of pertinent clinical and laboratory evidence for the syndrome of inappropriate secretion of ADH, it was thought that the most likely etiology of her hyponatremia was psychogenic polydipsia. It should be pointed out that this is a diagnosis of exclusion. It is important to identify preoperative hyponatremia as CPB itself can cause decreases in serum sodium, even in otherwise normal patients. Thus, if the patient suffers from a relative excess of free water (or sodium depletion) it may worsen during CPB.

Several techniques were used for the prevention of cerebral edema during CPB. In order to maintain plasma osmolarity during CPB, hypertonic saline was added to the pump prime. This was in addition to mannitol (50 ml, 25% solution), which is a routine constituent of the CPB prime at our institution. Any decline in serum sodium results in a reduction in plasma osmotic pressure that can lead to increases in brain water with elevations in ICP.[14] A beneficial

effect of hypertonic solutions to injured brain has been demonstrated previously.[15] It may have its main effect, however, in areas of the brain that are relatively uninjured. For example, although in an animal model of traumatic brain injury, administration of hypertonic LR compared to regular LR, leads to similar brain water retention in the region of the lesion, the non-lesioned hemisphere in the hypertonic LR group had a lower water content than the regular LR group.[16] As a result, this may decrease the overall ICP by reducing the volume of the normal tissue thus compensating for the 'swollen' injured tissue. However, in a rabbit model of traumatic brain injury, plasma oncotic pressure did not influence brain water content.[17,18]

During CPB, the effects of serum sodium changes on osmotic pressure appear to be more important than oncotic pressure influences with regard to cerebral edema formation during CPB. Hindman et al, using a rabbit model of CPB, found that colloid oncotic pressure did not affect brain water content during CPB.[19] The investigators concluded that blood–brain osmotic gradients, rather than oncotic gradients determine the net water movement during CPB in the presence of an intact BBB. McDaniel et al, using a normothermic pig CPB model, noted that hypertonic saline in dextran (a hyperosmotic, hyperoncotic solution) prevented elevation of ICP and reduced fluid requirements.[11] These data indicate that during CPB, in the presence of a brain lesion, maintenance of normal plasma osmolarity is essential for preventing further occurrence of cerebral edema and elevation of ICP.

As previously reported, dexamethasone has a positive effect by decreasing peritumoral BBB permeability and inhibition of VEGF action.[9,20] Although corticosteroids are routinely administered for most cerebral tumor surgeries at our institution they are not routinely administered to patients undergoing CPB – although it is routine at some centers. In this particular case we administered two doses of dexamethasone, the first at the onset of CPB, and the second following CPB, in order to minimize peritumoral edema that might be enhanced during CPB. The disadvantage of steroid administration, from a cerebral perspective, is the associated hyperglycemia that can result from the 'anti-insulin' effect of the steroids. This needs to be aggressively treated with intravenous insulin, as was the case with our patient.

Temperature management is very important when trying to modulate any type of cerebral injury. Hypothermia is a robust neuroprotectant in the laboratory, even though clinical trials have had mixed results. In the setting of CPB, however, hypothermia is still considered protective, even though its use may be associated with adverse effects. One of these relates to the need for subsequent rewarming. In our case, rewarming proceeded slowly, avoiding temperatures higher than 36°C. Although NP temperature is generally considered to be a good surrogate of cerebral temperature, it has been shown to underestimate jugular venous bulb temperature (another cerebral temperature surrogate). As a result, NP temperatures higher than 36°C (which would correspond to jugular bulb temperatures 2–3°C higher) could expose the CNS to hyperthermia and its associated detrimental effects on injured brain tissue.[21] Hyperthermia has been associated with impairment of cerebral autoregulation, aggravation of vasogenic brain edema, elevation of ICP, and worsened outcome after cerebral injury.[22]

Postoperative management should focus upon maintaining normal hemodynamics, avoiding hyperthermia, and maintaining normal serum glucose levels. Several clinical studies have reported adverse neurologic outcome when hyperglycemia occurred during a period of ischemic cerebral injury.[23,24] The mechanism of hyperglycemia-enhanced cerebral ischemic injury is not completely understood but its main effect is thought to be due to elevations in intracellular lactate production with concomitant acidosis.[25,26] We administered insulin during CPB but despite this, serum glucose levels remained elevated during the post CPB and immediate postoperative periods. Hyperglycemia can be very difficult to treat during CPB, particular in the setting of hypothermia where the insulin may not have the same effects due to pharmacodynamic changes induced with lower temperatures.

Special attention must also be directed towards post-operative fluid shifts that usually occur in the first 2–3 days after surgery. Insidious increases in intravascular volume can lead to increases in central venous pressure with subsequent ICP elevations. Attention to the onset of these changes and early intervention with diuresis may prevent this potential problem. Frequent and regular monitoring of neurologic status is very important as it may alert the medical team to any changes in mental status that may be associated with these ICP increases.

Conclusions and learning points

- The patient with a brain tumor who requires cardiac surgery with CPB presents a number of interesting and challenging considerations to the anesthesiologist caring for these patients.
- The interaction between ICP and changes in fluid and electrolytes associated with CPB expose the patient to the development of cerebral edema.
- During surgery, strict attention should be paid to temperature management and the maintenance of normoglycemia to prevent deterioration in neurologic status.

References

1. Arrowsmith JE, Grocott HP, Newman MF. Neurologic risk assessment, monitoring and outcome in cardiac surgery. *J Cardiothorac Vasc Anesth* 1999;**13**:736–43.

2. Harris DN, Bailey SM, Smith PL *et al*. Brain swelling in first hour after coronary artery bypass surgery. *Lancet* 1993;**342**:586–7.

3. Harris DN, Oatridge A, Dob D *et al*. Cerebral swelling after normothermic cardiopulmonary bypass. *Anesthesiology* 1998;**88**:340–5.

4. Murkin JM. Cardiopulmonary bypass and the inflammatory response: a role for serine protease inhibitors? *J Cardiothorac Vasc Anesth* 1997;**11**:19–23.

5. Philbin DM, Coggins CH, Wilson N, Sokoloski J. Antidiuretic hormone levels during cardiopulmonary bypass. *J Thorac Cardiovasc Surg* 1977;**73**:145–8.

6. Boulton AJ, Wilson N, Turnbull KW, Yip RW. Haemodynamic and plasma vasopressin responses

during high-dose fentanyl or sufentanil anaesthesia. *Can Anaesth Soc J* 1986;**33**:475–83.

7. Yamane Y, Yamadori Y, Umeda Y, Shiota T. Plasma ADH levels during heart surgery. *Jpn Circ J* 1979;**43**:263–75.

8. Hossmann KA, Wechsler W, Wilmes F. Experimental peritumorous edema. Morphological and pathophysiological observations. *Acta Neuropathol (Berl)* 1979;**45**:195–203.

9. Heiss JD, Papavassiliou E, Merrill MJ *et al.* Mechanism of dexamethasone suppression of brain tumor-associated vascular permeability in rats. Involvement of the glucocorticoid receptor and vascular permeability factor. *J Clin Invest* 1996;**98**:1400–8.

10. Provias J, Claffey K, delAguila *et al.* Meningiomas: role of vascular endothelial growth factor/vascular permeability factor in angiogenesis and peritumoral edema. *Neurosurgery* 1997;**40**:1016–26.

11. McDaniel LB, Nguyen T, Zwischenberger JB *et al.* Hypertonic saline dextran prime reduces increased intracranial pressure during cardiopulmonary bypass in pigs. *Anesth Analg* 1994;**78**:435–41.

12. Moody DM, Bell MA, Challa VR *et al.* Brain microemboli during cardiac surgery or aortography. *Ann Neurol* 1990;**28**:477–86.

13. Shapiro HM. Intracranial hypertension: therapeutic and anesthetic considerations. *Anesthesiology* 1975;**43**:445–71.

14. Zornow MH, Prough DS. Fluid management in patients with traumatic brain injury. *New Horiz* 1995;**3**:488–98.

15. Shackford SR, Bourguignon PR, Wald SL *et al.* Hypertonic saline resuscitation of patients with head injury: a prospective, randomized clinical trial. *J Trauma* 1998;**44**:50–8.

16. Zornow MH, Scheller MS, Shackford SR. Effect of a hypertonic lactated Ringer's solution on intracranial pressure and cerebral water content in a model of traumatic brain injury. *J Trauma* 1989;**29**:484–8.

17. Kaieda R, Todd MM, Warner DS. Prolonged reduction in colloid oncotic pressure does not increase brain edema following cryogenic injury in rabbits. *Anesthesiology* 1989;**71**:554–60.

18. Zornow MH, Todd MM, Moore SS. The acute cerebral effects of changes in plasma osmolality and oncotic pressure. *Anesthesiology* 1987;**67**:936–41.

19. Hindman BJ, Funatsu N, Cheng DC *et al.* Differential effect of oncotic pressure on cerebral and extracerebral water content during cardiopulmonary bypass in rabbits. *Anesthesiology* 1990;**73**:951–7.

20. Ostergaard L, Hochberg FH, Rabinov JD *et al.* Early changes measured by magnetic resonance imaging in cerebral blood flow, blood volume, and blood–brain barrier permeability following dexamethasone treatment in patients with brain tumors. *J Neurosurg* 1999;**90**:300–5.

21. Grocott HP, Newman MF, Croughwell ND *et al.* Continuous jugular venous versus nasopharyngeal temperature monitoring during hypothermic cardiopulmonary bypass for cardiac surgery. *J Clin Anesth* 1997;**9**:312–6.

22. Hosotani K, Katsumura H, Kabuto M *et al.* Effect of whole-body hyperthermia on the development of peritumoral brain oedema. *Int J Hyperthermia* 1993;**9**:25–36.

23. Candelise L, Landi G, Orazio EN, Boccardi E. Prognostic significance of hyperglycemia in acute stroke. *Arch Neurol* 1985;**42**:661–3.

24. Berger L, Hakim AM. The association of hyperglycemia with cerebral edema in stroke. *Stroke* 1986;**17**:865–71.

25. Kraig RP, Chesler M. Astrocytic acidosis in hyperglycemic and complete ischemia. *J Cereb Blood Flow Metab* 1990;**10**:104–14.

26. Pulsinelli WA, Waldman S, Rawlinson D, Plum F. Moderate hyperglycemia augments ischemic brain damage: a neuropathologic study in the rat. *Neurology* 1982;**32**:1239–46.

4

Cardiothoracic trauma: a case of traumatic aortocoronary saphenous vein graft occulsion

Eric Jacobsohn and Trevor WR Lee

Introduction

Approximately 25% of all trauma deaths are due to chest injuries.[1] Both blunt and penetrating chest trauma contribute to the wide variety of injuries encountered. Of these two categories of injury, blunt chest trauma is the more frequent cause of cardiac injury, occurring in approximately 900 000 cases annually in the USA.[2] Motor vehicle accidents account for more than 70% of blunt chest injuries with an associated mortality rate of approximately 5%.[1] Clinical presentations of cardiac injuries include hemopericardium with tamponade, cardiac chamber rupture, cardiac lacerations and contusions, aortic dissection, valvular damage, and ventricular and atrial septum injuries.[3] Most cardiac injuries present acutely, but delayed presentation as a result of a cardiac injury can occur.[4] These may present as valvular regurgitation, cardiomyopathies, ateriovenous fistulae, arteriocameral fistulae, atrial septal defects, ventricular septal defects, and retained cardiac foreign bodies.[5]

Damage to native coronary arteries is also a well-described presentation of blunt chest and penetrating chest trauma. However, the occlusion of aorto-coronary vein grafts has rarely been documented.[6,7]

Case history

A 48-year-old male was admitted to the emergency department after he was involved in a two-vehicle collision. The patient's vehicle was struck on the driver's side by the second vehicle while proceeding through an intersection. He was thrown against the steering wheel and sustained multiple injuries, including a head injury and blunt chest trauma. In addition, he experienced a transient loss of consciousness, lasting approximately 3–5 minutes. The passenger, who was the driver's daughter, was unharmed. The patient was transported by the emergency medical service to the hospital.

The patient's daughter revealed that her father was a relatively healthy person who was not suffering from chest pain before the accident. However, his past medical history did include a coronary artery bypass operation (CABG) 5 years previously for unstable angina. The procedure consisted of a left internal mammary artery graft to the left anterior descending (LAD) artery for mild diffuse disease of the proximal LAD artery, and a saphenous vein graft to the proximal right coronary artery (RCA) for a tight proximal RCA stenosis. Subsequent to his CABG operation, he had a postoperative echocardiogram that showed normal biventricular function and no regional wall motion abnormalities. The patient had no cardiac symptoms after his operation and participated in strenuous daily exercise.

On arrival to the emergency department, the patient complained of severe left-sided chest pain that was aggravated by deep breathing. The primary trauma survey revealed a spontaneously breathing patient with an oxygen saturation of 98% on high-flow face-mask oxygen, a blood

Past medical history	CABG
Regular medications	Aspirin EC 325 mg OD.
Examination	**Primary survey:** Spontaneous respiration. SaO$_2$ 98% on supplemental oxygen. Trachea central. Reduced left basal breath sounds. Pulse 60. BP 120/75 mmHg. Heart sounds normal. **Secondary survey:** GCS 14/15. Retrograde amnesia. Minor forehead contusion. Spine – normal. Severe left posterolateral chest wall pain on palpation.
Investigations	[Na$^+$] 143 mmol l^{-1}, [K$^+$] 4.3 mmol l^{-1}, [Cl$^-$] 103 mmol l^{-1}, [HCO$_3^-$] 25 mmol l^{-1}, urea 5.7 mmol l^{-1}, creatinine 0.8 mg dl^{-1} (72 µmol l^{-1}), anion gap 13 mmol l^{-1}, ALT 25 u l^{-1}, AST 26 u l^{-1}, LDH 192 u l^{-1}, CK 210 u l^{-1} (NR < 175), CK-MB 23 u l^{-1} (NR < 21), Hb 16.2 g dl^{-1}, PT 13 s, aPTT 28 s **CXR:** Left hemothorax and multiple rib fractures. **Spinal X-rays:** Normal. **CT chest:** Pulmonary contusion. No evidence of aortic dissection or pericardial effusion. **CT head:** Normal. **ECG:** Third degree heart block. Junctional escape rhythm 50 beats min^{-1}. Atrial rate 100 beats min^{-1}. 2 mm ST elevation in leads II, III and aVF and 2 mm ST depression and T wave inversion in leads V$_1$, V$_2$ and V$_3$.

pressure of 120/75 mmHg in both arms, and a regular heart rate of 60 beats per minute. The heart sounds were normal. The anterior breath sounds were normal bilaterally, but there was a slight decrease in the left base and the patient was splinting on inspiration. The trachea was not deviated. The secondary trauma survey revealed a Glasgow coma scale (GCS) of 14. Although he had only a minor contusion to his left forehead, he had no recall for the accident or any events of that day. Palpation of his cervical, thoracic, and lumbar spine was normal, and there was no evidence of long bone fractures. Palpation of his chest showed severe pain over his middle and lower ribs posterolaterally on the left, consistent with the patient's complaints. The rest of the secondary trauma survey was unremarkable.

Radiological studies in the emergency department included a chest X-ray that showed a small left hemothorax, and evidence of fractured fourth, seventh, and eighth ribs. There was no evidence of a pneumothorax. The lung fields were clear. Because of concern regarding a possible widened mediastinum on chest X-ray, a contrast-enhanced CT scan of the chest was obtained. This showed moderate bilateral pulmonary contusions, multiple rib fractures, and a small left hemothorax. There was no evidence of an aortic dissection or pericardial

effusion. A CT scan of his head was normal, as were X-rays of the cervical, lumbar, and thoracic spine. The admission electrocardiogram (ECG) showed complete heart block and evidence of inferior-posterior injury. (Figure 4.1) After 15 minutes the atrioventricular block spontaneously resolved. The patient was admitted to the critical care unit. Based on the history of blunt chest trauma, absence of chest pain before the collision, past history of CABG surgery, and the appearance of the initial electrocardiogram, an acutely occluded vein graft was suspected. An emergency transthoracic echocardiogram (TTE) showed an akinetic posterior and inferior wall, with the left ventricular ejection fraction estimated to be 40%. There was no evidence of a pericardial effusion, and all of the valves were normal.

The admission arterial blood gas on 100% facemask revealed; pH 7.35, PO$_2$ 101 mmHg (13.3 kPa), PCO$_2$ 47 mmHg (6.2 kPa), and HCO$_3^-$ 29 mmol l^{-1}. There was mild elevation of creatine kinase (CK) with a CK-MB fraction of 11%. Troponin testing was not available at the time of this accident.

After admission to the ICU, the patient continued to complain of persistent left-sided chest pain, aggravated by deep breathing. In order to confirm the suspicion of an acutely occluded

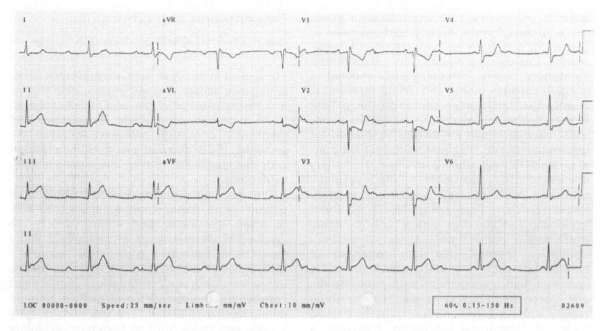

Figure 4.1

Admission 12-lead electrocardiogram, showing complete heart-block and evidence of inferior-posterior myocardial injury.

vein graft to the right coronary artery, an arch aortogram and coronary angiography were performed. The aortogram showed no evidence of an aortic dissection. The native left coronary system showed mild diffuse disease, and the left internal mammary artery graft to the left anterior descending artery was patent. The native right coronary vessel was occluded at its origin. The vein graft to the proximal right coronary artery was occluded about 6-cm distal to the aortic anastomosis (Figure 4.2). A cardiac surgery consult was obtained. Because of the associated closed head injury, pulmonary contusions, and left hemothorax, the cardiovascular surgeon declined to perform a redo CABG operation. The invasive cardiology team felt that the risks of percutaneous revascularization, which would also require some heparin administration, outweighed the potential benefits. In addition, in the event of a major complication of percutaneous revascularization, cardiopulmonary bypass would be required. Conservative medical management with aspirin, metoprolol, and a nitroglycerin infusion was instituted. The patient's chest wall pain was treated with patient-controlled morphine infusion. Serial electrocardiograms showed an evolving inferior–posterior myocardial infarction. The total creatine kinase peaked at 1 840 u l⁻¹, with a peak CK-MB of 250 u l⁻¹ (13.6%).

The patient clinically deteriorated over the next 12 hours, becoming increasingly tachypneic. His chest X-ray showed the progressive changes of

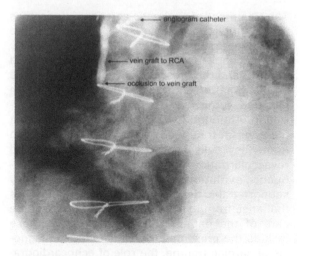

Figure 4.2

Coronary angiogram, showing occlusion of the right coronary artery vein graft 6 cm distal to the aortic anastomosis.

bilateral pulmonary contusions. Despite excellent analgesia from a thoracic epidural, used to control the pain from the fractured ribs, his respiratory status continued to deteriorate. Pulmonary artery catheterization showed a normal cardiac index and filling pressures. Twenty-four hours after admission the patient further decompensated and required endotracheal intubation and mechanical ventilation for respiratory failure. A transesophageal echocardiogram (TEE) was then performed. This study confirmed the previously noted akinetic segments with the left ventricular ejection fraction assessed as being 45–50 %. Right ventricular function was normal, and the aortic examination ruled out aortic dissection. Continued medical treatment consisted of metoprolol, aspirin, a nitroglycerin infusion, judicious fluid management, early mobilization, and deep breathing exercises. His condition rapidly improved, and he was extubated after 36 hours of mechanical ventilation. Following a predischarge exercise stress-test which showed no evidence of ongoing ischemia, the patient was discharged from the hospital 7 days later. Two months later he was asymptomatic and had returned to work.

Discussion

The treatment of traumatic coronary injuries has to be individualized and will depend on the hemodynamic stability of the patient, the type and mechanism of the injury, other associated injuries, and the presence of contraindications to anticoagulation. Suggested therapies have included surgical and percutaneous revascularization. Although it was clear to the authors that there was a traumatic occlusion to the RCA vein graft, they believed that the risks of attempted revascularization were not justified. The subsequent evolution of the pulmonary injury supported this decision. There are several issues that arise from this case that are important in the care of the patient with chest trauma. These include the presentation and differential diagnosis of cardiac trauma, the role of echocardiography in the acute setting, and the consideration of the benefits and risks of CPB in the multisystem trauma patient.

Presentation and differential diagnosis of cardiac trauma

The patient in this case scenario presented to the emergency department with multisystem trauma and severe chest pain that was initially believed to be secondary to multiple rib fractures and myocardial contusion. However, because the screening ECG showed changes inconsistent with that diagnosis, further investigations were carried out.

Thoracic injury occurs in about 15–30% of patients with major trauma, and in 30–50% of these, the heart and major vessels are involved.[8,9] Several types of myocardial injury have been described after chest trauma.[10] Myocardial contusion, the most common cardiac injury, results from compression of the heart between the thoracic vertebrae and the sternum during rapid deceleration. The spectrum of injury is wide and varies from an asymptomatic injury to cardiogenic shock. Pathologically, contusion consists of anatomic changes in the myocardium with patchy areas of necrosis and interstitial hemorrhage. The serum level of CK-MB is usually elevated. However, in a retrospective study by Healey et al, only 38% of patients with blunt cardiac trauma and a CK-MB greater than 200 u l[-1] developed any cardiac complications.[11] Measurements of blood troponin-T, a cardiac specific enzyme, has more recently been used for the diagnosis of traumatic cardiac injury.[12–14] Troponin I, another enzyme normally restricted to myocardium, has also been used to diagnose myocardial contusion more specifically. Adams et al prospectively investigated 44 patients after incurring blunt chest trauma.[15] In this study, using a cut-off value of 3.5 ng ml[-1], there was no overlap in troponin I values in the cardiac injury group versus the no-injury group. Whereas conventional diagnostic imaging studies are often unhelpful, TEE may be an important diagnostic tool for the evaluation of these injuries.[16] The most common complications of myocardial contusions are impaired ventricular function and arrhythmias. These arrhythmias usually resolve within a few hours, and most myocardial contusions resolve without any definitive therapy.

Other cardiac injuries occur less frequently. Traumatic acute valvular incompetence can occur from either direct or indirect injury. Injury to the aortic valve is the most common.[9,17] Acute aortic regurgitation leads to an increase in left ventricular wall tension which is not well tolerated, and acute pulmonary edema often follows. Tricuspid and mitral valve injuries are less common but are more often fatal.[18] Deep and superficial penetrating injuries of the ventricular free walls present as pericardial tamponade. In addition, traumatic rupture of the ventricular and atrial septa have also been described.[19] Septal rupture may be acute at the time of impact or can be delayed because of myocardial necrosis after septal contusion. Infarction of the septum, caused by traumatic coronary artery occlusion, can result in late septal rupture. Occurrences such as cardiac cavity rupture are usually instantly fatal.

Coronary artery injuries occur infrequently. Acute myocardial infarction can be caused by penetrating and blunt chest trauma.[5,20–23] Because of its anterior location, the most frequently injured coronary artery is the native LAD artery.[24] More rarely, the circumflex or the RCA is injured.[25] The RCA is vulnerable during systole when the proximal portion of the vessel moves anteriorly.[26]

The initial clinical findings of coronary artery injury are usually those of chest pain (often not very helpful) and ECG evidence of acute myocardial infarction. A variety of coronary artery lesions can be found after chest trauma, including coronary dissection, thrombosis, and spasm.[27–30] Material from the aorta may embolize, and aortic dissection may also involve the coronary arteries. The least frequent but most often fatal lesion is coronary artery rupture, due to secondary hemopericardium.

The traumatic occlusion of an aortocoronary vein graft differs from that of a native coronary artery. In addition to the anterior location of these vessels which makes them more susceptible to injury, the wall of a vein graft is also markedly different from that of a native coronary artery.[30] Over time, the adaptation mechanism of a vein placed in the arterial system consists of medial thickening and infiltration with fibroblasts and myocytes. As in the case presentation described above, it is likely that chest trauma caused dislodgment or rupture of such an atherosclerotic plaque causing subsequent graft occlusion. Other mechanisms of graft occlusion such as vein dissection rarely occur, because veins lack the typical layers of an arterial wall that can be prone to dissection.

Echocardiography in chest trauma

Echocardiography is useful as a screening modality in chest trauma for the array of cardiac injuries, as well as aortic and mediastinal injuries. The role of echocardiography in blunt and penetrating chest trauma is well established.[9,31–34] As illustrated in our own case study above, echocardiography enabled the physicians to verify that the ECG changes represented an evolving myocardial infarction caused by traumatic coronary occlusion. Although it did not change the management in this patient, it was essential in formulating a diagnosis and avoiding the risks associated with systemic heparinization and CPB.

Several studies have evaluated the use of echocardiography in the immediate diagnosis of cardiac injury. Approximately 25% patients with an abnormal echocardiogram develop cardiac complication requiring treatment, whereas only 1–3% of those with a normal echocardiogram develop complications.[31,35] Transesophageal imaging may be more effective in making the diagnosis of cardiac injury when compared to TTE, because the incidence of suboptimal studies is lower with TEE. However, laryngeal and esophageal injuries have to be excluded before a TEE study can be performed. Which patients with blunt chest trauma should have TEE? In considering the role of TEE in major trauma, a consensus panel of trauma surgeons suggested that it was probably useful only in the certain cases with hemodynamic instability.[36]

When selecting an imaging method for the investigation of suspected traumatic cardiac lesions such as aortic dissection, the efficacy and efficiency of the study to obtain necessary diagnostic information must be considered. This includes the ability of the test to detect the extent of the dissection, the involvement of the ascending aorta, the site of the entry and re-entry, thrombosis in the false lumen, branch vessel involvement, aortic insufficiency, pericardial effusion, and coronary artery involvement. Other factors affecting selection include rapid availability, local expertise, cost, contraindications to the use of intravenous contrast agents, and whether it is invasive or non-invasive. Diagnostic imaging methods for evaluation of suspected aortic dissections were reviewed by Cigarroa et al.[37] The sensitivity of TEE for detecting dissection is about 99%, with a specificity of 97%. Although the evaluation of the aortic valve is good, evaluation of the branch vessels and the coronary arteries is not optimal with TEE. Contrast-enhanced CT scanning has a sensitivity of 83–100% and a specificity of 90–100%. In comparison, aortography has an overall sensitivity of 88% and a specificity of 94%. However, aortography can very accurately identify complications at the dissection site such as aortic insufficiency, involvement of branch vessels, thrombosis, and involvement of the proximal coronary arteries. Magnetic resonance imaging is an excellent non-invasive modality to be considered. It can be very accurate in diagnosing aortic dissection, with a sensitivity of 96% and a specificity of 100%. Unfortunately, it cannot yet identify aortic insufficiency, and does not reliably provide information about involvement of the coronary arteries.

Cardiopulmonary bypass in the multisystem trauma patient

As in all cases, the potential risks and benefits associated with extensive and invasive procedures must be carefully assessed. The multisystem trauma patient provides a particular challenge when being evaluated for a surgical procedure that may require CPB. The effects of systemic heparinization in a patient with a variety of active or potential sites of hemorrhage (such as a closed head injury, multiple rib fractures, pulmonary contusion, and a known hemothorax) are potentially catastrophic. However, the introduction of heparin-bound CPB circuits and oxygenators has markedly decreased the amount of systemic heparinization required to safely establish CPB. In addition to requiring less heparinization, these circuits are associated with less fibrinolysis during CPB.[38] It is therefore now possible to perform surgical procedures requiring CPB in patients with multiple trauma, with less

associated risk than before. Most commonly, these circuits are used in the case of traumatic aortic injuries. Cardiopulmonary bypass also activates the complement cascade and the kinin systems.[39] These systems are already activated in a patient with major trauma. When there is the additional insult of pulmonary contusion, the institution of CPB and subsequent further activation of the complement cascade could certainly compound lung injury and make recovery much more problematic.

Minimally invasive approaches to coronary artery bypass operations can also be utilized in multiple-trauma patients in whom the coronary angiogram clearly shows a discrete occlusion. In these cases, CPB is not usually required.[40] However, heparin is still required, but in smaller doses than full CPB. Median sternotomy is also associated with a high incidence of wound complications in the patient with extensive chest trauma.[41] The practitioner must also determine whether the patient may benefit from medical management alone. For example, the Coronary Artery Surgery Study (CASS) documented no advantage of 'bypass' surgery in patients with single-vessel coronary artery disease.[42]

Lateral thoracotomy in the Emergency Department in the chest trauma patient?

Penetrating trauma is more likely than blunt trauma to require emergency thoracotomy. Emergency lateral thoracotomy in the Emergency Department is infrequently life saving. In one study by Millham et al, emergency department thoracotomy was associated with only a 14% overall survival in 'all comers'. If the patient had no recordable vital signs in the field or on arrival in the Emergency Department, the prognosis for meaningful recovery was zero.[43] Although some authors have strongly argued for using Emergency Department thoracotomies, their data is descriptive and cannot be used to suggest that it improves survival.[44] Additional disadvantages of an emergency lateral thoracotomy are that it provides relatively poor access to the anterior surface of the heart (the most likely surface to be injured during trauma), and it is not the optimal approach for cannulation if CPB is required.

Conclusions and learning points

- Cardiac injury is a relatively common occurrence in major chest trauma.
- All cardiac structures can be injured, and although most cardiac injuries present acutely, delayed presentations can occur.
- The diagnostic work-up and management plan of the patient with cardiac trauma must be individualized.
- Troponin I or T may be more specific markers for cardiac contusion.
- Transesophageal echocardiography is very sensitive for cardiac and aortic injuries that require treatment.
- The role of Emergency Department lateral thoracotomy is still unclear.
- Cardiopulmonary bypass with full heparinization after major trauma may have serious consequences. Heparin bonded circuits may be useful in diminishing the degree of anticoagulation required. Off-pump procedures may also have a role to play in this situation.

References

1. Pezzella TA, Silva WE, Lancey RA. Current problems in surgery: cardiothoracic trauma. *Curr Probl Surg* 1998;**35**:656–67.

2. Tenzer ML. The spectrum of myocardial contusion. A review. *J Trauma* 1985;**25**: 620–7.

3. Liedtke AJ, De Muth WE Jr. Non-penetrating cardiac injuries. A collective review. *Am Heart J* 1973;**86**:687–97.

4. Baum VC. The patient with cardiac trauma. *J Cardiothorac Vasc Anesth* 2000;**14**:71–81.

5. Abbott JA, Cousineau M, Cheitlin M *et al*. Late sequelae of penetrating cardiac wounds. *J Thorac Cardiovasc Surg* 1978;**75**:510–8.

6. Esplugas E, Barthe J, Sabate J, Fontanillas C. Obstruction of aortocoronary bypass grafts due to blunt chest trauma. *Int J Cardiol* 1983;**3**:311–4.

7. Jacobsohn E, Shields K, Aronson S, Albertucci M. Case 6-1996: traumatic aortocoronary saphenous vein graft occlusion. *J Cardiothorac Vasc Anesth* 1996;**10**:950–6.

8. Charbonnier B, Desveaux B, Cosnay P *et al*. Les infarctes myocardiques traumatiques [Traumatic myocardial infarction. Apropos of 2 cases]. *Arch Mal Coeur Vaiss* 1984;**77**:273–82.

9. Pretre R, Chilcott M. Blunt trauma to the heart and great vessels. *N Engl J Med* 1997;**336**:626–32.

10. Mattox KL, Feliciano DV, Burch J *et al*. Five thousand seven hundred sixty cardiovascular injuries in 4459 patients. Epidemiologic evolution 1958 to 1987. *Ann Surg* 1989;**209**:698–707.

11. Healey MA, Brown R, Fleiszer D. Blunt cardiac trauma: is this diagnosis necessary? *J Trauma* 1990;**30**:137–46.

12. Ferjani M, Droc G, Dreux S *et al*. Circulating cardiac troponin T in myocardial contusion. *Chest* 1997;**111**:427–33.

13. Helm M, Hauke J, Lampl L. Diagnostic value of troponin T as a biochemical marker of myocardial contusion. *Anesthesiology* 1998;**89**:A467.

14. Helm M, Hauke J, Weiss A, Lampl L. [Cardiac troponin T as a biochemical marker of myocardial injury early after trauma. Diagnostic value of a qualitative bedside test]. *Chirurg* 1999;**70**:1347–52.

15. Adams JE 3rd, Davila-Roman VG, Bessey PQ *et al*. Improved detection of cardiac contusion with cardiac troponin I. *Am Heart J* 1996;**131**:308–12.

16. O'Connor C. Chest trauma: the role of transesophageal echocardiography. *J Clin Anesth* 1996;**8**:605–13.

17. German DS, Shapiro MJ, Wilman VL. Acute aortic valvular incompetence following thoracic-deceleration injury: case report. *J Trauma* 1990;**30**:1411–2.

18. Werne C, Sagraves SG, Costa C. Mitral and tricuspid valve rupture from blunt trauma sustained during a motor vehicle collision. *J Trauma* 1989;**29**:113–5.

19. Stajer D, Kariz S. Ventricular septal rupture following blunt chest trauma after a long delay: a case report. *Int J Cardiol* 1994;**47**:187–8.

20. Mattox KL, Koch LV, Beall AC Jr, DeBakey ME. Logistic and technical considerations in the treat-

ment of the wounded heart. *Circulation* 1975;**52(2 Suppl)**:I210–4.

21. Anonymous. Traumatic injury of the heart. *Lancet* 1990;**356**:1287–9.

22. Kahn JK, Buda AJ. Long-term follow-up of coronary occlusion secondary to blunt chest trauma. *Am Heart J* 1987;**113**:207–10.

23. Mairesse GH, Timmermans P. Post traumatic myocardial infarction. *Acta Clin Belg* 1993;**48**:128–31.

24. Stern T, Wolf RY, Reichart B *et al.* Coronary artery occlusion resulting from blunt trauma. *JAMA* 1974;**230**:1308–9.

25. Shapiro MJ, Wittgen C, Flynn *et al.* Right coronary artery occlusion secondary to blunt trauma. *Clin Cardiol* 1994;**17**:157–9.

26. Oliva PB, Hilgenberg A, McElroy D. Obstruction of the proximal right coronary artery with acute inferior infarction due to blunt chest trauma. *Ann Intern Med* 1979;**91**:205–7.

27. Watt AH, Stephens MR. Myocardial infarction after blunt chest trauma incurred during rugby football that later required cardiac transplantation. *Br Heart J* 1986;**55**:408–10.

28. Merek A, Rey J, Larry G *et al.* Myocardial infarction caused by closed thoracic injury. Pathogenic and angiographic aspects. Apropos of four cases and review of the literature. *Ann Cardiol Angiol* 1991;**40**:111–21.

29. Vlay SC, Blumenthal DS, Shoback *et al.* Delayed acute myocardial infarction after blunt chest trauma in a young woman. *Am Heart J* 1980;**100**:907–16.

30. Campeau L, Enjalbert M, Lesperance *et al.* Atherosclerosis and late closure of aortocoronary saphenous vein grafts: sequential angiographic studies at 2 weeks, 1 year, 5 to 7 years, and 10 to 12 years after surgery. *Circulation* 1983;**68**:II1–7.

31. Karalis DG, Victor MF, Davis GA *et al.* The role of echocardiography in blunt chest trauma: a transthoracic and transesophageal echocardiographic study. *J Trauma* 1994;**36**:53–8.

32. Kearney PA, Smith DW, Johnson SB *et al.* Use of transesophageal echocardiography in the evaluation of traumatic aortic injury. *J Trauma* 1993;**34**:696–703.

33. Brooks SW, Young JC, Cmolik B *et al.* The use of transeophageal echocardiography in the evaluation of chest trauma. *J Trauma* 1992;**32**:761–8.

34. Thakur RK, Aufderheide TP, Boughner DR. Emergency echocardiographic evaluation of penetrating chest trauma. *Can J Cardiol* 1994;**10**:374–6.

35. Reif J, Justice JL, Olsen WR, Prager RL. Selective monitoring of patients with suspected blunt cardiac injury. *Ann Thorac Surg* 1990;**50**:530–3.

36. Pasquale M, Fabian TC. Practice management guidelines for trauma from the Eastern Association for the Surgery of Trauma. *J Trauma* 1998;**44**:941–57.

37. Cigarroa JE, Isselbacher EM, DeSanctis RW, Eagle KA. Diagnostic imaging in the evaluation of suspected aortic dissection. Old standards and new directions. *N Engl J Med* 1993;**328**:35–43.

38. Steinberg BM, Grossi EA, Schwartz DS *et al.* Heparin bonding of bypass circuits reduces cytokine release during cardiopulmonary bypass. *Ann Thorac Surg* 1995;**60**:525–9.

39. Kirklin JK, Westaby S, Blackstone EH *et al.* Complement and the damaging effects of cardiopulmonary bypass. *J Thorac Cardiovasc Surg* 1983;**86**:845–57.

40. Moshkovitz Y, Lusky A, Mohr R. Coronary artery bypass without cardiopulmonary bypass: analysis of short-term and mid-term outcomes in 220 patients. *J Thorac Cardiovasc Surg* 1995;**110**:979–87.

41. Boyd DA. Chest wall trauma. In: Hood RM, Boyd AD, Culmford AT (eds) *Thoracic Trauma.* Philadelphia: WB Saunders, 1989; 101–32.

42. CASS Principal Investigators and their Associates. Myocardial infarction and mortality in the coronary artery surgery (CASS) randomized trial. *N Engl J Med* 1984;**310**:750–8.

43. Millham FH, Grindlinger GA. Survival determinants in patients undergoing emergency room thoracotomy for penetrating chest injury. *J Trauma* 1993;**34**:332–6.

44. Asensio JA, Berne JD, Demetriades D *et al.* One hundred five penetrating cardiac injuries: a 2-year prospective evaluation. *J Trauma* 1998;**44**:1073–82.

5
Severe aortic atheromatous disease in cardiac surgery

Gary W Roach

Introduction

Severe aortic atheromatous disease continues to pose serious risks to the patient undergoing cardiac surgery despite many technical advances in cardiac surgical, anesthetic, and perfusion techniques. The determination of severity of proximal aortic atherosclerosis may require alterations in standard anesthetic or surgical techniques in the hope of decreasing the high rate of perioperative complications.

Case history 1

An 80-year-old woman presented with a 3-week history of unstable angina. Following coronary angiography she was referred for coronary artery bypass surgery.

The patient was premedicated with morphine sulfate (MS) 7 mg and midazolam 4 mg intramuscularly. Following placement of routine monitors

including radial arterial and pulmonary arterial catheters, anesthesia was induced with sufentanil 250 µg, midazolam 3 mg, and pancuronium 7 mg, and then maintained with isoflurane 0.5–1.0% in 60% oxygen. Following tracheal intubation, transesophageal echocardiographic (TEE) examination revealed normal cardiac valve and myocardial function, but a large mobile atheromatous plaque was noted at the junction of the ascending aorta and aortic arch. Epiaortic scanning subsequently demonstrated an area of the ascending aorta that was relatively free of disease. The aorta was cannulated in this site and cardiopulmonary bypass (CPB) was initiated with systemic cooling to 28°C. With TEE it was demonstrated that the plaque was intact after these manipulations. The proximal vein grafts were anastomosed to the LIMA to avoid further manipulation of the aorta, using ventricular fibrillation, rather than cardioplegic arrest for myocardial protection.

Saphenous vein grafts were placed to the posterior descending artery and the first obtuse marginal artery. The left internal mammary

Past medical history	Hypertension
Regular medications	Atenolol 50 mg OD, isosorbide dinitrate 20 mg TDS, glyceryl trinitrate 0.3 mg PRN.
Examination	Weight 72 kg. BP 162/94. Left carotid bruit.
Investigations	Hb 11.2 g dl⁻¹ (all other laboratory values were normal). **Carotid ultrasound:** Bilateral internal carotid artery stenoses (< 30%). **Cardiac catheterization:** 90% stenosis of the left anterior descending artery and 60% stenosis of the circumflex coronary artery. Left ventricular ejection fraction 73% without regional wall motion abnormalities.

artery (LIMA) was anastomosed to the left anterior descending artery. The proximal ends of the vein grafts were anastomosed to the LIMA to avoid further manipulation of the aorta.

Following rewarming, the patient defibrillated easily and was weaned from CPB with infusion of dobutamine 5 µg kg^{-1} min^{-1}. At this time TEE demonstrated good ventricular function, but a portion of the aortic atheroma was noted to be missing. The patient was transferred to the cardiovascular intensive care unit in stable condition with good hemodynamics. The dobutamine was weaned over the next 3 hours. On the first postoperative day, the patient was noted to be unresponsive with right hemiparesis. Computerized axial tomography revealed a large left hemispheric stroke with cerebral edema, ventricular compression, and midline shift consistent with occlusion of the left middle cerebral artery. She failed to improve, demonstrating evidence of clinical brain death and expired 3 days after surgery.

Case history 2

A 67-year-old diabetic male presented for an elective CABG.

On the morning of surgery, the patient was premedicated with morphine sulfate 9 mg and midazolam 6 mg. Following intravenous, radial arterial and pulmonary arterial cannulation, anesthesia was induced with sevoflurane 1–6% in oxygen, sufentanil 50 µg and pancuronium 9 mg. Anesthesia was maintained with sevoflurane 1–2% (end-tidal concentration) in 60% oxygen. TEE demonstrated thickening of the aortic arch

and descending aorta, with suggestion of calcification in the ascending aorta. Surgical palpation of the ascending aorta confirmed severe circumferential calcification or 'porcelain' aorta. After discussion between the surgeon and the anesthesiologist, a decision was made to proceed with an off-pump coronary artery bypass (OPCAB) surgery to avoid aortic manipulation.

The patient was given heparin 17 000 iu (~200 iu kg^{-1}) to maintain the activated clotting time at >300 seconds. Using a myocardial stabilization device, the LIMA and a saphenous vein graft were anastomosed to the LAD and the posterior descending artery respectively. The proximal end of the right coronary vein graft was anastomosed to the LIMA to avoid any aortic manipulation. Following completion of the anastomoses and a check for bleeding, the heparin was reversed with protamine 150 mg.

At the completion of the procedure neuromuscular blockade was reversed with neostigmine 2.5 mg and glycopyrrolate 0.5 mg. When the patient was awake and breathing spontaneously with an end-tidal CO_2 of 38–43 mmHg (5.1–5.7 kPa), the endotracheal tube was removed. He was transferred to the cardiovascular ICU neurologically intact and in stable condition. His subsequent recovery was unremarkable, with discharge from the intensive care unit on postoperative day 1, and discharge from the hospital on postoperative day 4.

Discussion

Atherosclerosis of the ascending aorta and the aortic arch has increasingly been recognized as a

Past medical history	Hypertension, hyperlipidemia, type II diabetes mellitus, peripheral vascular disease. 82 pack-year history of smoking.
Regular medications	Metoprolol 50 mg BD, diltiazem 30 mg TDS, isosorbide dinitrate 10 mg QDS, tolazamide 500 mg OD.
Examination	Weight 86 kg. BP 154/90.
Investigations	Glucose 230 mg dl^{-1} (12.8 mmol l^{-1}) All other laboratory values were normal.
Cardiac catheterization:	95% LAD stenosis, 80% RCA stenosis and <50% stenosis of the first obtuse marginal artery. LVEF 47% with mild hypokinesis of the mid-anterior wall. LVEDP 26 mmHg.

major cause of morbidity associated with cardiac surgery. Cardiac surgeons have recognized calcification of the aorta as a risk factor for adverse neurologic outcomes following cardiac surgery for many years. Gardner and colleagues analyzed 3279 consecutive patients undergoing CABG, finding severe atherosclerosis of the ascending aorta to be a major risk factor.[1] More recently, a multicenter study found proximal aortic atherosclerosis, as determined by the surgeon at the time of surgery, to be associated with a four-fold increase in the risk of adverse cerebral outcomes in CABG patients.[2] Similarly, the same group of investigators found proximal aortic atherosclerosis to significantly increase the risk of cerebral dysfunction in patients undergoing combined CABG and valve procedures.[3] Not surprisingly, atherosclerosis of the ascending aorta has also been associated with renal dysfunction, mortality, and long-term neurologic events following cardiac surgery.[4,5]

Surgical palpation has historically been the primary method of detecting aortic atherosclerosis, however many studies have shown that palpation seriously underestimates the presence and severity of disease. When compared to epiaortic scanning, palpation of the aorta detected only 17–46% of significant atheromatous plaques.[6–8] Compared to epiaortic scanning, TEE provides much less reliable images of the ascending aorta.[9,10] TEE imaging of the descending aorta and aortic arch, however, has good predictive value for the presence of ascending aortic disease with excellent sensitivity, and a low false negative rate although the specificity is only fair. The combination of TEE and surgical palpation improves predictive value with further diminution of the false negatives.[11] Risk factors for moderate to severe aortic atherosclerosis include age, smoking, and a history of peripheral vascular disease.[12] Patients presenting with these risk factors should have both surgical palpation and a TEE examination of their aorta. If significant plaques are found, epiaortic scanning should be performed to further identify the nature of the plaques, as well as to locate less severely diseased areas of the aorta that may be suitable for manipulations such as aortic cannulation, and placement of aortic clamps and grafts.

Numerous variations in surgical techniques have been espoused for the patient with signifi-

cantly diseased aortas. These include use of single cross-clamp technique;[13] changing the location of cannulation, clamp and graft sites; and in some cases ascending aortic replacement or endarterectomy utilizing circulatory arrest[7] More recently, it has been suggested that the use of OPCAB with anastomosis of the proximal grafts to an arterial inflow other than the aorta may decrease the likelihood of adverse cerebral outcomes.[14] Unfortunately, while some of these approaches may seem intuitively beneficial, none has been tested in prospective, randomized trials. Likewise, techniques that may seem to work at one institution, such as replacement of the ascending aorta, have been associated with worse outcomes when applied at other institutions.[15] Thus, it is difficult to make firm recommendations for the surgical management of these patients.

Similarly, there is little data to suggest that variations in the anesthetic or perfusion management of these patients can improve outcomes. Data from a prospective, randomized trial at Cornell suggested that maintaining mean arterial pressure >80 mmHg during CPB was associated with a decrease in the *combined* incidence of death, myocardial infarction, and stroke.[16] However, others have found little evidence that higher arterial pressure during bypass can improve neurologic outcomes.[17] Although hypothermia has clearly been demonstrated to be neuroprotective, its role during CPB remains controversial and there are no specific recommendations for temperature management in patients with significant aortic atherosclerosis.[18–20] Despite numerous attempts at pharmacological neuroprotection, there remains no evidence that any clinically available drugs provide significant protection. Recently, the N-methyl-D-aspartate (NMDA) antagonist remacemide hydrochloride has been reported to improve global neuropsychological scores.[21] Further investigation is necessary to determine if it also improves neurologic outcomes.

The two cases presented here, with different manifestations of aortic atherosclerosis, demonstrate that adverse outcomes can occur despite reasonable precautions, and that in some cases adverse neurologic sequelae can be avoided. In the first case, the area of diseased aorta was located and alterations in the surgical technique were made. Despite these precautions, however, a portion of the large mobile atheroma embolized to the middle cerebral artery resulting in a massive and ultimately fatal stroke. In the second case, a more classical situation of 'porcelain aorta' was discovered intraoperatively leading to the decision to perform off-pump CABG and avoid manipulation of the aorta. The result in this case was an excellent neurologic outcome despite the high-risk profile of the patient. Although early results from OPCAB are encouraging, the lack of adequate controls and long-term follow-up mandates some healthy skepticism regarding the utility of the procedure in patients with moderate to severe aortic atherosclerosis.

In summary, aortic atherosclerosis of the ascending aorta and aortic arch is associated with a marked increase in adverse cerebral outcomes following cardiac surgery. The gold standard for defining the severity of disease is epiaortic ultrasonographic scanning, although TEE plus palpation is a reasonable screen. Surgical palpation alone is woefully inadequate in the detection of aortic plaques. A wide range of alterations in surgical technique in patients with significant aortic atherosclerosis has been proposed, but none has withstood the scrutiny of prospective, randomized trials. Currently, it would seem prudent to minimize aortic manipulations while still providing adequate revascularization and myocardial protection for this group of patients. Although the anesthesiologist plays a critical role in ascertaining the presence or absence of aortic plaques and risk stratification, we have no proven therapeutic options available at this time.[22] Pharmacologic neuroprotection may be an available option in the near future.

Learning points

- Aortic atheroma is associated with a significant increase in the risk of cerebral injury following cardiac surgery.
- The identification of severe atheromatous disease of the descending aorta by TEE is predictive of significant disease in the ascending aorta.
- Epiaortic ultrasonography is the gold standard for assessing the severity of proximal aortic atheromatous disease.

- The efficacy of modifications to surgical technique proposed in patients with severe aortic atheroma have yet to determined in prospective, randomized studies.

References

1. Gardner TJ, Horneffer PJ, Manolio TA et al. Stroke following coronary artery bypass grafting: a ten-year study. Ann Thorac Surg 1985;40:574–81.

2. Roach GW, Kanchuger M, Mangano CM et al for the Multicenter Study of Perioperative Ischemia Research Group and the Ischemia Research and Education Foundation Investigators. Adverse cerebral outcomes after coronary bypass surgery. N Engl J Med 1996;335:1857–63.

3. Wolman RL, Nussmeier NA, Aggarwal A et al for the Multicenter Study of Perioperative Ischemia Research Group (McSPI) and the Ischemia Research Education Foundation (IREF) Investigators. Cerebral injury after cardiac surgery: identification of a group at extraordinary risk. Stroke 1999;30:514–22.

4. Davila-Roman VG, Kouchoukos NT, Schechtman KB, Barzilai B. Atherosclerosis of the ascending aorta is a predictor of renal dysfunction after cardiac operations. J Thorac Cardiovasc Surg 1999;117:111–6..

5. Davila-Roman VG, Murphy SF, Nickerson NJ et al. Atherosclerosis of the ascending aorta is an independent predictor of long-term neurologic events and mortality. J Am Coll Cardiol 1999;33:1308–16.

6. Katz ES, Tunick PA, Rusinek H et al. Protruding aortic atheromas predict stroke in elderly patients undergoing cardiopulmonary bypass: experience with intraoperative transesophageal echocardiography. J Am Coll Cardiol 1992;20:70–7.

7. Wareing TH, Davila-Roman VG, Barzilai B et al. Management of the severely atherosclerotic ascending aorta during cardiac operations. A strategy for detection and treatment. J Thorac Cardiovasc Surg 1992;103:453–62.

8. Nicolosi AC, Aggarwal A, Almassi GH, Olinger GN. Intraoperative epiaortic ultrasound during cardiac surgery. J Card Surg 1996;11:49–55.

9. Konstadt SN, Reich DL, Quintana C, Levy M. The ascending aorta: how much does transesophageal echocardiography see? Anesth Analg 1994;78:240–4.

10. Davila-Roman VG, Phillips KJ, Daily BB *et al.* Intraoperative transesophageal echocardiography and epiaortic ultrasound for assessment of atherosclerosis of the thoracic aorta. *J Am Coll Cardiol* 1996;**28**:942–7.

11. Tissot M, Kanchuger M, Grossi E *et al.* The prevalence of atheromatous diseases of the ascending aorta and its relationship to such disease in the aortic arch. *Anesthesiology* 1994;**81**:A167.

12. Davila-Roman VG, Barzilai B, Wareing TH *et al.* Atherosclerosis of the ascending aorta. Prevalence and role as an independent predictor of cerebrovascular events in cardiac patients. *Stroke* 1994;**25**:2010–6.

13. Aranki SF, Sullivan TE, Cohn LH. The effect of the single aortic cross-clamp technique on cardiac and cerebral complications during coronary bypass surgery. *J Card Surg* 1995;**10**:498–502.

14. Anderson RE, Li TQ, Hindmarsh T *et al.* Increased extracellular brain water after coronary artery bypass grafting is avoided by off-pump surgery. *J Cardiothorac Vasc Anesth* 1999;**13**:698–702.

15. Stern A, Tunick PA, Culliford AT *et al.* Protruding aortic arch atheromas: risk of stroke during heart surgery with and without aortic arch endarterectomy. *Am Heart J* 1999;**138**:746–52.

16. Gold JP, Charlson ME, Williams-Russo P *et al.* Improvement of outcomes after coronary artery bypass. A randomized trial comparing intraoperative high versus low mean arterial pressure. *J Thorac Cardiovasc Surg* 1995;**110**:1302–11.

17. Govier AV, Reves JG, McKay RD *et al.* Factors and their influence on regional cerebral blood flow during nonpulsatile cardiopulmonary bypass. *Ann Thorac Surg* 1984;**38**:592–600.

18. Mora CT, Henson MB, Weintraub WS *et al.* The effect of temperature management during cardiopulmonary bypass on neurologic and neuropsychologic outcomes in patients undergoing coronary revascularization. *J Thorac Cardiovasc Surg* 1996;**112**:514–22.

19. Plourde G, Leduc AS, Morin JE *et al.* Temperature during cardiopulmonary bypass for coronary artery operations does not influence postoperative cognitive function: a prospective, randomized trial. *J Thorac Cardiovasc Surg* 1997;**114**:123–8.

20. McLean RF, Wong BI, Naylor CD *et al.* Cardiopulmonary bypass, temperature, and central nervous system dysfunction. *Circulation* 1994;**90**:II250–5.

21. Arrowsmith JE, Harrison MJ, Newman SP *et al.* Neuroprotection of the brain during cardiopulmonary bypass: a randomized trial of remacemide during coronary artery bypass in 171 patients. *Stroke* 1998;**29**:2357–62.

22. Newman MF, Wolman R, Kanchuger M *et al* for the Multicenter Study of Perioperative Ischemia (McSPI) Research Group. Multicenter preoperative stroke risk index for patients undergoing coronary artery bypass graft surgery. *Circulation* 1996;**94**:II74–80.

6
Anesthesia for transmyocardial laser revascularization

Hilary P Grocott

Introduction

The later part of the twentieth century saw the development of a number of novel techniques for the management of severe and otherwise inoperable coronary artery disease. One of these was the development (and approval by health regulatory agencies) of transmyocardial laser revascularization (TMLR). With this procedure, new transmural channels are created in the myocardium using an epicardially placed laser thereby allowing oxygen and other blood-borne nutrients to reach otherwise compromised myocardial tissue. The transmural channels act as conduits for the flow of oxygenated blood from the chamber of the left ventricle into the ischemic myocardium. Although it is a relatively new procedure, its development took several decades, yet despite this time, its exact mechanism for patient benefit is much disputed. The use of TMLR has presented the anesthesiologist with a number of unique considerations, several of which are outlined in the case and discussion to follow.

Case history

A 51-year-old male presented to his cardiologist with increasing exertional angina. He had undergone coronary artery bypass grafting (CABG) 6 years previously but continued to have some residual angina within months after surgery. This had been increasing with him experiencing, at the time of presentation, several anginal episodes daily brought on by minimal exertion. A coronary angiogram revealed occlusion of a saphenous vein graft to his right coronary artery (RCA), a patent left internal mammary artery (LIMA) to his left anterior descending (LAD) artery, and significant disease in his circumflex distribution. It was felt that the distal circulation in the circumflex artery was not amenable to myocardial revascularisation via repeat CABG.

A myocardial viability study and ^{201}Tl single-positron emission computed tomography (^{201}Tl-SPECT) were performed which demonstrated viable myocardium in the distribution of the circumflex coronary artery (lateral wall).

Past medical history	Previous CABG.
Regular medications	Metoprolol 50 mg BD, isosorbide dinitrate 30 mg TDS, enalapril 10 mg BD, aspirin 80 mg OD.
Examination	Weight 92 kg. BMI 31.5 kg.m^{-2}.
Investigations	**CXR**: Consistent with previous CABG. Otherwise unremarkable. **Coronary angiography**: Patent LIMA graft to LAD. Occluded RCA graft. Severe native circumflex coronary artery disease. **TTE**: Lateral hypokinesia. Left ventricular ejection fraction 40%.

Transthoracic echocardiography revealed impaired left ventricular function. He was referred for consideration for TMLR with the intent of improving the blood flow in the ischaemic distribution of his lateral myocardial wall.

The patient was admitted to hospital on the day of proposed TMLR and was premedicated with diazepam 10 mg and methadone 10 mg orally 90 minutes before transfer to the operating room. On arrival an intravenous cannula was sited under local anesthesia. Midazolam 2 mg and fentanyl 50 μg were administered prior to placement of a thoracic epidural at the T_6 interspace. This was followed by cannulation of the right radial arterial and right internal jugular vein under local anesthesia with insertion of a pulmonary artery (PA) catheter.

Anesthesia was induced with fentanyl 500 μg, thiopental 275 mg, and vecuronium 10 mg. A 39 French left-sided double-lumen endotracheal tube was placed without difficulty and the lungs ventilated with isoflurane (0.6–1.5% inspired) in an oxygen/air mixture. The patient was positioned in the right lateral semi-decubitus position and 'prepped' for a left anterior thoracotomy. A transesophageal echocardiography (TEE) probe was inserted for imaging of the myocardium and confirmation of the upcoming laser strikes. Preservative-free bupivicaine, 3 ml 0.5%, was injected through the epidural catheter followed by an infusion of bupivicaine 0.125% and fentanyl 2.5 μg ml^{-1} at 3 ml hour^{-1} throughout the case.

Following left lung deflation, a left anterior thoracotomy was performed and the pericardium opened to expose the lateral wall of the left ventricle. Targets for the CO_2 laser 'hits' were identified using the previous viability study as a guide. Successful penetration of 16/17 'hits' was confirmed by TEE. After obtaining hemostasis, the pericardium was closed, the lung reinflated, and the thoracotomy closed. After repositioning the patient into the supine position, the double-lumen tube was exchanged for a single-lumen endotracheal tube and the patient was transferred to the ICU in stable condition. He was weaned from mechanical ventilation and the trachea extubated approximately 1.5 hours after arrival. The epidural catheter remained in place until the third postoperative day after which he was treated with oral analgesics.

On return to the outpatient department for his 6-week follow-up, his angina had improved significantly having experienced only one episode of angina per week, with much improved exercise tolerance. He continues on his medical regimen although with lower doses of isosorbide dinitrate.

Discussion

Direct myocardial revascularization using laser-based technologies has at its origins the utilization of several anatomical features of the heart that allow blood to flow directly from the ventricle into the myocardium, in effect, 'bypassing' diseased coronary arteries. In the eighteenth century, Adrian Christian Thebesius described a network of intramyocardial connections to the ventricular cavity that now bear his name.[1] Pratt, in 1898 demonstrated that blood perfused directly from the ventricle into the myocardium could keep a cat alive, presumably utilizing the Thebesian system to deliver the nutrient-rich blood to the myocardium.[1] Further evidence for the rationale of TMLR takes its inspiration from reptilian myocardial anatomy where the myocardium is completely dependent upon a complex network of myocardial sinusoids allowing the flow of oxygenated blood directly from the left ventricle (LV) in the absence of any significant coronary arteries. In 1933, Wearns confirmed the presence of similar myocardial sinusoids in humans, and the ability of the heart to perfuse itself from the ventricular chamber.[2] It is this system of intramyocardial sinusoids that allows for the distribution of intraventricular blood that flows into the myocardium after establishing TMLR channels.

TMLR is not the only method developed to use intramural myocardial sinusoids to improve regional myocardial blood flow. In the early days of coronary artery surgery, Vineberg established a procedure that involved implantation of the internal mammary artery directly into the myocardium.[3] From this source, oxygenated blood was delivered to previously ischemic tissue. Techniques more closely related to the TMLR came in the form of myocardial acupuncture, reported by Sen, who inserted a probe through the myocardium into the cavity of the LV thereby creating a transmural channel for the flow of blood into ischemic myocardium.[4–6]

Although not the exclusive precursors to TMLR, these procedures offered a new understanding of myocardial blood flow pathways that allowed Mirhoseini in 1981 to first report the use of a low-power laser to create transmural myocardial channels.[7, 8] Mirhoseini, a pioneer in this field, reported the first TMLR in a human in 1983.[9] Since that time, research and development of TMLR has expanded dramatically with the application of several types of lasers in numerous different clinical situations. The most common used systems utilize either a CO_2 or an yttrium aluminum garnet (YAG) laser.

Although the ultimate effect of the TMLR is to reduce ischemia by augmenting myocardial blood flow, and in doing so, reduce patient symptoms, improve quality of life (and potentially longevity), the exact mechanism(s) by which this occurs is incompletely understood. There are several theories as to its efficacy. Post mortem imaging studies by both Cooley[10] and Mirhoseini[11] have revealed that patients who died from non-cardiac causes after TMLR had intact transmyocardial channels. They demonstrated in pathologic specimens that the TMLR channels remained patent from 3 months to 4 years after the procedure. Other investigators have suggested that the mechanism of action is more complex than simply creating myocardial conduits with each laser strike. Stimulation of some other form of myocardial protection has been postulated, including ventricular remodeling and ischemic preconditioning. The most intriguing work relates to the potential of TMLR to stimulate angiogenensis. Indeed, neorevascularization may be the main mechanism by which ischemia and symptoms are improved.[12–14] This mechanism corresponds best to the 3–6 month period that it generally takes to see significant improvement in symptoms.

The most commonly used and well-studied system is the Heart Laser (PLC Medical Systems, Inc., Milford, MA, USA). It is a CO_2 laser that delivers 800 watts of peak power during laser strikes. The laser strikes are timed to coincide with the R wave on the electrocardiogram thereby ensuring that the myocardium is struck when the ventricle is not only maximally dilated (and thinnest) at diastole, but more importantly, electrically silent. This minimizes the risk of both collateral damage and the induction of dysrhythmias.

During the actual laser procedure, the surgeon places a hand-held laser probe (brought into the surgical field via an articulated arm with a sterile cover on it) onto the epicardium. Depending on the area to be revascularized, approximately 15–50 laser strikes are fired on the epicardial surface, targeting the viable hibernating myocardium below. Between each of the strikes, any residual epicardial bleeding is tamponaded by direct digital compression or, uncommonly, a purse-string suture. Successful transmyocardial penetration following the laser strike is confirmed by TEE with the appearance of characteristic intraventricular 'bubbles'.

The principle indication for TMLR is coronary artery disease (CAD) that is symptomatic despite maximal medical therapy, and also is not amenable to conventional revascularization procedures. However, patients on submaximal therapy but with disabling side-effects should also be considered for TMLR. Other patients with severe saphenous vein graft disease postCABG and in whom poor conduits exist but distal vessels are present (making repeat CABG not possible) have also been proposed as candidates for TMLR. Patients with contraindications to CPB such as recent hemorrhagic stroke might also be considered. Severe allograft CAD in the postheart transplant recipients has also been treated with TMLR.

Percutaneous myocardial laser revascularization (PMLR) is a relatively non-invasive technique for TMLR has recently been developed and is undergoing clinical trials. With this technique, a percutaneous catheter-based approach is used in the interventional cardiology laboratory.[15] This technique has not yet undergone the rigorous evaluation of the open technique, but may prove useful in addition to avoiding the hazards and complications of the surgery. The avoidance of one lung anesthesia and the ability to reach the interventricular septum make PMLR attractive. Another approach that is less invasive than thoracotomy is thoracoscopic TMLR.[16, 17]

Preoperative evaluation

Before surgery, most patients will have undergone investigation to determine the extent of coronary artery disease (coronary angiography), overall left ventricular function (multigated

Table 6.1 Typical preoperative clinical characteristics of 132 patients undergoing transmyocardial laser revascularization. (Modified and reproduced from Allen et al[22] with permission)

Males	75%
Age (mean ±SD years)	60 ±10
Left ventricular ejection fraction (mean ±SD)	47 ±11%
Hypertension	70%
Diabetes mellitus	46%
Previous myocardial infarction	64%
History of smoking	72%
Hypercholesterolemia	79%
History of congestive cardiac failure	17%
Previous coronary angioplasty (PTCA)	48%
Previous coronary artery surgery (CABG)	86%
Previous PTCA and CABG	92%

acquisition radionuclide ventriculography (MUGA), standard echocardiography or dobutamine stress echocardiography) and myocardial viability (positron emission tomography (PET) or TI[201]-SPECT). Most series report left ventricular ejection fractions (LVEF) between 35 and 68%.[18–23] A LVEF <35% and/or moderate mitral insufficiency represent relative contraindications for TMLR due to the higher incidence of associated adverse cardiac events.[19]

The typical clinical characteristics of the TMLR patient are listed in Table 6.1. This represents the preoperative findings with TMLR patients with the target trial (to date) of TMLR versus medical therapy.[22] Approximately 50% of patients are diabetic, up to 65% have had a previous myocardial infarction, 75% have hypertension; a past history of tobacco use is also very common. A past history of congestive heart failure (CHF) has been reported in up to 15% of patients although current CHF is a relative contraindication for TMLR. Almost all (>90%) have had undergone prior percutaneous transluminal coronary angioplasty (PTCA) and/or CABG.

Intraoperative management

Table 6.2 describes the intraoperative considerations for the TMLR patient. Overall, the anesthetic must be geared towards a comfortable awakening and an ability to breathe effectively with the goals of early mobilization and minimizing the myocardial demands of tachycardia and hypertension. We have advocated placement of a thoracic epidural prior to anesthesia, whenever possible, to minimize the need for intraoperative anaesthetic requirements as well as to provide for later postoperative analgesia.

In general, the patient may be brought to the operating room (with or without premedication) and made comfortable with small doses of narcotics and benzodiazepines during placement of thoracic epidural, radial artery and PA catheters. At our center, we commonly use an oximetric PA catheter in order to follow the mixed venous oxygen saturation. There can be considerable hemodynamic instability during pericardial dissection, one lung ventilation and other operative maneuvers. The tolerance of the heart to this and the subsequent laser surgery injury is monitored using this indirect indicator of myocardial performance. Although the oximetric PA catheter serves this purpose well, other monitoring modalities can also be utilized. If the TMLR is undertaken in the previous CABG patient, then the ability to use internal paddles may be limited by mediastinal and pericardial adhesions. Placement of adhesive external defibrillator pads may facilitate management of ventricular dysrhythmias induced by surgical maneuvers.

The patient is positioned in a partial lateral position allowing access for the left anterior thoracotomy. Temperature maintenance is important to facilitate prompt emergence and extubation. It also assists in preventing the increases in myocardial oxygen consumption

Table 6.2 Anesthetic considerations for patients undergoing transmyocardial laser revascularization

Thoracic epidural analgesia	
Monitoring	Pulmonary artery pressure
	± Continuous cardiac output
	± mixed venous saturation
Lateral position	
Transesophageal echocardiography	
External and internal defibrillation capability	
Temperature maintenance	
Anesthetic agents (avoidance of nitrous oxide)	
Lung isolation and one lung ventilation	
Laser safety	

and potential resulting ischemia coincident with intrinsic rewarming efforts (i.e. shivering) by the patient. We use a forced air convective heating system placed over the lower body to allow maintenance of normothermia.

Lung isolation is essential for adequate exposure of the heart and can be obtained with many different techniques. Following induction of anesthesia, we commonly use a double lumen endotracheal tube after which, a TEE probe is also inserted. Anesthesia can be maintained by numerous methods. It is desirable to avoid nitrous oxide in order to reduce myocardial depression and prevent expansion of bubbles generated by laser vaporization of blood and myocardial tissue. Neurologic morbidity — either stroke of neuropsychiatric dysfunction — has not been reported in the small series available, but hundreds of gaseous emboli have been detected in the middle cerebral artery during TMLR.[24]

Transesophageal echocardiography is an essential part of TMLR for monitoring of myocardial function, mitral valve integrity and to assess laser ventricular wall penetration. As the surgeon attempts to create multiple laser channels through salvageable myocardium, transmyocardial penetration of each laser strike is confirmed by the appearance of bubbles in the left ventricular cavity.[24] The mitral apparatus must be examined for evidence of any newly ruptured chords and mitral insufficiency. Regional myocardial function is also be monitored by TEE.

Postoperative care

Most patients can be extubated at the end of surgery or soon after admission to the ICU. At the outset, it should be recognised that the intraoperative creation of laser channels does not mean instantaneous myocardial revascularization. The improvement in myocardial perfusion and function develops over the first 3–6 months postoperatively. Therefore the patient will awaken from the procedure in the same (or worse) condition than existed preoperatively. Myocardial ischemia and dysfunction may be anticipated in the postoperative period compounded by the problems of postthoraco-

tomy pain and fluid management. Up to 50% of patients may show evidence for myocardial ischemia in the immediate postoperative period. The majority of this ischemia may be silent making the diagnosis difficult and dependent upon serial or continuous ECG monitoring.[23]

Table 6.3 summarizes the incidence of mortality and morbidity associated with TMLR. The long-term benefits for TMLR are still under investigation. However, it appears that the primary benefit relates to the reduction in patient symptoms, reduced hospital readmissions, and quality of life (Figure 6.1).[21, 22, 25] At the present time, a clear overall mortality benefit has not been demonstrated (Figure 6.2).[22, 25]

Table 6.3 Observed mortality and morbidity in 132 patients undergoing transmyocardial laser revascularization. (Modified and reproduced from Hughes et al[22] with permission)

Mortality (in-hospital or 30-day)	5%
Atrial fibrillation	10%
Ventricular dysrhythmia	12%
Non-Q wave myocardial infarction	5%
Congestive cardiac failure	4%
Q wave myocardial infarction	1%
Respiratory failure	3%

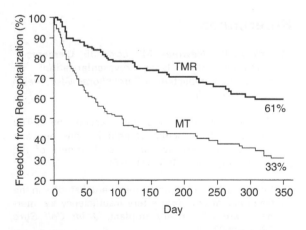

Figure 6.1

Kaplan–Meier estimates of 1-year freedom from cardiac-related rehospitalization (reproduced from Allen et al[22] with permission).

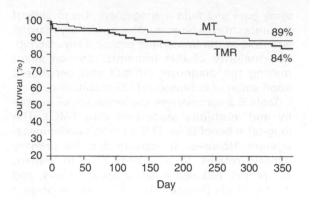

Figure 6.2

Kaplan–Meier estimates of 1-year survival demonstrating no significant longevity (mortality) benefit of TMLR (reproduced from Allen et al[22] with permission).

Summary

- TMLR presents the anesthesiologist with a clinical challenge unique from the 'mundane' traditional method of direct coronary artery bypass grafting (i.e. operative CABG).
- TMLR represents one of the many newer procedures in cardiac surgery that are defining novel approaches to this seemingly ever-present medical problem.

References

1. Grocott HP, Newman MF, Lowe JE, Clements F. Transmyocardial laser revascularization: an anesthetic perspective. *J Cardiothorac Vasc Anesth* 1997;**11**:206–10.

2. Wearn J, Mettier S, Klumpp T, Zschiesche L. The nature of the vascular communications between the coronary arteries and the chambers of the heart. *Am Heart J* 1933;**9**:143–64.

3. Vineberg A. Clinical and experimental studies in the treament of coronary artery insufficiency by internal mammary artery implant. *J Int Coll Surg* 1954;**22**:503–18.

4. Sen P, Udwadia T, Kinare S, Parulkar G. Transmyocardial acupuncture. *J Thorac Cardiovasc Surg* 1965;**50**:181–9.

5. Sen P. Studies in myocardial revascularization. *Ind J Med Res* 1969;**57**:415–33.

6. Sen PK, Daulatram J, Kinare SG *et al*. Further studies in multiple transmyocardial acupuncture as a method of myocardial revascularization. *Surgery* 1968;**64**:861–70.

7. Mirhoseini M, Cayton MM. Revascularization of the heart by laser. *J Microsurg* 1981;**2**:253–60.

8. Mirhoseini M, Muckerheide M, Cayton MM. Transventricular revascularization by laser. *Lasers Surg Med* 1982;**2**:187–98.

9. Mirhoseini M, Fisher JC, Cayton M. Myocardial revascularization by laser: a clinical report. *Lasers Surg Med* 1983;**3**:241–5.

10. Cooley DA, Frazier OH, Kadipasaoglu KA *et al*. Transmyocardial laser revascularization. Anatomic evidence of long-term channel patency. *Tex Heart Inst J* 1994;**21**:220–4.

11. Mirhoseini M, Shelgikar S, Cayton M. Clinical and histological evaluation of laser myocardial revascularization. *J Clin Laser Med Surg* 1990;**8**:73–7.

12. Hughes GC, Abdel-aleem S, Biswas SS *et al*. Transmyocardial laser revascularization: experimental and clinical results. *Can J Cardiol* 1999;**15**:797–806.

13. Hughes GC, Lowe JE, Kypson AP *et al*. Neovascularization after transmyocardial laser revascularization in a model of chronic ischemia. *Ann Thorac Surg* 1998;**66**:2029–36.

14. Horvath KA. Transmyocardial laser revascularization. *Adv Card Surg* 1998;**10**:141–54.

15. Kornowski R, Bhargava B, Leon MB. Percutaneous transmyocardial laser revascularization: an overview. *Catheter Cardiovasc Interv* 1999;**47**:354–9.

16. Milano A, Pratali S, De Carlo M *et al*. Transmyocardial holmium laser revascularization: feasibility of a thoracoscopic approach. *Eur J Cardiothorac Surg* 1998;**14 (Suppl 1)**:S105–10.

17. Horvath KA. Thoracoscopic transmyocardial laser revascularization. *Ann Thorac Surg* 1998;**65**:1439–41.

18. Cooley DA, Frazier OH, Kadipasaoglu KA *et al*. Transmyocardial laser revascularization: clinical experience with twelve-month follow-up. *J Thorac Cardiovasc Surg* 1996;**111**:791-7; discussion 797–9.

19. Frazier OH, Cooley DA, Kadipasaoglu KA *et al.* Myocardial revascularization with laser. Preliminary findings. *Circulation* 1995;**92**:II58–65.

20. Horvath KA, Mannting F, Cummings N *et al.* Transmyocardial laser revascularization: operative techniques and clinical results at two years. *J Thorac Cardiovasc Surg* 1996;**111**:1047–53.

21. Frazier OH, March RJ, Horvath KA. Transmyocardial revascularization with a carbon dioxide laser in patients with end-stage coronary artery disease. *N Engl J Med* 1999;**341**:1021–8.

22. Allen KB, Dowling RD, Fudge TL *et al.* Comparison of transmyocardial revascularization with medical therapy in patients with refractory angina [see comments]. *N Engl J Med* 1999;**341**:1029–36.

23. Hughes GC, Landolfo KP, Lowe JE *et al.* Diagnosis, incidence, and clinical significance of early postoperative ischemia after transmyocardial laser revascularization. *Am Heart J* 1999;**137**:1163–8.

24. Grocott HP, Amory DW, Lowry E *et al.* Cerebral embolization during transmyocardial laser revascularization. *J Thorac Cardiovasc Surg* 1997;**114**:856–8.

25. Schofield PM, Sharples LD, Caine N *et al.* Transmyocardial laser revascularisation in patients with refractory angina: a randomised controlled trial. *Lancet* 1999;**353**:519–24 (erratum in *Lancet* 1999;**353**:1714).

7
Port-Access cardiac surgery

Colleen Gorman Koch and Michelle J Capdeville

Introduction

Some of the earliest interventions for the treatment of diseased heart valves utilized 'Port'-Access surgery. In the early 1920s Evarts Graham and Duff Allan invented a cardioscope to directly visualize diseased heart valves. The device consisted of a scope with a lens attachment at the tip, and a knife attached alongside the tube that was intended to come into direct contact with heart valve.[1]

Since its introduction in the mid-1990s, Port-Acess cardiac surgery with the use of the Endovascular Cardiopulmonary Bypass System (EndoCPB; Heartport, Inc., Redwood City, CA, USA) has enabled cardiac surgeons to perform a variety of cardiac procedures without the conventional median sternotomy incision and central cannulation. The Heartport cannula/catheter provides cardiopulmonary bypass (CPB) using endovascular cannulae and cardioplegic arrest of the heart with both antegrade and retrograde cardioplegia delivery using endovascular catheters via percutaneous access. Surgery is performed through small or 'port' incisions with the use of modified surgical instruments and/or video assistance. The ultimate goal of Port-Access surgery is to allow for less invasive surgical incisions thereby reducing tissue trauma, patient discomfort, recovery time and hospital stay. A 'Port-Access' approach to surgery expands the role of the cardiothoracic anesthesiologist with regard to patient monitoring and anesthetic management.

Case history

A 60-year-old man was referred to the Cleveland Clinic for surgical evaluation of known valvular heart disease.

Past medical history	None significant.
Regular medications	Paroxetine, atenolol. No known drug allergies.
Examination	Weight 75 kg. Height 1.88 m. Grade 2/6 ejection systolic murmur best heard at the left sternal border.
Investigations	Routine laboratory values within normal limits. **TTE:** Mild left atrial enlargement. Moderate to severe left ventricular dilation with normal systolic function. Moderate to severe myxomatous mitral valve disease with severe thickening of both the anterior and posterior mitral leaflets. Prolapse of the anterior and posterior mitral leaflets with a moderately severe jet of mitral regurgitation and a blunted pulmonary venous waveform pattern. **Coronary angiography:** Normal coronary arteries. **CXR:** Normal pulmonary vascularity with scattered granulomata. **ECG:** Normal sinus rhythm with frequent unifocal premature ventricular contractions

On the day of surgery the patient was premedicated with intramuscular lorazepam 5 mg prior to transfer to the operating room. Standard ASA intraoperative monitors (i.e. continuous ECG, pulse oximetry, inspired oxygen and end-tidal carbon dioxide concentration, and temperature) were utilized. Using local anesthesia, a peripheral intravenous line and both right radial and left brachial arterial lines were placed on arrival to the operating room. Anesthesia was induced with fentanyl 1 mg, pancuronium 10 mg and midazolam 4 mg, and the trachea intubated with a #37 left-sided double-lumen tube. Correct positioning of the tube was verified with a fiberoptic bronchoscope. The stomach was emptied of its contents with an orogastric tube and a multiplane transesophageal echocardiography (TEE) probe was placed within the esophagus. Following the administration of heparin 100 u kg^{-1}, the Endocoronary Sinus Catheter (ESC) and the Endopulmonary Vent (EPV) catheter were placed through introducer sheaths in the right internal jugular vein. Under TEE guidance and with the aid of hemodynamic waveform and pressure measurements, the ESC catheter was guided into the coronary sinus. The EPV catheter was similarly guided into position in the pulmonary artery. Anesthesia was maintained with isoflurane 1% in oxygen with intermittent doses of pancuronium for muscle relaxation.

Single lung ventilation was instituted and a small right anterior thoracotomy was performed in the fourth intercostal space. The right common femoral vein was dissected out and prepared for cannulation and a further 300 u kg^{-1} heparin administered to achieve a Celite activated clotting time (ACT) $\geq$480 s. Epsilon aminocaproic acid 10 g was then administered and followed by an infusion at 1 g hour^{-1}. Through a 1-cm diameter port, placed in the right anterior chest in the first intercostal space, a Heartport transthoracic aortic cannula was introduced into the ascending aorta under direct vision. Under TEE guidance the femoral venous and the transthoracic Heartport aortic cannulae were then maneuvered into the correct position. Following the institution of cardiopulmonary bypass (CPB), the endoaortic balloon clamp was inflated and Buckberg cardioplegia solution administered via the endoaortic clamp and then via the ESC. TEE and continuous monitoring of bilateral brachial artery and aortic root pressures were used to detect any migration of the endoaortic balloon. A left atriotomy was performed and a mitral valve repair involving a quadrilateral resection of the middle scallop of the posterior mitral valve leaflet was performed. Calcium was debrided from the posterior annulus and a 30-mm Cosgrove–Edwards annuloplasty ring was placed. The heart was de-aired, the atriotomy closed and atrial pacing instituted. The patient was then weaned from CPB without difficulty. TEE demonstrated a competent valve repair with the remainder of the examination unchanged from baseline. The heparin was reversed with protamine sulfate. The double-lumen endotracheal tube was changed to a single-lumen endotracheal tube prior to transfer to the ICU. Nine hours later the patient was weaned from mechanical ventilation without difficulty and the trachea extubated. He was transferred to a regular nursing floor the following day and discharged to home on the fifth postoperative day.

Discussion

Utilization of the Heartport EndoCPB system can initially be both labor intensive and technically challenging for the cardiothoracic anesthesiologist. Not only should they be skilled in the management of one lung ventilation, the use of TEE, and placement of invasive monitoring but also be intimately familiar with the components of Heartport EndoCPB. The system consists of three catheters and two cannulae that are utilized to facilitate cardiac surgical procedures, avoiding central cannulation via the median sternotomy approach. The anesthesiologist, with the aid of TEE and/or fluoroscopy and monitoring of pressures and waveform patterns, is paramount for positioning and monitoring the proper function of these catheters. The anesthesiologist is required to place two catheters percutaneously through introducer sheaths, commonly from the right internal jugular approach after the patient is partially anticoagulated. The EPV catheter is placed through a 9-French introducer sheath and is floated into the main pulmonary artery via a 5-French flow-directed balloon catheter similar to the Swan–Ganz catheter. The EPV is attached to the pulmonary artery vent line to allow decompression of the heart during CPB. The ESC is passed through an 11-French introducer sheath with the guidance of the TEE and/or fluoroscopy and pressure monitoring and advanced approximately 2 cm into the coronary sinus. A separate pressure-monitoring port on the ESC allows monitoring of coronary sinus pressure during retrograde cardioplegia administration. The other cannulae and catheter are placed by the cardiac surgeon with the aid of TEE and/or fluoroscopy. Prior to placing the Endovenous Drainage (EVD) cannula the patient is fully anticoagulated. The EVD cannula is advanced from the femoral vein over a guidewire and is positioned at the junction of the right atrium and superior vena cava. The Endoarterial Return Cannula (EARC) is placed with guidewire assistance via the femoral artery and is connected to the arterial line of the bypass circuit. It has another lumen to allow passage of the Endoaortic Clamp (EAC), which is advanced into the ascending aorta and positioned, just above the sinotubular junction. The EAC has three lumina: a lumen for balloon inflation for aortic occlusion, a lumen for delivery of antegrade cardioplegia and aortic root venting and a lumen for aortic root pressure measurements. Alternatively, a transthoracic aortic cannula can be introduced through a port placed via an anterior thoracotomy at the level of the first intercostal space. Confirmation and maintenance of proper positioning of the EVD cannula and EARC with the endoaortic clamp require TEE and/or fluoroscopy. Figure 7.1 illustrates the components of the Heartport EndoCPB system in their anatomically correct positions. Table 7.1

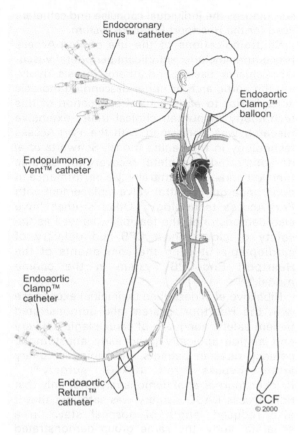

Figure 7.1

The components of the Heartport EndoCPB system in their anatomically correct positions. Transfemoral, rather than transthoracic, placement of the endoaortic clamp catheter is shown. Reproduced by courtesy of Cleveland Clinic Foundation.

Table 7.1 Catheter position and function with the Heartport Endovascular Cardiopulmonary Bypass System. TEE: transesophageal echocardiography; SVC: superior vena cava; RA: right atrium; CPB: cardiopulmonary bypass

Device	Position	Function
Endopulmonary Vent Catheter (EPV)	TEE, fluoroscopic and/or waveform guidance into the main pulmonary artery	Decompression of the heart
Endocoronary Sinus Catheter (ESC)	TEE, fluoroscopic and/or waveform guidance into the coronary sinus	Delivery of retrograde cardioplegia
Endovenous Drainage Cannula (EVD)	TEE and/or fluoroscopic guidance from the femoral vein to SVC-RA junction	Venous drainage for CPB
Endoarterial Return Cannula and Endoaortic Clamp (EARC / EAC)	TEE and/or fluoroscopic guidance of guidewire/endoaortic clamp into ascending aorta	Arterial return cannula for CPB, antegrade cardioplegia, aortic root pressure and venting

summarizes the individual cannulae and catheters used for the Heartport EndoCPB system.

Contraindications to the use of Port-Access procedures include: significant peripheral vascular occlusive disease and atherosclerosis involving the aortic arch or upper descending thoracic aorta.[2] Prior to early clinical application of this technology in human clinical trials, extensive research was performed with the Port-Access technology in the canine model. Schwartz et al demonstrated complete recovery of cardiac function and normal mitral valve performance in dogs undergoing mitral valve replacement with Port-Access technology.[3] Other studies have also demonstrated the feasibility, as well as the safety of closed-chest CPB and delivery of cardioplegia utilizing the components of the Heartport EndoCPB system in the canine model.[4, 5]

Ribakove et al described their initial experience with the Heartport system and demonstrated patient safety, adequacy of cardioplegia delivery and angiographically good early anastomotic patency rates in patients undergoing coronary artery bypass graft (CABG) surgery.[6, 7] Reichenspurner et al demonstrated not only that Port-Access CABG surgery was safe, but that it also reduced length of hospital stay.[8] In a separate study, the same group demonstrated good postoperative valve function following Port-Access mitral valve procedures.[9] Their results were comparable to conventional cardiac surgery with a lower incidence of postoperative atrial fibrillation. Groh demonstrated the reliability, low postoperative morbidity and mortality rates and decreased length of hospital stay in patients with multivessel coronary artery disease who underwent myocardial revascularization utilizing Port-Access technology.[10] In a study of patients undergoing mitral valve surgery using either a conventional or port-access technique, Glower et al reported that the patients undergoing Port-Access procedures returned to normal activity more rapidly than those undergoing the standard median sternotomy.[11] Similar studies of Port-Access CABG and mitral valve procedures demonstrate patient safety, reproducible graft patency rates, and good postoperative valve function with minimal patient morbidity and mortality rates.[12–15]

No specific recommendations are made about the choice of anesthetic agents other than to mention that most centers advocate the use of a technique that permits extubation in the operating room or shortly after admission to the intensive care unit. The anesthetic preparation for Port-Access cardiac surgery can, at least initially, be fairly arduous. In a small retrospective study, Ostrowski et al demonstrated that an individual anesthesiologist's mean anaesthesia time decreased after 10 cases, reflective of the learning curve involved with the placement of the catheters.[16] A double-lumen endotracheal tube or a bronchial blocker is utilized for one lung ventilation (right lung ventilation for CABG procedures, left lung ventilation for mitral valve procedures). Additional monitoring must be utilized for patients undergoing Port-Access surgery. Because of the potential for cannula migration additional monitors are required to detect a change in the EAC position. Bilateral upper limb arterial monitoring, transcranial and carotid Doppler sonography, and electroencephalography have all been use to detect brachiocephalic artery occlusion caused by EAC migration toward the arch vessels. Direct palpation of the EAC balloon by the surgeon, measurement of balloon pressure and comparison of aortic root and systemic arterial pressures can also be use to detect EAC migration. Figure 7.2 demonstrates the position of the EAC in relation to the aortic valve and the arch vessels. Siegel et al used the following monitors to detect EAC migration: TEE, pulsed-wave Doppler of the right carotid artery, measurement of balloon pressure, comparison of aortic root and right radial artery pressures and fluoroscopy. They were able to detect EAC migration toward the aortic valve with inadequate balloon inflation. EAC movement toward the arch vessels during administration of antegrade cardioplegia was detected by the cessation of carotid artery flow.[17]

In a study of the utility of TEE in Port-Access, minimally invasive cardiac surgery, Applebaum et al were able to use the technique as the primary imaging technique to assist in the placement of catheters and cannulae.[18] The authors stress the need for a comprehensive examination to exclude pathology that might preclude the use of the Port-Access system or indicate the need for an alteration in surgical technique. Particular attention should be paid to the degree of atherosclerotic plaque within the

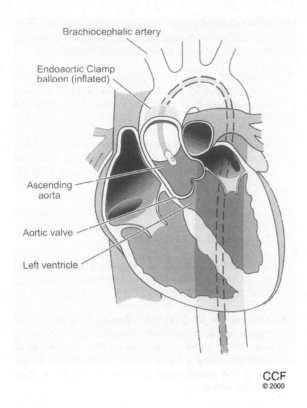

Brachiocephalic artery

Endoaortic Clamp
balloon (inflated)

Ascending
aorta

Aortic valve

Left ventricle

CCF
© 2000

Figure 7.2

Correct positioning of the endoaortic balloon clamp.
Reproduced by courtesy of Cleveland Clinic Foundation.

descending and ascending thoracic aorta. Dense or mobile plaque can be dislodged during instrumentation or by inflation of the EAC balloon. TEE can detect the presence of right atrial thrombus that may be dislodged during EVD cannula placement. Finally, the presence of aortic insufficiency can preclude the use of antegrade cardioplegia delivery. Fluoroscopy was only found useful as an aid to TEE during placement of the ESC.

The use of TEE during Port-Access surgery can be summarized as follows: the pre-CPB TEE examination should consist of a complete two-dimensional, Doppler and color Doppler examination of the heart. Assessment should be made of the size of the ascending aorta, presence of aortic insufficiency or atrial septal defect, and degree of atherosclerotic plaque of the ascending and descending aorta. TEE imaging of the coronary sinus assists in the placement of the ESC, imaging

of the right ventricular outflow tract assists in the positioning of the EPV catheter. Visualization of the guidewires aids in positioning of both the EVD cannula and the EAC. During CPB the EAC is continuously monitored for potential migration. TEE monitoring in the post-CPB period consists of assisting in the deairing process, assessing the adequacy of valve repair/replacement and monitoring the heart for regional left ventricular wall motion abnormalities with coronary grafting procedures. The aorta is examined for potential injury, for example, aortic dissection and a complete post-CPB examination is completed.

Reported complications of Port-Access surgery have included the following: endoaortic balloon clamp migration,[19] right ventricular perforation with the ESC guidewire,[20] endoaortic balloon rupture,[21] EPV catheter entrapment by atrial sutures,[22] and retrograde aortic and femoral artery dissection.[8, 23]

The increased cost of Port-Access surgery unfortunately does not offset many of the purported benefits, including reduced length of hospital stay.[24] The increased material costs and increased operating room time are major factors. Earlier return to work may be the most important finding to support continued use of the Port-Access approach.[25]

Conclusions and learning points

- While the technique is initially technically challenging, familarity with the Heartport EndoCPB system will result in improved efficiency over time.
- The anesthesiologist is responsible for the accurate placement of the ECS and EPV catheters with the assistance of TEE, and invasive pressure and waveform monitoring.
- There are known potential catheter-related complications. The anesthesiologist needs to be aware of what these are for each catheter and how to monitor for and detect catheter-related problems.
- Many pharmacologic agents have been utilized to provide anesthesia for patients undergoing Port-Access cardiac surgery. An anesthetic that will allow extubation in the operating room or soon after in the intensive care unit is optimal.

Heartport, Port-Access, Endovascular Cardiopulmonary Bypass (EndoCPB) System, Endocoronary Sinus Catheter (ESC), Endopulmonary Vent (EPV), Endovenous Drainage (EVD), Endoarterial Return Cannula (EARC), Endoaortic Clamp (EAC) are trademarks of Heartport Inc., Redwood City, CA, USA.

References

1. Development of surgery for valvular heart disease. In: Westaby S, Bosher C (eds). *History of Cardiac Surgery*. Oxford: Oxford University Press. 1997; 139–85.

2. *Port-Access™ minimally invasive cardiac surgery training manual*. Redwood City, CA: Heartport Inc. 1997.

3. Schwartz DS, Ribakove GH, Butteheim PM *et al*. Minimally invasive mitral valve replacement: port-access technique, feasibility, and myocardial functional preservation. *J Thorac Cardiovasc Surg* 1997;**113**:1022–30.

4. Peters WS, Siegel LC, Stevens JH *et al*. Closed-chest cardiopulmonary bypass and cardioplegia: basis for less invasive cardiac surgery. *Ann Thorac Surg* 1997;**63**:1748–54.

5. Pompili MF, Stevens JH, Burdon TA *et al*. Port-Access mitral valve replacement in dogs. *J Thorac Cardiovasc Surg* 1996;**112**:1268–74.

6. Ribakove GH, Galloway AC, Grossi EA *et al*. Port-Access coronary artery bypass grafting. *Semin Thorac Cardiovasc Surg* 1997;**9**:312–19.

7. Ribakove GH, Miller JS, Anderson RV *et al*. Minimally invasive port-access coronary artery bypass grafting with early angiographic follow-up: initial clinical experience. *J Thorac Cardiovasc Surg* 1998;**115**:1101–10.

8. Reichenspurner H, Gulielmos V, Wunderlich J *et al*. Port-access coronary artery bypass grafting with the use of cardiopulmonary bypass and cardioplegic arrest. *Ann Thorac Surg* 1998;**65**:413–9.

9. Reichenspurner H, Wilz A, Gulielmos V *et al*. Port-Access cardiac surgery using endovascular cardiopulmonary bypass: theory, practice and results. *J Card Surg* 1998;**13**:275–80.

10. Groh MA. Port-Access coronary artery bypass grafting: technical strategies for multivessel complete revascularization. *J Card Surg* 1998;**13**:297–301.

11. Glower DD, Landolfo KP, Clements F *et al*. Mitral valve operation via Port-Access versus median sternotomy. *Eur J Cardiothorac Surg* 1998;**14 (Suppl 1)**: S143–7.

12. Galloway AC, Ribakove GH, Grossi EA *et al*. Port-Access coronary artery bypass grafting: technical considerations and results. *J Card Surg* 1998;**13**: 281–5.

13. Fann JI, Pompili MF, Burdon T *et al*. Minimally invasive mitral valve surgery. *Semin Thorac Cardiovasc Surg* 1997;**9**:320–30.

14. Colvin SB, Galloway AC, Ribakove G *et al*. Port-Access mitral valve surgery: summary of results. *J Card Surg* 1998;**13**:286–9.

15. Gulielmos V, Wagner FM, Waetzig B *et al*. Clinical experience with minimally invasive coronary artery and mitral valve surgery with the advantage of cardiopulmonary bypass and cardioplegic arrest using the port-access technique. *World J Surg* 1999;**23**:480–5

16. Ostrowski JW, Cutler WM, Grossi EA *et al*. Experience improves anesthesia time in port access cardiac surgery. *Anesth Analg* 1999; **88(4S)**: SCA126.

17. Siegel LC, St Goar FG, Stevens JH *et al*. Monitoring considerations for port-access cardiac surgery. *Circulation* 1997;**96**:562–8.

18. Applebaum RM, Cutler WM, Bhardwaj N *et al*. Utility of transesophageal echocardiography during port-access minimally invasive cardiac surgery. *Am J Cardiol* 1998;**82**:183–8.

19. Grocott HP, Stafford SM, Glower DD, Clements FM. Endovascular aortic balloon clamp malposition during minimally invasive cardiac surgery. Detection by transcranial Doppler monitoring. *Anesthesiology* 1998;**88**:1396–9.

20. Abramson DC, Giannoti AG. Perforation of the right ventricle with a coronary sinus catheter during preparation for minimally invasive cardiac surgery. *Anesthesiology* 1998;**89**:519–21.

21. Hesselvik JF, Ortega RA, Treanor P, Shemin RJ. Intraoperative rupture of the endoaortic clamp balloon in a patient undergoing port-access mitral

valve repair. *J Cardiothorac Vasc Anesth* 1999;**13**: 462–5.

22. Deneu S, Coddens J, Deloof T. Catheter entrapment by atrial suture during minimally invasive port-access cardiac surgery. *Can J Anaesth* 1999;**46**:983–6.

23. Mohr FW, Falk V, Diegeler A *et al.* Minimally invasive port-access mitral valve surgery. *J Thorac Cardiovasc Surg* 1998;**115**:567–76.

24. Watson DR, Duff SB. The clinical and financial impact of port-access coronary revascularization. *Eur J Cardiothorac Surg* 1999;**16 (Suppl 1)**:S103–6.

25. Arom KV, Emery RW, Kshettry VR, Janey PA. Comparison between port-access and less invasive valve surgery. *Ann Thorac Surg* 1999;**68**: 1525–8.

8
Off-pump coronary artery bypass

Neville M Gibbs

Introduction

Coronary artery bypass grafting (CABG) without cardiopulmonary bypass (CPB) is becoming increasingly popular, particularly for patients who are at high risk of cerebral injury. It might be expected that avoidance of CPB simplifies anesthetic management. However, off-pump surgery presents new challenges for both the surgeon and the anesthetist. This is especially so for high-risk patients who require multiple bypass grafts.

Case history

An 80-year-old Caucasian male with increasing angina and severe triple vessel coronary artery disease presented for elective CABG. Due to the high risk of cerebral injury in this age group,[1]

and the suggestion that the risk might be reduced by avoiding CPB,[2] off-pump surgery was planned, despite a requirement for five bypass grafts.

Aspirin was stopped 3 days prior to surgery. On the evening before surgery, subcutaneous heparin (5000 iu BD) was commenced as prophylaxis against deep venous thrombosis. Anesthetic premedication consisted of lorazepam 2 mg PO 2 hours before induction of anesthesia. Initial monitoring consisted of ECG, direct radial artery pressure, pulse oximetry, and end-tidal carbon dioxide ($_{ET}CO_2$). After establishing peripheral venous access, and preoxygenating for 3 minutes, anesthesia was induced with intravenous midazolam 3 mg, fentanyl 500 µg, and propofol 80 mg. Muscle relaxation was achieved with rocuronium 50mg. Anesthesia was maintained with isoflurane 0.5–1.0% in oxygen-enriched air, and increments of fentanyl (total 500 µg). Following tracheal intubation, intermittent positive pressure ventila-

Past medical history	Severe coronary artery disease. Hypertension. Osteoarthritis.
Regular medications	Metoprolol 50 mg BD, pravastatin 20 mg OD, aspirin 100 mg OD, glyceryl trinitrate spray PRN.
Examination	A fit-looking elderly man. Weight 68 kg. Height 171 cm. Heart rate 70 bpm. BP 120/70 mmHg.
Investigations	Hb 13.2 g dl^{-1}, platelets 267 × 10^9 l^{-1}. [Na$^+$] 140 mmol l^{-1}, [K$^+$] 4.5 mmol l^{-1}, bicarbonate 24 mmol l^{-1}, urea 9.3 mmol l^{-1}, creatinine 1.1 mg dl^{-1} (99 µmol l^{-1}). **ECG:** Sinus rhythm with non-specific lateral ST segment depression. **Coronary angiography:** Discrete stenoses (99–100%) of the proximal right, mid-left anterior descending (LAD), second diagonal, and first obtuse marginal coronary arteries. Diffuse disease of the circumflex coronary artery. Left ventricular function within normal limits.

tion was established maintaining the $_{ET}CO_2$ at 30–35 mmHg (4–4.7 kPa). A nasogastric tube was passed and an indwelling urinary catheter was inserted. A thermodilution cardiac output pulmonary artery catheter was inserted through an introducer placed in the right internal jugular vein. In addition, a triple lumen central venous catheter was placed in the right subclavian vein. Infusions of glyceryl trinitrate (GTN), epinephrine, and noradrenaline were prepared. To minimize heat loss, all intravenous fluids were warmed and warm air was circulated over the patient's head and neck.

After induction of anesthesia, but before surgical incision, noradrenaline 2-5 µg min^{-1} was required to maintain the systolic blood pressure (BP) above 100 mmHg. At this time the central venous pressure (CVP) was 12 mmHg, the pulmonary capillary wedge pressure (PCWP) 14 mmHg, and cardiac index (CI) 2.0 l min^{-1} m^{-2}. Following median sternotomy, the systolic BP increased to 120 mmHg, and the CI to 2.2 l min^{-1} m^{-2}. The left internal mammary artery (LIMA) was dissected out and saphenous vein was harvested. The pericardium was opened and the coronary vessels were identified. Heparin 100 mg was given IV resulting in an activated clotting time (ACT) of 318s. Two further boluses of heparin 25 mg were required over the next hour to maintain the ACT >300 s. Prior to each distal coronary anastomosis, ischemic preconditioning was conducted by proximally occluding the target artery for 3–5 minutes. An OCTOPUS II device (Medtronics DPL, Grand Rapids, MI, USA) was used to stabilize the heart over each anastomosis site. During each anastomosis, the target artery was again occluded and a humidified carbon dioxide blower was used to prevent blood obscuring the arteriotomy. The first two anastomoses were the LIMA end to side to the LAD with a side-to-side 'skip' to the first diagonal. During this time, 2–3 mm ST segment elevations were noted on leads II and V$_5$ of the ECG, but the cardiac output and blood pressure remained stable. The ECG changes resolved upon re-establishment of flow. The heart was then rotated using stay sutures and packs to allow access to the obtuse marginal arteries on the lateral aspect. The operating table was also rotated toward the surgeon to improve the surgical view. These maneuvers were associated with a reduction in systolic BP to 60 mm Hg, and CI to 1.1 l min^{-1} m^{-2}. At this stage, considera-

tion was given to converting to on-pump surgery using CPB. However, over the next few minutes the BP and CI were improved by positioning the patient slightly head down, administering a fluid bolus of 500 ml of colloid solution, and commencing epinephrine 3–5 µg min^{-1} IV. After completing the distal end-to-side anastomosis of a saphenous vein graft (SVG) to the second obtuse marginal (with a side to side 'skip' to the first obtuse marginal), the position of the heart was adjusted to expose the posterior descending artery (PDA) on the inferior aspect. In this position, which required steep head-down tilt, the apex of the heart was outside the thorax pointing toward the ceiling. However, the BP and cardiac output were surprisingly well maintained, and the distal end-to-side anastomosis of the SVG to the PDA was completed without incident. No surgical intracoronary shunts were required. The patient was then returned to the horizontal position. Prior to performing the proximal SVG anastomoses to the aorta, the systolic BP was reduced to 90 mmHg using GTN 25–50 µg min^{-1} IV, thus ensuring that the aortic side-biting clamps did not slip or damage the aorta. Following the completion of the two SVG proximal anastomoses, protamine 75 mg was administered. Prior to closure of the thorax, surgical drains were placed in left pleural cavity, pericardial cavity, and mediastinum, and atrial pacing wires were positioned and tested. The time taken from surgical incision to closure was 3 hours, and from commencing the first distal anastomosis to completing the last proximal anastomosis was 1 hour and 45 minutes. The total volume of intravenous fluids administered was 3500 ml crystalloid and 500 ml colloid. Estimated blood loss was 1000 ml. At the end of the procedure the patient's systolic BP was 110 mmHg, CVP 11 mmHg, PCWP 13 mmHg, CI 2.9 l min^{-1} m^{-2}, temperature 35.9 °C, ACT 132s, and Hb 9 g dl^{-1}.

Postoperatively the patient was transferred to an intensive care unit (ICU) where he required mechanical ventilation for 9 hours. The reason for the delay in extubation was persistent bleeding. Laboratory tests were not suggestive of a coagulopathy and the hemorrhage was self-limiting, although transfusion of 2 units of allogeneic packed red cells was required. The patient remained hemodynamically stable and his urine output remained satisfactory. The serum creatine kinase concentration 24 hours after surgery was only marginally increased at 223 u l^{-1} (normal <167 u l^{-1}) and the creatinine concentration increased to a peak of 2.3 mg dl^{-1} (205 µmol l^{-1}) on the third postoperative day. In other respects the postoperative course was uneventful. In particular, there were no overt signs of neurological injury or cognitive dysfunction. The patient was discharged home 6 days after surgery and was well and symptom free when reviewed 6 weeks later.

Discussion

Off-pump coronary artery bypass surgery (OPCAB) is not a new procedure. However, until recently it was used only in a few centers, and only for high-risk patients. The introduction of minimally invasive direct coronary artery bypass (MIDCAB) through a left anterior small thoracotomy (LAST) renewed interest in off-pump surgery, particularly as the short-term and mid-term results appeared satisfactory.[3, 4] The MIDCAB approach was improved by the use of devices to stabilize the target vessels.[5] Nevertheless, a major limitation of MIDCAB through a LAST incision is that access is usually limited to the LAD and proximal RCA. Moreover, it soon appeared that the benefit of MIDCAB was due mostly to the avoidance of CPB rather than the less invasive surgical approach. This resulted in an increase in popularity of the OPCAB through a full or limited median sternotomy.[6–8] This enabled lessons learned from single vessel bypass to be applied to multiple vessels. With better access and the introduction of improved stabilization techniques, grafts are now theoretically possible on all target vessels.

Although it is now established that multiple vessel coronary artery bypass can be performed off-pump, there is considerable divergence of opinion about whether it *should* be performed off-pump.[9] The main issues for off-pump surgery are whether the long-term graft patency rates are as good as on-pump techniques, and whether reduced mortality and morbidity can be demonstrated. Being a relatively new technique, there are no long-term outcome studies that address these issues, let alone randomized controlled trials. Nevertheless, some early results have been promising. Calafiore *et al* reported their

early angiographic results in 67 patients who underwent off-pump coronary revascularization with two or more arterial conduits.[10] At 1 month, the overall graft patency rate was at >98%.[10] More recently, Cremer *et al* reported a short-term global patency rate of 97.8%.[11] Satisfactory risk-adjusted short-term mortality rates for off-pump surgery compared to on-pump surgery have also been reported.[8, 10–12] Intensive care unit and in-hospital stay have also been reduced.[6–8] However, there is a need for well controlled randomized trials to determine whether off-pump surgery is as safe as on-pump surgery in the intermediate and longer term.

It is possible that the avoidance of CPB may have practical advantages in reducing costs, ICU stay, and length of hospital stay. However, the main attraction of off-pump surgery is the potential reduction of the neurological and neuropsychological complications associated with CPB. A recent multicenter study indicated that over 6% of patients undergoing CABG surgery with CPB have an adverse cerebral outcome.[1] Approximately half of these are focal neurological deficits, with the remainder being deterioration in intellectual function. The mechanism by which CPB causes cerebral injury is most likely multifactorial, but embolic phenomena are most frequently implicated.[13] These may be due to gaseous microemboli during CPB, or particulate micro-emboli caused by the application of aortic clamps, especially in patients who have atherosclerosis of the proximal aorta. The introduction of air during insertion of arterial cannula may also contribute to cerebral injury. The other potential cause of cerebral injury during CPB is the inflammatory response to the artificial surfaces which may explain the development of cerebral edema.[13] In any event, most of these are avoided by avoiding CPB.

Early results suggest that the incidence of neurological injury might be reduced by avoiding CPB.[2] A lower incidence of stroke and neuropsychological dysfunction have been reported,[2, 14–16] as well as reduced postoperative serum S100b protein levels.[17–19] A significant reduction in cerebral microemboli as detected by transcranial Doppler sonography has also been documented.[16,20] However, not all studies have found an improvement in neurological outcome with off-pump surgery.[17, 21] This has highlighted the need for randomized controlled studies to determine whether improved neurological outcome is a real benefit of off-pump surgery.[22–25]

Until recently there has been a tendency to consider all off-pump cases as a homogenous group. However, there is a clear difference between single vessel arterial revascularizations and multivessel revascularizations requiring aorto-coronary saphenous vein grafts. The latter requires the application of aortic side-biting clamps that could dislodge aortic atheroma and contribute to neurological morbidity. Moreover multivessel revascularizations are more extensive procedures and are usually associated with greater hemodynamic instability. These differences should be considered when comparing outcome.

Anesthetists may be forgiven for hoping that off-pump surgery would simplify anesthetic management. However, it became apparent very early that this was not the case.[26] It is true that difficulties weaning from CPB are avoided, but most other aspects are more challenging than on-pump surgery. The main difference for the anesthetist is that it is no longer possible to rely on CPB for the maintenance of hemodynamic stability during manipulations of the heart and anastomosis of grafts. The causes of hemody-namic compromise during off-pump surgery include impairment of venous return due to chamber compression or abnormal positioning, and pump failure due to direct ventricular compression or ischemia during arterial occlu-sion. The reduction in venous return and chamber compression are mostly encountered when attempting to graft vessels on the lateral or posterior aspects of the heart. These problems are compounded in patients with preoperative ventricular dysfunction, such that severe left ventricular dysfunction may be considered a relative contraindication to off-pump surgery. Arrhythmias may develop: notably bradycardia, multifocal ectopics, and even ventricular fibrilla-tion. If the proximal right coronary is occluded, there is a risk of heart block due to ischemia of the atrioventricular node. Surgical intracoronary shunts can be used in selected vessels if neces-sary. Despite the many sources of hemodynamic instability, it is imperative that cardiac output and blood pressure are maintained in order to ensure adequate cerebral and coronary perfu-sion. If adequate hemodynamic parameters cannot be maintained it is necessary to convert to an on-pump technique. Facilities for immedi-ate conversion to CPB should always be avail-able.

The case described illustrates many of the features and problems associated with OPCAB. The patient, being 80 years old, had a high risk of adverse cerebral outcome.[1] At present, some surgical units only perform OPCAB on high-risk cases. However, OPCAB is becoming increas-ingly popular for a wide range of patients, including low-risk patients. The number of grafts was greater than usual for off-pump surgery, but illustrates that with appropriate surgical and anesthetic planning, five or more grafts can be performed safely. As expected, most of the hemodynamic instability was encountered during grafts to vessels on the lateral or poste-rior aspects of the heart. This was severe and persistent, but with appropriate anesthetic inter-ventions, conversion to on-pump surgery was not required. The patient was also typical in displaying no overt signs of neurological injury or cognitive dysfunction postoperatively.

The anticipation of hemodynamic instability dictates the need for invasive monitoring. In addition to routine monitoring and direct measurement of blood pressure, cardiac output monitoring is advisable, particularly if multiple grafts are required. In the case reported, intermit-tent thermodilution cardiac output measurements gave valuable information and provided a guide to appropriate therapy. Non-invasive beat to beat cardiac output measurement would be even more helpful, but the accuracy and reliability of currently available non-invasive continuous cardiac output monitors, although promising, have not been fully validated. Transesophageal echocardiography (TEE) may be helpful before and after the anastomoses are performed, but during grafting there is often a loss of image due to distraction of the heart away from the esopha-gus. Although TEE was not used in the case described, it would have been useful for the detection or exclusion of new regional wall motion abnormalities following revascularization. Five-lead ECG monitoring is mandatory, but may be less reliable when the heart is in an abnormal orientation, and the signal becomes attenuated by an interface of air or surgical packs.

The other point illustrated in this case is that patients undergoing OPCAB still have the poten-tial for significant blood loss. In this case aspirin was discontinued 3 days before surgery, but many patients continue to receive aspirin until the day of surgery. In contrast to conventional CABG surgery, the dose of heparin administered during OPCAB is reduced, but is often only partially reversed, in order to protect the coronary grafts. Therefore there is still a potential for perioperative bleeding, although the development of a coagulopathy is less likely due to the avoidance of CPB. There is also less scope to scavenge blood from the surgical field because there is no cardiotomy suction. For this reason, cell salvage may be beneficial if multiple grafts are performed.

Another issue for off-pump surgery is the question of early extubation, and the related question of postoperative analgesia. It can be argued that off-pump surgery is ideally suited to early, or even 'on-table' extubation. However, the extent of surgery is similar whether it is performed off-pump or on-pump. The only real difference being the use of CPB. Therefore, there is no more compelling case for early extubation in off-pump cases than for on-pump cases, and each case should be assessed on its merits. Similarly the issue of epidural analgesia should be considered on a case-by-case basis, rather than assuming that off-pump surgery provides a compelling indication. Furthermore, attention should be paid to maintaining body temperature as close to normal as possible so that early extubation is possible. This requires early active warming, because there is no option for 'rewarming' using CPB. If active warming is undertaken it is important to monitor nasopharyngeal temperature to ensure that patients are not overheated. In practice, this is rarely possible. In the case described, early extubation was not planned due to the patient's age. Nevertheless, the patient's temperature of 35.9°C on transfer to the ICU was not a limiting factor.

In summary, the case report describes many features that are typical of multivessel OPCAB. Given appropriate training, expertise, and planning, there are few limitations to performing coronary artery bypass off-pump. The results of long-term outcome studies and randomized controlled trials comparing off-pump to on-pump surgery are keenly awaited. Nevertheless, it is possible that in the future, OPCAB might become the technique of choice for coronary artery bypass, and CPB might be used only for those patients who do not tolerate surgery off-pump.

Conclusions and key learning points

- Off-pump coronary artery bypass (OPCAB) is becoming more popular.
- Unlike MIDCAB, OPCAB through a median sternotomy allows access to multiple vessels.
- Short-term and mid-term graft patency rates for OPCAB appear to be similar to on-pump surgery, but long-term patency rates are not known at present.
- The main theoretical benefit of OPCAB is a lower incidence of neurological injury and cognitive dysfunction due to the avoidance of CPB, but this benefit has not been proven as yet.
- Anesthesia for OPCAB is often more challenging than for on-pump surgery.
- Hemodynamic instability should be anticipated during periods of ischemia, and when grafting lateral and posterior vessels.
- Cardiac output monitoring is required, especially if grafts to lateral and posterior vessels are planned.
- Pre-emptive fluid loading and positioning minimizes hemodynamic changes during grafting. Vasopressor or inotropic support may be required.
- Facilities for cardiac pacing and conversion to on-pump surgery should be immediately available.
- OPCAB lends itself to early extubation, but each case should be assessed on its merits
- Prospective randomized controlled trials are required to compare long-term outcome following on-pump and off-pump coronary artery surgery.

References

1. Roach GW, Kanchuger M, Mangano CM *et al.* Adverse cerebral outcomes after coronary bypass surgery. Multicenter Study of Perioperative Ischemia Research Group and the Ischemia Research and Education Foundation Investigators. *N Engl J Med* 1996;**335**:1857–63.

2. Murkin JM, Boyd WD, Ganapathy S *et al.* Beating heart surgery: why expect less central nervous system morbidity? *Ann Thorac Surg* 1999;**68**:1498–501.

3. Calafiore AM, Giammarco GD, Teodori G *et al.* Left anterior descending coronary artery grafting via left anterior small thoracotomy without cardiopulmonary bypass. *Ann Thorac Surg* 1996;**61**:1658–63.

4. Calafiore AM, Di Giammarco G, Teodori G *et al.* Midterm results after minimally invasive coronary surgery (LAST operation). *J Thorac Cardiovasc Surg* 1998;**115**:763–71.

5. Calafiore AM, Vitolla G, Mazzei V *et al.* The LAST operation: techniques and results before and after the stabilization era. *Ann Thorac Surg* 1998;**66**:998–1001.

6. Bergsland J, Hasnan S, Lewin AN *et al.* Coronary artery bypass grafting without cardiopulmonary bypass—an attractive alternative in high risk patients. *Eur J Cardiothorac Surg* 1997;**11**:876–80.

7. Calafiore AM, Di Giammarco G, Teodori G *et al.* Recent advances in multivessel coronary grafting without cardiopulmonary bypass. *Heart Surg Forum* 1998;**1**:335–89 (http://www.hsforum.com/journal/ vol1/issue1).

8. Turner WF, Jr. 'Off-pump' coronary artery bypass grafting: the first 100 cases of the Rose City experience. *Ann Thorac Surg* 1999;**68**:1482–5.

9. Bonchek LI, Ullyot DJ. Minimally invasive coronary bypass: a dissenting opinion. *Circulation* 1998;**98**:495–7.

10. Calafiore AM, Teodori G, Di Giammarco G *et al.* Multiple arterial conduits without cardiopulmonary bypass: early angiographic results. *Ann Thorac Surg* 1999;**67**:450–6.

11. Cremer JT, Wittwer T, Boning A *et al.* Minimally invasive coronary artery revascularization on the beating heart. *Ann Thorac Surg* 2000;**69**:1787–91.

12. Arom KV, Flavin TF, Emery RW *et al.* Safety and efficacy of off-pump coronary artery bypass grafting. *Ann Thorac Surg* 2000;**69**:704–10.

13. Murkin JM. Etiology and incidence of brain dysfunction after cardiac surgery. *J Cardiothorac Vasc Anesth* 1999;**13**:12–7.

14. Ricci M, Karamanoukian HL, Abraham R *et al.* Stroke in octogenarians undergoing coronary artery surgery with and without cardiopulmonary bypass. *Ann Thorac Surg* 2000;**69**:1471–5.

15. Murkin JM, Boyd WD, Ganapathy S *et al.* Postoperative cognitive dysfunction is significantly less after coronary revascularization without cardiopulmonary bypass. *Ann Thorac Surg* 1999;**68**:1469–72.

16. Diegeler A, Hirsch R, Schneider F *et al.* Neuromonitoring and neurocognitive outcome in off-pump versus conventional coronary bypass operation. *Ann Thorac Surg* 2000;**69**:1162–6.

17. Lloyd CT, Ascione R, Underwood MJ *et al.* Serum S-100 protein release and neuropsychologic outcome during coronary revascularization on the beating heart: a prospective randomized study. *J Thorac Cardiovasc Surg* 2000;**119**:148–54.

18. Anderson RE, Hansson LO, Vaage J. Release of S100B during coronary artery bypass grafting is reduced by off-pump surgery. *Ann Thorac Surg* 1999;**67**:1721–5.

19. Westaby S, Johnsson P, Parry AJ *et al.* Serum S100 protein: a potential marker for cerebral events during cardiopulmonary bypass. *Ann Thorac Surg* 1996;**61**:88–92.

20. Watters MP, Cohen AM, Monk CR *et al.* Reduced cerebral embolic signals in beating heart coronary surgery detected by transcranial Doppler ultrasound. *Br J Anaesth* 2000;**84**:629–31.

21. Kshettry VR, Flavin TF, Emery RW *et al.* Does multivessel, off-pump coronary artery bypass reduce postoperative morbidity? *Ann Thorac Surg* 2000;**69**:1725–30.

22. Alston RP. Off-pump coronary artery surgery and the brain. *Br J Anaesth* 2000;**84**:549–52.

23. Ali ZA, Large SR. Key outcomes '99: gone west? *Ann Thorac Surg* 2000;**69**:336.

24. Arrowsmith JE, Large SR. Off-pump revascularization and the brain. *Br J Anaesth* 2000;**85**:492–3.

25. Haxby E, Khan N, De Souza A, Pepper J. Off-pump revascularization and the brain. *Br J Anaesth* 2000;**85**:492.

26. Maslow AD, Park KW, Pawlowski J *et al.* Minimally invasive direct coronary artery bypass grafting: changes in anesthetic management and surgical procedure. *J Cardiothorac Vasc Anesth* 1999;**13**:417–23.

9
Mediastinitis

Gregory R McAnulty

Case history

A 58-year-old Caucasian male presented for coronary artery bypass surgery. Fourteen months before surgery he had an inferior myocardial infarction (peak creatine kinase 3647 u l⁻¹) for which he received TPA (tissue-type plasminogen activatior) thrombolysis. Two months later he was experiencing exertional angina after walking 2 km on level ground. The patient had diabetes mellitus, diagnosed 17 years before this presentation, treated with insulin for 14 years. He had also suffered from ulcerative colitis for 21 years. The symptoms from this latter condition, apart from occasional exacerbations, were controlled with an aminosalicylate, antispasmodics and episodic topical steroids.

The patient was symptom-free on admission. 'Sliding scale' soluble insulin and 5% glucose infusions were prescribed from midnight on the day before surgery. Capillary glucose concentrations were maintained between 83 and 123 mg dl⁻¹ (4.6–6.8 mmol l⁻¹).

Cephradine 1 g IV was given at induction of anesthesia for surgery. Two further doses were prescribed for 8 and 16 hours postinduction. At surgery three coronary artery bypass grafts (saphenous vein grafts to the intermediate branch of the left anterior descending (LAD) and left ventricular (LV) branch of right carotid artery (RCA), and left internal mammary artery to LAD) were fashioned during cardiopulmonary bypass (CPB) at 28°C using cold antegrade blood cardioplegia. Left ventricular function was noted to be good following separation from CPB. The sternum was closed with nine interrupted stainless steel wires.

Immediately after surgery the patient was stable, remained in sinus rhythm and did not require inotropic support. Serum glucose

Past medical history	Coronary artery disease. Myocardial infarction. Insulin dependent type II diabetes mellitus. Hypercholesterolemia. Transient ischemic attack 7 years before. Ulcerative colitis. No known drug allergies.
Regular medications	Insulin (human zinc suspension 20 iu morning, 18 iu evening; human soluble insulin 12 iu morning, 8 iu evening), diltiazem SR 90 mg BD, sulfasalazine 1 g QDS, mebeverine 135 mg TDS, atenolol 25 mg OD, simvastatin 10 mg OD
Examination	Weight 80.5 kg. BP 120 / 70. No carotid bruits.
Investigations	Hb 14.1 g dl⁻¹, WBC 9.5 × 10⁹ l⁻¹, platelets 182 × 10⁹ l⁻¹, [Na⁺] 138 mmol l⁻¹, [K⁺] 4.2 mmol l⁻¹, urea 5.5 mmol l⁻¹, creatinine 0.8 mg dl⁻¹ (71 µmol l⁻¹). Random glucose 205 mg dl⁻¹ (11.4 mmol l⁻¹). HbA1c 7.8%. **CXR:** Heart size normal, lungs clear. **ECG:** Sinus rhythm 82 min⁻¹. Q wave (5 mm) in lead III. **Cardiac catheter:** Good overall left ventricular function. Stenotic lesions (> 70%) of the LAD, intermediate branch of the LCA and the RCA.

concentrations were controlled between 101 and 198 mg dl^{-1} (5.6–11.0 mmol l^{-1}) with a 'sliding scale' prescription of soluble insulin (1–6 iu hour^{-1}) and 50% glucose (10 ml hour^{-1}). The patient was weaned from mechanical ventilation and the trachea extubated 9 hours after the completion of surgery. The following morning he was discharged to the ward receiving oxygen 2 l min^{-1} via a Hudson mask. The blood pressure was 120/60 mmHg, pulse rate 95 (sinus rhythm). The blood glucose was 180 mg dl^{-1} (10.0 mmol l^{-1}) and he was not acidemic.

The glucose and insulin infusions were continued until the patient began taking oral nutrition. The insulin infusion was then continued, alone, with 2-hourly capillary glucose estimations. Tight glycemic control, however, was difficult to achieve on the ward for the following 5 days after the re-establishment of a subcutaneous insulin regimen. Capillary blood glucose concentrations varied between 83 and 396 mg dl^{-1} (4.6–22.0 mmol l^{-1}).

On the fourth postoperative day the patient developed fast atrial fibrillation. He was given digoxin 750 µg in divided doses. As he reverted to sinus rhythm within 12 hours the digoxin was not continued. Apart from a low-grade temperature (maximum 37.8°C) the patient remained otherwise well and was discharged home on the sixth postoperative day. The white blood cell (WBC) count was 7.2 × 10^9 l^{-1} and capillary glucose concentrations were consistently between 108 and 180 mg dl^{-1} (6–10 mmol l^{-1}) on the day before discharge.

On the tenth postoperative day the patient became aware of a dull pain which radiated to the back and which changed in character with change in his position. This was associated with moderate dyspnea and a general feeling of being unwell. He presented to the Accident and Emergency department of the hospital where he had undergone cardiac surgery. On arrival he was noted to be pale and clammy.

The patient was readmitted to the ward. As a small pericardial effusion revealed by transthoracic echocardiography was thought unlikely to be causing tamponade a putative diagnosis of 'postpericardotomy syndrome' was made with a differential diagnosis of left lower lobe pneumonia. Supplemental oxygen 8 l min^{-1} was administered via a Hudson mask, boluses of frusemide 50 mg IV and diclofenac 75 mg IM given, and ceftazidime 1 g IV administered 8 hourly. The patient was transferred to the ICU 8 hours after readmission because of increasing arterial hypotension and metabolic acidosis (base excess –4.8 mmol l^{-1}). Invasive hemodynamic monitoring revealed; central venous pressure (CVP) 20 mmHg, and significant (>30 mmHg) pulsus paradoxus (MAP 40–70 mmHg). Transthoracic

Medications on readmission	Aspirin 150 mg OD, simvastatin 40 mg OD, sulfasalazine 1 g QDS, mebeverine 135 mg TDS, insulin (human zinc suspension 20 iu morning, 18 iu evening; human soluble insulin 12 iu morning, 8 iu evening).
Examination	Temperature 36.5°C. Respiratory rate 18. Sinus tachycardia 130 min^{-1}. BP 118/80 mmHg. Heart sounds normal in volume and character – no murmurs audible. Bilateral basal inspiratory crackles. Sternal wound unremarkable. No sternal instable.
Investigations	Hb 11.8 g dl^{-1}, WBC 18.5 × 10^9 l^{-1}, platelets 563 × 10^9 l^{-1}, [Na$^+$] 129 mmol l^{-1}, [K$^+$] 5.0 mmol.l^{-1}, urea 4.7 mmol.l^{-1}, creatinine 1.0 mg.dl^{-1} (85 µmol.l^{-1}). Glucose 16.3 mmol.l^{-1} **CXR:** Consistent with left lower lobe collapse—consolidation and pleural effusion. (Left lung volume reduced. Left hemidiaphragm obscured. Blunting of left costophrenic angle. **ECG:** Sinus tachycardia 126 min^{-1}. ST segment elevation (< 1 mm) in inferior and lateral leads. **TTE:** Small posterolateral pericardial effusion. (Study made difficult by tachycardia and recent surgery. Poor views of atria and right ventricle obtained.)

echocardiography (TTE) again revealed a small posterolateral pericardial effusion. As before, this was considered to be consistent with recent cardiac surgery and unlikely to be causing tamponade. The ventricular dimensions were normal. An attempt was made to perform a transesophageal echocardiography (TEE) but it was felt that it was unsafe to proceed without tracheal intubation and ventilation.

A pulmonary artery catheter was then inserted. The initial measurements were: pulmonary capillary wedge pressure (PCWP) 12 mmHg; cardiac index (CI) 1.9 l min^{-1} m^{-2}, systemic vascular resistance (SVR) 1258 dyne s cm$^{-5;}$ pulmonary vascular resistance (PVR) 274 dyne s cm^{-5}; SvO$_2$ 41%. At this point gelatine colloid solution (Gelofusine; Braun; Melsungen, Germany) 750 ml IV was given and intravenous infusions of epinephrine 2.7 µg min^{-1} and dobutamine 5.2 µg kg^{-1} min^{-1} started. The degree of pulsus paradoxus decreased. Measurements from the pulmonary artery catheter improved to: PCWP 16 mmHg, CI 2.5 l min^{-1} m^2; SVR 906 dyne s cm^{-5}; PVR 227 dyne s cm^{-5}; SvO$_2$ 48%. Urine output remained above 30 ml hour^{-1}. Twelve hours after readmission the WBC count had risen to 18.5 × 10^9 l^{-1}. Blood cultures were taken and blood was sent for urgent serum amylase and *Mycoplasma*, *Legionella* and cytomegalovirus serology. Erythromycin 1 g IV QDS was added to the antibiotic regimen. Over the following 3 hours the SVR fell to 550 dyne s cm^{-5}. The dobutamine infusion was discontinued and replaced with noradrenaline to a maximum of 0.1 µg kg^{-1} min^{-1}.

Ten hours after admission to the ICU the patient was sedated, the trachea intubated and the lungs ventilated so that TEE could be safely performed. This revealed a considerable posterolateral pericardial fluid collection, which was producing atrial collapse during the inspiratory phase of the ventilator cycle. Based on these findings, a decision was made to proceed immediately to surgery.

A left anterior thoracotomy via a left submammary incision (thereby avoiding the original sternotomy) was undertaken. Six hundred millilitres of 'straw-coloured' fluid was found in the left pleural cavity and 300 ml purulent fluid was drained after opening the pericardium. Fenestrated tube drains (28 G) were left in the pericardial and left pleural space. The wound was closed in layers. Urgent microbiological examination revealed that the pericardial fluid contained polymorphs and Gram-positive cocci.

On return from the operating room the patient remained tachycardic. Infusions of epinephrine (2.66 µg min^{-1}) and noradrenaline (4.6 µg kg^{-1} min^{-1}) were continued. In view of the microbiological findings erythromycin was discontinued and vancomycin 1 g IV (at intervals determined by subsequent drug levels) and rifampicin 600 mg IV BD commenced. Subsequent culture and sensitivities revealed that the organism was *Staphylococcus aureus* sensitive to flucloxacillin, fusidic acid and erythromycin. Flucloxacillin 2 g IV QDS and fusidic acid 500 mg PO TDS were prescribed to replace the vancomycin and rifampicin. Ceftazidime was continued until Gram-negative organism infection could be excluded by negative cultures.

Blood glucose concentrations were between 267 and 339 mg dl^{-1} (14.8–18.8 mmol l^{-1}) for the first 4 hours after return from the operating room but became well controlled with infusions of 'sliding scale' insulin (1 iu hour^{-1}) and 50% glucose (20 ml hour^{-1}). The 50% glucose infusion was discontinued once nasogastric feed absorption was established. The patient was weaned from mechanical ventilation and the trachea extubated 3 hours after surgery. Inotropic support was gradually withdrawn over the following 48 hours and the patient was discharged to the ward on the third postoperative day where, except for a sinus tachycardia (110 min^{-1}), he was hemodynamically stable. *Legionella* and cytomegalovirus serology were found to be negative. The serum amylase was normal.

The drains continued to drain purulent fluid for 10 days after which they were removed. Flucloxacillin was continued for 2 weeks intravenously and a further 2 weeks by mouth. Fusidic acid was continued for 4 weeks by mouth. The WBC count returned to normal 3 weeks after the drainage procedure. Apart from a small area of sternal wound breakdown inferiorly, which responded to local dressings, the patient made a full recovery.

Discussion

Mediastinal infection after cardiac surgery has an incidence of between 1.3 and 2.3 %.[1–3] Reported mortality rates vary according to how the complication is defined but are as high as 29–51% for patients who are found to have deep mediastinitis rather than superficial mediastinal infection.[3, 4] However, mortality is generally quoted as being in the order of 5%.[5]

Perioperative risk factors for both superficial and deep mediastinal infections include diabetes mellitus, use of bilateral internal mammary grafts, re-sternotomy for postoperative bleeding, duration of surgery, obesity and acute renal failure.[3, 5, 6] Early re-exploration for bleeding,[7] increased adherence to strict asepsis protocols,[8] irrigation of the wound with Povidone iodine solution[9, 10] and, perhaps, interpositioning of a pericardial flap between the heart and sternum during wound closure[11] may reduce the incidence of this serious complication. The value of antibiotic prophylaxis, with agents active against Gram-positive bacteria, has been demonstrated convincingly in cardiac surgery patients.[12] Whether prophylaxis is a single dose, or continued for up to 3 days postoperatively, does not seem to matter.[13, 14]

Causative organisms are predominantly staphylococcal species (*S. aureus* and *S. epidermidis*). Gram-negative bacteria and yeasts are cultured in 5–23% of cases. This spectrum appears to have changed little over the last decade.[1, 15] One French report suggests that coinfection with CMV is common amongst patients with mediastinal infection following cardiac surgery and this coinfection is associated with persistence of local infection, more prolonged hospitalization, and increased late mortality.[16]

Poststernotomy mediastinal infection may present with fever, leukocytosis, erythema of the skin over or purulent discharge from the sternal wound, sternal or deeper chest pain of a 'pleuritic' nature, cardiac arrhythmias or signs of systemic sepsis. The onset is usually insidious but may be more dramatic where there is mediastinal pus.

Investigations that may indicate or confirm the diagnosis of deep mediastinitis following cardiac surgery may include chest X-ray, TTE, TEE, computer tomography, magnetic resonance imaging and, occasionally, radio labeled WBC scan techniques.[17] The choice will depend upon the presentation of the complication. The diagnosis may well be made late; for example upon re-exploration of an apparently superficially infected sternal wound. Patients who present with overwhelming sepsis of unknown origin present a particular problem in the ICU and an appropriate and efficient investigative strategy must be followed at the same time as resuscitative measures are being instigated. Where there are signs of raised atrial pressures, low cardiac output and pulsus paradoxus, tamponade from a pericardial collection or constriction, must be considered. In this case TTE failed to elucidate the diagnosis and led to an unwarranted complacency. TEE allows unimpeded views of the posterior aspect of the heart, particularly of the atria and posterior pericardium.

Operative treatment of apparent superficial mediastinitis may reveal more extensive infection and involvement of major structures. Unexpected, and occasionally catastrophic bleeding may occur and cardiopulmonary bypass may need to be established precipitously. The prudent anesthetist will plan for the worst case, establish full invasive monitoring, obtain substantial intravenous access and alert perfusion and intensive care staff.

Infective complications are more common in diabetic patients in all types of surgery.[18] However, improving perioperative glycemic control with insulin infusions has been shown to reduce the incidence of deep sternal wound infection following cardiac surgery in diabetic patients.[19] This may be explained, in part, by the observation that neutrophil function in diabetic cardiac surgery patients is better preserved in patients receiving insulin infusions rather than intermittent therapy.[20]

'Postpericardotomy syndrome' is an autoimmune disorder which presents with fever, pleuritic chest pain and dyspnea and is associated with pleural effusions and eosinophilia. It generally responds to anti-inflammatory therapy.[21] In the early stages, late-presenting mediastinal sepsis may mimic this condition. A full blood count and echocardiography should clarify the diagnosis. Constrictive pericarditis following cardiac surgery is well described.[22]

Summary

This case demonstrates that deep mediastinitis following cardiac surgery may present without classical signs of wound infection. Cardiac arrhythmias and raised atrial pressures point to a diagnosis of pericardial constriction. Where a clear diagnosis cannot be made by TTE, a TEE investigation or other imaging is required. Diabetics are at increased risk of infective postoperative complications. Attention to improving both preoperative and postoperative glycemic control will reduce this risk.

Key learning points

* Deep mediastinitis may present insidiously and is not always associated with sternal wound infection.
* Low cardiac output, dysrhythmia and raised atrial pressures may indicate cardiac constriction.
* The most appropriate immediate investigation is echocardiography. TEE may reveal posterior collections invisible on transthoracic views.
* Improving perioperative glycemic control of diabetic cardiac surgical patients will reduce the risk of mediastinitis.

References

1. Antunes PE, Bernardo JE, Eugenio L et al. Mediastinitis after aorto-coronary bypass surgery. Eur J Cardiothorac Surg 1997;**12**:443–9.

2. Stahle E, Tammelin A, Bergstrom R et al. Sternal wound complications: incidence, microbiology and risk factors. Eur J Cardiothorac Surg 1997;**11**:1146–53.

3. Milano CA, Kesler K, Archibald N et al. Mediastinitis after coronary artery bypass graft surgery. Risk factors and long-term survival. Circulation 1995;**92**:2245–51.

4. Rutledge R, Applebaum RE, Kim BJ. Mediastinal infection after open heart surgery. Surgery 1985;**97**:88–92.

5. Zacharias A, Habib RH. Factors predisposing to median sternotomy complications. Deep vs superficial infection. Chest 1996;**110**:1173–8.

6. Chertow GM, Levy EM, Hammermeister KE et al. Independent association between acute renal failure and mortality following cardiac surgery. Am J Med 1998;**104**:343–8.

7. Talamonti MS, LoCicero J 3rd, Hoyne WP et al. Early re-exploration for excessive postoperative bleeding lowers wound complication rates in open heart surgery. Am Surg 1987;**53**:102–4.

8. Ferrazzi P, Allen R, Crupi G et al. Reduction of infection after cardiac surgery: a clinical trial. Ann Thorac Surg 1986;**42**:321–5.

9. Angelini GD, Lamarra M, Azzu AA, Bryan AJ. Wound infection following early repeat sternotomy for postoperative bleeding. An experience utilizing intraoperative irrigation with povidone iodine. J Cardiovasc Surg (Torino) 1990;**31**:793–5.

10. Klovekorn WP, Meisner H, Sebening F. Ten years experience with povidone-iodine in heart surgery. J Hosp Infect 1985;**6 (Suppl A)**:117–21.

11. Nugent WC, Maislen EL, O'Connor GT et al. Pericardial flap prevents sternal wound complications. Arch Surg 1988;**123**:636–9.

12. Fong IW, Baker CB, McKee DC. The value of prophylactic antibiotics in aorta-coronary bypass operations: a double-blind randomized trial. J Thorac Cardiovasc Surg 1979;**78**:908–13.

13. Nooyen SM, Overbeek BP, Brutel de la Riviere A et al. Prospective randomised comparison of single-dose versus multiple-dose cefuroxime for prophylaxis in coronary artery bypass grafting. Eur J Clin Microbiol Infect Dis 1994;**13**:1033–7.

14. Sisto T, Laurikka J, Tarkka MR. Ceftriaxone vs cefuroxime for infection prophylaxis in coronary bypass surgery. Scand J Thorac Cardiovasc Surg 1994;**28**:143–8.

15. Verkkala K. Occurrence of and microbiological findings in postoperative infections following open-heart surgery. Effect on mortality and hospital stay. Ann Clin Res 1987;**19**:170–7.

16. Domart Y, Trouillet JL, Fagon JY et al. Incidence and morbidity of cytomegaloviral infection in patients with mediastinitis following cardiac surgery. Chest 1990;**97**:18–22.

17. Bitkover CY, Gardlund B, Larsson SA et al. Diagnosing sternal wound infections with 99mTc-labeled monoclonal granulocyte antibody scintigraphy. Ann Thorac Surg 1996;**62**:1412–6

18. Hickman MS, Schwesinger WH, Page CP. Acute cholecystitis in the diabetic. A case-control study of outcome. Arch Surg 1988;**123**:409–11.

19. Furnary AP, Zerr KJ, Grunkemeier GL, Starr A. Continuous intravenous insulin infusion reduces the incidence of deep sternal wound infection in diabetic patients after cardiac surgical procedures. *Ann Thorac Surg* 1999;**67**:352–60.

20. Rassias AJ, Marrin CA, Arruda J *et al*. Insulin infusion improves neutrophil function in diabetic cardiac surgery patients. *Anesth Analg* 1999;**88**:1011–6.

21. Prince SE, Cunha BA. Postpericardiotomy syndrome. *Heart Lung* 1997;**26**:165–8.

22. Killian DM, Furiasse JG, Scanlon PJ *et al*. Constrictive pericarditis after cardiac surgery. *Am Heart J* 1989;**118**:563–8.

10
Perioperative transesophageal echocardiography

Bernhard JCJ Riedel, A Timothy Lovell and Shane J George

Introduction

Transesophageal echocardiography (TEE) is a semi-invasive, low-risk procedure[1] that provides both diagnostic and continuous monitoring capabilities during cardiac surgery without encroaching on the operative field. The detailed extra- and intracardiac anatomical and functional information provided by TEE allows physicians (a) to confirm or modify the preoperative diagnosis and thereby adapt anesthetic and surgical strategies; (b) monitor the perioperative hemodynamic status (loading conditions, systolic and diastolic function); (c) diagnose the cause of perioperative complications (e.g. ischemia, ventricular failure, tamponade); (d) assess the efficiency of therapeutic maneuvers instituted for these complications; and (e) evaluate the adequacy of the corrective procedure immediately following cessation of CPB.

Perioperative complications that result in a low cardiac output/hypotensive state may arise at separation from CPB or in the early postoperative period. This complication is more commonly seen in patients with pre-existing ventricular dysfunction or where problems of myocardial protection, reperfusion injury, inadequate revascularization or surgical repair occur. Most causes of a low cardiac output/hypotensive state following cardiac surgery are easily identified on TEE and the early diagnosis and management of these causes may reduce associated morbidity and mortality. The following case report aims to highlight how intraoperative TEE may contribute to the reduction in the incidence of morbidity and mortality associated with cardiac surgery.

Case history

A 53-year-old Caucasian male presented with mitral stenosis for mitral valve repair or replacement. Preoperative symptoms included chest pain (CCS grade I), dyspnea (NYHA grade III), episodic paroxysmal nocturnal dyspnea and deteriorating exercise tolerance. There was no other medical or surgical history of relevance. On examination, a loud first heart sound accompanied by a diastolic (grade 2/4) murmur with presystolic accentuation was auscultated in the apical region.

Preoperative work-up included a chest X-ray (CXR), transthoracic echocardiogram (TTE) and cardiac catheterization. Findings were consistent with mitral stenosis, with characteristics of pulmonary venous hypertension and mild interstitial pulmonary edema on CXR and thickened mitral leaflet cusps and chordae tendinae on TTE. Transmitral Doppler demonstrated a prolonged pressure half-time ($P_{1/2}t$ = 270 ms) therefore estimating the mitral valve area (MVA = $220/P_{1/2}t$) at 0.8 cm^2.[2] TTE also demonstrated trivial mitral and tricuspid regurgitation. Tricuspid regurgitation was however insufficient to allow a Doppler estimate of the RA–RV pressure difference and therefore an estimate of systolic pulmonary artery (sPA) pressure (where sPA = sRV pressure = RV-RA pressure difference + RA pressure) was not possible.[3] However, right heart catheterization confirmed pulmonary hypertension (pulmonary artery pressure (PAP) 80/40 mmHg, mean 56 mmHg; pulmonary capillary wedge pressure (PCWP) a wave 36 mmHg, v wave 56 mmHg, mean 36 mmHg). Left heart catheterization revealed normal coronary arteries on angiography and preserved left ventricular function (left ventricular end-diastolic pressure (LVEDP) 12 mmHg; left ventricular ejection fraction (LVEF) 68%) on ventriculography. The gradient between PCWP and LVEDP, as an estimate of the transvalvular (mitral) pressure gradient, was 20 mmHg.

The operative period was uneventful. Cardiopulmonary bypass (CPB; total duration 94 minutes) was instituted using bicaval and aortic cannulation. During aortic cross-clamping (total duration 74 minutes) antegrade cold blood cardioplegia was used for myocardial preservation. Direct examination of the mitral valve revealed a rigid stenotic valve with calcification of the anterior leaflet and part of the posterior leaflet annulus. These findings were compatible with rheumatic valve disease. The valve was not amenable to repair and therefore the decision was made to proceed to mitral valve replacement. Following excision of the anterior leaflet, with preservation of the posterior leaflet and chordae tendinae, a standard Carbomedics 33-mm bileaflet prosthetic valve (Sulzer Carbomedics, Austin, TX, USA) was inserted using an interrupted suturing technique. On completion of surgery the patient was weaned from CPB without difficulty and required only minimal inotropic support (dopamine 6 µg kg⁻¹ min⁻¹). Intraoperative TEE was not available for post-CPB evaluation of the adequacy of surgical replacement, however, based on clinical experience the surgeon was satisfied with the procedure.

The early postoperative period was complicated by a low cardiac output state requiring increased inotropic support (dopamine 6 μg kg^{-1} min^{-1}, epinephrine 0.15 μg kg^{-1} min^{-1}, norepinephrine 0.15 μg kg^{-1} min^{-1}, and enoximone 1.25 μg kg^{-1} min^{-1}) and intra-aortic balloon pump (IABP) augmentation. A PA catheter was inserted (PCWP 20 mmHg, cardiac index (CI) 3.8 l min^{-1} m^{-2}, (systemic vascular resistance indexed, SVRI) 1041 dyne s cm^{-5} m^{-2}) and TEE performed. TEE revealed good function of the prosthetic valve with an acceptable peak LA–LV pressure gradient (8 mmHg during diastole) and a normal diastolic filling pattern (where passive ventricular diastolic velocity (E wave) $\geq$ atrial systolic velocity (A wave)). Characteristic of this type of prosthetic valve, normal wash jets (small central regurgitant jets within the sewing ring; see Figure 10.1) were seen during systole. However, in addition

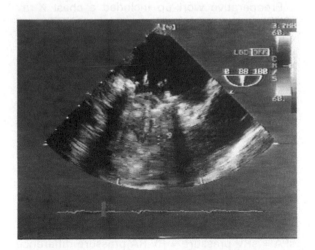
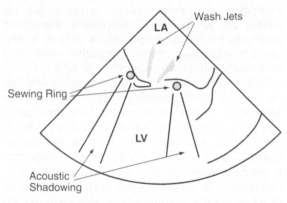

Figure 10.1

Mid-esophageal two-chamber (LA–LV long axis (90°)) view demonstrating normal wash jets of a prosthetic valve. This view demonstrates the typical 'signature' of a bileaflet prosthetic mitral valve, with two normal regurgitant (wash) jets occurring on the inside of the sewing ring. Up to six jets can be seen and these are designed to facilitate closure of the leaflet during systole as well as to keep the low flow atrial surface free of thrombus. Note acoustic shadowing on the ventricular side of the valve caused by the very echo-dense sewing ring of the valve.

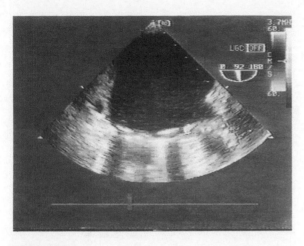 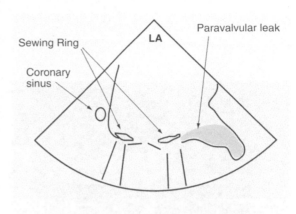

Figure 10.2

Mid-esophageal two-chamber (LA–LV long axis (90°)) view demonstrating a paravalvular leak on color flow mapping. Characteristically a plume of mosaic coloring originates from outside the sewing ring of a prosthetic valve. In this case it is directed into the atrial appendage.

two paravalvular jets (peripheral regurgitant jets outside the sewing ring) were seen on the midesophageal four-chamber transverse (0°) and mid-esophageal two-chamber (LA-LV long axis; Figure 10.2) views — a mild regurgitant jet at the medial border along the atrial septal wall and a moderate regurgitant jet at the lateral border that was directed into the left atrial appendage (Figure 10.2). Transgastric examination revealed global impairment of LV function (LVEF ~ 40%). The hemodynamic influence of these regurgitant jets on pulmonary venous return to the LA was evaluated by pulse-wave Doppler of the pulmonary vein. This revealed absent filling of the left atrium during systole (no S waves) from the pulmonary veins, consistent with moderate mitral (or paravalvular) regurgitation.[4]

In view of the high-risk status of the patient (hemodynamic instability and postoperative impaired LV function) the decision was made not to return to surgery to repair the paravalvular leaks but rather to opt for conservative treatment using inotropic support and diuretic therapy in an attempt to decrease LA pressure and promote forward flow. The patient responded favorably to conservative management with improvement of the low cardiac output state. Repeat TEE revealed a reduction in the paravalvular jet size and it was now estimated as mild regurgitation

(< 4 cm^2), together with a partial return of LA filling during ventricular systole as shown by blunted S waves on pulmonary venous flow patterns (Figure 10.3).

Further intensive care unit (ICU) management was complicated by a requirement for prolonged inotropic support and difficulty in weaning from mechanical ventilation. Despite good gas exchange on pressure support and continuous positive airway pressure (CPAP) the patient failed a trial of extubation on postoperative day 8 and required reintubation for tachypnea and exhaustion. Following a further period of extensive diuresis the patient was extubated successfully on postoperative day 11 and discharged from the ICU on postoperative day 12. Further postoperative recovery was uneventful and the patient was discharged from hospital on postoperative day 20.

At long-term follow-up (2 years following surgery) the patient was relatively stable but still required diuretic and angiotensin-converting enzyme inhibitor therapy. A complaint of amaurosis fugax was investigated by TEE to exclude a source of emboli from within the left atrium. TEE failed to find a source of emboli but demonstrated persistence of the mild regurgitant paravalvular jets and an increase in left atrial dimensions.

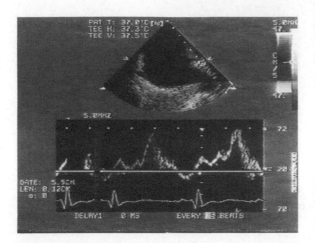
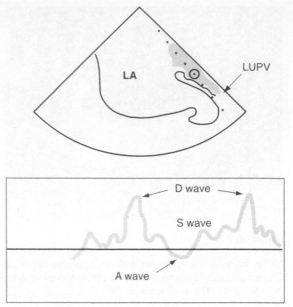

Figure 10.3

Doppler display of pulmonary venous flow pattern. This pulsed wave Doppler spectral display of pulmonary venous flow demonstrates depression of the systolic component (S wave) of venous return to the left atrium and is characteristic of mild to moderate mitral regurgitation. In the absence of mitral regurgitation (normal pattern) the velocity of the systolic flow component should equal to or be greater than that of the early diastolic flow component (D wave), with flow reversal down the pulmonary veins during atrial contraction (A wave). In severe mitral regurgitation, flow reversal may also occur in the systolic component (a negative S wave).

Discussion

TEE is an expensive but useful intraoperative diagnostic tool that can alter surgical and anesthetic management with tremendous potential benefit to both the cardiac surgical patient and to health-care resources. Potential cost-effectiveness of intraoperative TEE is obtained through avoidance of unnecessary surgery and a reduction in the risk of complications such as delayed re-operation and stroke in selected cardiac surgical populations. Alternatively, the failure to use intraoperative TEE may increase perioperative morbidity and mortality following cardiac surgery.

This case report demonstrates how the failure to use intraoperative TEE to evaluate the adequacy of the surgical procedure following CPB resulted in a delayed diagnosis of a hemodynamically significant paravalvular leak. The diagnosis was only made in the ICU following hemodynamic deterio-

ration — at which point it was decided that the patient was too high-risk for reoperation and repair of the paravalvular lesions. In contrast, had the diagnosis been established immediately following cessation of CPB then an immediate return to CPB for repair could have prevented the low cardiac output state that ensued in the postoperative period. It may therefore be argued that timely surgical intervention (i.e. immediately following CPB) could have resulted in improved patient quality of life and a vast cost saving effect through a reduction in the lengths of ICU and hospital stay by approximately 8 and 12 days, respectively. A further argument could be made for potential cost saving of health-care resources by reducing the requirement of long-term follow-up and chronic medication in this patient.

TEE permits immediate detection of an inadequate surgical procedure. In one series, 8% of patients scheduled for mitral valve repair (MVR) had problems discovered on intraoperative TEE following CPB that warranted further surgery during the same thoracotomy.[5] Paravalvular regurgitation is an uncommon complication of MVR. Most cases of severe paravalvular regurgitation are almost always repaired immediately when recognized during surgery. Little data is however available on the conservative management of patients with mild and moderate paravalvular regurgitation. In a study by Movsowitz et al,[6] eight patients with either mild (n = 6) or moderate (n = 2) paravalvular regurgitation, identified by TEE at the time of MVR, were treated conservatively and followed-up for a mean period of 16 months. A third of patients with mild and all of those with moderate paravalvular regurgitation at the time of MVR had deteriorated clinically and echocardiographically over time. The authors suggested that moderate paravalvular regurgitation should be corrected at the time of valve-replacement surgery, if this can be performed without high operative risk, and that mild paravalvular regurgitation should probably also be repaired, if this can be performed at low risk, because some will progress. Those patients left with mild paravalvular regurgitation after surgery, or patients in whom paravalvular regurgitation is recognized only after surgery, should be followed up carefully with serial clinical and echocardiographic examinations.

Evaluating the costs and outcomes associated with TEE during and after cardiac surgery Benson and Cahalan[7] showed that patients undergoing surgery for congenital heart disease derived the greatest overall benefit: around $600 cost saving per case studied. Patients undergoing valvular repair surgery derived the next greatest benefit: around $450 per case studied. In contrast patients having valve replacement had an overall *cost* of around $150 per case studied. Patients having surgery for coronary artery disease also derived an overall benefit: around $100–300 per case studied, dependent on the assumptions regarding the role of TEE in intraoperative stroke prevention. In this study liberal estimates of the direct and indirect costs (including the complications of TEE) and conservative estimates of positive outcomes: (money and lives saved) were used. Similarly, Murphy[8] reported that TEE was instrumental in diagnosing inadequate surgical repair in 20% of pediatric cardiac patients, with potential savings estimated between $30 000 and $70 000 per patient. In a study of high-risk

patients undergoing myocardial revascularization, intraoperative TEE was responsible for alterations in surgical management in 33% of patients and alterations in anesthetic management in 51% of patients. These alterations resulted in a reduction in the overall mortality of this group of patients, however because of the small study population, this finding did not reach statistical significance.[9] These studies clearly support the notion that intraoperative TEE is a cost-effective tool for cardiac surgery, especially for valvular and congenital heart repairs, where the financial benefits of TEE are substantial and frequently outweigh costs.

Whatever the reason for failure to examine this patient intraoperatively (unavailability of TEE facilities, inexperienced operator) intraoperative TEE would have facilitated the decision not to contemplate a repair (as evidenced by extensive calcification of both leaflets, annulus and chordae tendinae), or should a repair have been feasible it would have guided the surgeon as to the type of repair required and allowed evaluation of the adequacy of repair on weaning from CPB. Following MVR, postCPB echocardiography would have revealed significant paravalvular leaks resulting in hemodynamic embarrassment of pulmonary venous return. Safe and rapid reinstitution of CPB and accurate repair of the paravalvular leaks would have followed.

It is however essential to provide accurate and reproducible information about the precise location of valvular or paravalvular lesions in order to facilitate surgical intervention. A systematic examination improves the assessment of the mitral valve and reduces the incidence of diagnostic errors. Lambert et al[10] have recently published an excellent description of a six-step systematic TEE examination of the mitral valve. In brief, it is essential that all modalities of TEE (2-D examination, color flow mapping and Doppler) be used when assessing the mitral valve and that an attempt should be made to provide the surgeon with the pathological mechanism, as well as the grade of severity of the lesion(s). The simplest way of evaluating the severity of mitral valvular or paravalvular regurgitation is to use a semiquantitative estimate by color flow mapping to determine regurgitant jet length, regurgitant jet size, regurgitant jet width and the ratio of jet area to LA size. Other more advanced and more quantitative measures in determining the severity of mitral regurgitation include: mitral regurgitant orifice size and mitral regurgitant fraction. The PISA (proximal isovelocity surface area) technique, also known as flow convergence, is used to estimate the mitral regurgitant orifice size.[11] In this technique, color Doppler is used to calculate the surface area of a hemisphere of flow converging on the narrowed mitral orifice. The velocity at this hemisphere, where aliasing (V_{alias}) occurs, is known and equals the so-called Nyquist limit. Multiplying this velocity by the surface area allows determination of flow at the zone of convergence. Substituting the flow at the convergence zone and the maximal velocity (V_{max}) at the orifice (by continuous-wave Doppler) into the continuity equation [MVA = 2π $r^2.(\alpha/180) \times (V_{alias})/(V_{max})$] allows the regurgitant orifice area to be determined according to the law of conservation of mass (flow). Regurgitant orifice areas greater than 0.3 cm^2 are regarded significant. Furthermore, mathematical integration of the Doppler velocity–time profile (velocity–time integral; VTI) of the regurgitant jet on a spectral display provides an estimate of the distance travelled by the blood of the regurgitant jet in one cardiac cycle. Multiplying the VTI (cm) with the size of the regurgitant orifice (cm^2) through which the jet travels allows an estimate of the regurgitant volume (cm^3) per beat. Expressing the regurgitant volume as a ratio to the stroke volume would in

turn allow calculation of the regurgitant fraction. A regurgitant fraction >30% is associated with increased PCWP, reduced LVEF and cardiac output and increased long-term morbidity and mortality and should be addressed surgically.

Conclusions and learning points

- Intraoperative TEE is a cost-effective strategy that may reduce perioperative morbidity and mortality associated with cardiac surgery.
- Timely assessment for adequacy of the surgical procedure is important and should be done 'electively' following cessation of CPB – rather than at the time of hemodynamic deterioration in the postoperative period.
- Following mitral valve repair, evaluate for;
  - Residual mitral regurgitation
  - Induced or residual mitral stenosis
  - Systolic anterior motion of the mitral valve causing left ventricular out flow obstruction (Figure 10.4).
- Following mitral valve replacement, evaluate for;
  - Paravalvular leaks (Figure 10.2).
  - Normal leaflet motion of the mechanical prosthesis (Figure 10.5(a–c))

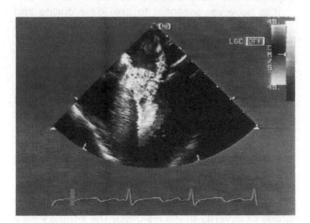

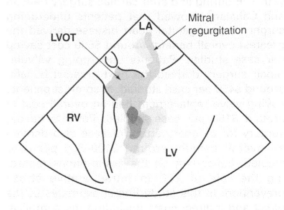

Figure 10.4

Mid-esophageal four-chamber view (0°) demonstrating left ventricular outflow tract (LVOT) obstruction. Color flow mapping demonstrates turbulent flow within the LVOT. This turbulence causes systolic anterior motion (SAM) of the mitral valve into the LVOT therefore worsening the obstruction, as well as distorting the mitral valves line of co-aptation — resulting in an eccentric mitral regurgitant jet, as shown here. LVOT obstruction can be caused by either a dynamic narrowing of the left ventricular outflow tract secondary to ventricular septal hypertrophy (e.g. hypertrophic obstructive cardiomyopathy, HOCM) or by a fixed narrowing secondary to a subaortic fibrous ring or following mitral valve repair.

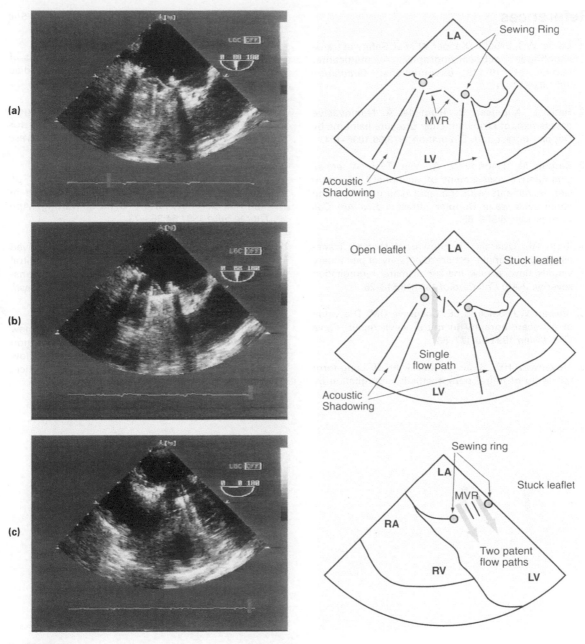

Figure 10.5

Mid-esophageal two-chamber (LA–LV long axis (90°)) views demonstrating an entrapped leaflet of a prosthetic mitral valve. (a and b) The prosthetic mitral valve appears normal in the systolic position, with two leaflets abutting the sewing ring. (a) However, during diastole only one leaflet moves to the open position (b). This will result in an elevated pressure gradient across the mitral valve with residual mitral stenosis and may be a cause of failure to wean from CPB. Commonly, the cause of failed leaflet opening is entrapment within the preserved subvalvular apparatus (e.g. chordae tendinae). Following return to CPB, the mitral valve was removed from the sewing ring and hence the two leaflets are now seen in a mid-esophageal four-chamber view (0°) (c). Both leaflets are now in the open position during diastole, thus creating two paths for forward flow through the mitral orifice.

References

1. Daniel WG, Erbel R, Kasper W *et al*. Safety of trans-esophageal echocardiography. A multicenter survey of 10 419 examinations. *Circulation* 1991;**83**:817–21.

2. Hatle L, Angelsen B, Tromsdal A. Noninvasive assessment of atrioventricular pressure half-time by Doppler ultrasound. *Circulation* 1979;**60**:1096–104.

3. Berger M, Haimowitz A, Van Tosh A *et al*. Quantitative assessment of pulmonary hypertension in patients with tricuspid regurgitation using continuous wave Doppler ultrasound. *J Am Coll Cardiol* 1985;**6**:359–65.

4. Klein AL, Obarski TP, Stewart WJ *et al*. Trans-esophageal Doppler echocardiography of pulmonary venous flow: a new marker of mitral regurgitation severity. *J Am Coll Cardiol* 1991;**18**:518–26.

5. Stewart WJ, Salcedo EE, Cosgrove DM. The value of echocardiography in mitral valve repair. *Cleve Clin J Med* 1991;**58**:177–83.

6. Movsowitz HD, Shah SI, Ioli A *et al*. Long-term follow-up of mitral paraprosthetic regurgitation by transesophageal echocardiography. *J Am Soc Echocardiogr* 1994;**7**:488–92.

7. Benson MJ, Cahalan MK. Cost-benefit analysis of transesophageal echocardiography in cardiac surgery. *Echocardiography* 1995;**12**:171–83.

8. Murphy PM. Pro: intraoperative transesophageal echocardiography is a cost-effective strategy for cardiac surgical procedures. *J Cardiothorac Vasc Anesth* 1997;**11**:246–9.

9. Savage RM, Lytle BW, Aronson S *et al*. Intraoperative echocardiography is indicated in high-risk coronary artery bypass grafting. *Ann Thorac Surg* 1997;**64**:368–73.

10. Lambert AS, Miller JP, Merrick SH *et al*. Improved evaluation of the location and mechanism of mitral valve regurgitation with a systematic trans-esophageal echocardiography examination. *Anesth Analg* 1999;**88**:1205–12.

11. Bargiggia GS, Tronconi L, Sahn DJ *et al*. A new method for quantitation of mitral regurgitation based on color flow Doppler imaging of flow convergence proximal to regurgitant orifice. *Circulation* 1991;**84**:1481–9.

11
Transesophageal echocardiography: its role in assessing the hypotensive patient undergoing cardiac surgery

A Timothy Lovell, Andrew D Shaw, Shane J George and Bernard JCJ Riedel

Introduction

The majority of patients undergoing cardiac surgery separate from cardiopulmonary bypass (CPB) with little trouble and their cardiac performance steadily improves in the postoperative period. However, difficulties resulting in a low cardiac output/hypotensive state may arise either at separation from CPB or in the early postoperative period following off-pump cardiac surgery in patients with pre-existing ventricular dysfunction, myocardial ischemia or those in whom technical problems occur. Traditional cardiovascular measurements (e.g. electrocardiogram (rate, rhythm), intravascular pressures, cardiac output measurement by thermodilution and direct inspection of the heart during surgery) undoubtedly provide useful information about cardiac function; however, the data is often incomplete and lacks detailed anatomical and regional functional information and often leaves the clinician with a differential diagnosis only. This is especially the case in valvular heart surgery. In contrast, transesophageal echocardiography (TEE) provides detailed extra- and intracardiac anatomical as well as functional information that may be extremely useful in this group of patients — allowing the clinician to rapidly reach a diagnosis and assess the effect of therapeutic maneuvres.

TEE is a semi-invasive procedure[1] capable of producing excellent quality images that allow continuous intra- and early postoperative monitoring without encroaching on the operative field. It carries a low risk of serious complica-tions[2-4] and, with the exception of esophageal stricture or tumors and recent esophageal or gastric surgery, few contraindications exist to TEE examination.[5] As a result TEE has expanded from the first tentative steps by Frazin and colleagues in 1976[6] to the extent that it is now used routinely in the perioperative period in a number of cardiac centers. This increase in usage of perioperative TEE has led to the publi-cation of a report on practice guidelines for perioperative TEE by the American Society of Anesthesiologists (ASA) and the Society of Cardiovascular Anesthesiologists (SCA) task force on TEE[7] and guidelines for performing a comprehensive intraoperative multiplane TEE examination by the American Society of Echocardiography (ASE) and the SCA.[5] These guidelines describe a set of standard views in an attempt to standardize terminology used in the perioperative setting and have subsequently been reinforced by various national bodies.[8]

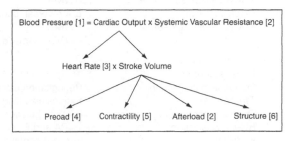

Figure 11.1

The factors that contribute to blood pressure.

Recognizing the importance of information derived from a TEE examination for the successful management of patients with a low cardiac output/hypotensive state following cardiac surgery,[7, 9, 10] the ASA and SCA guidelines (1996)[7] describe this condition as a category I indication (i.e. proven to influence clinical management for TEE).

Figure 11.1 depicts factors that contribute to blood pressure and thereby allows a simplified breakdown of common causes of a low output/hypotensive state following cardiac surgery, as presented in Table 11.1.

Common causes of immediate hypotension/low cardiac output resulting in failure to wean from CPB include myocardial ischemia, valvular dysfunction and aortic dissection. Common causes of delayed hypotension/low cardiac output state presenting in the ICU include myocardial ischemia, left and/or right ventricular failure, hypovolemia, cardiac tamponade and dynamic obstruction of the left ventricular outflow tract (LVOT). These causes will be discussed individually below using illustrative examples to describe the role of TEE.

Table 11.1 Assessment and treatment of hypotension/low cardiac output state. DC: direct current; FAC: fractional area change; IABP: intra-aortic balloon pump; IV: intravenous; LV: left ventricle; LVAD: left ventricular assist device; LVEDA: left ventricular end diastolic area; LVH: left ventricular hypertropy; LVOT: left ventricular outflow tract; MR: mitral regurgitation; NO: nitric oxide; PEEP: positive end expiratory pressure; PGI_2: prostaglandin I_2; RA: right atrium; RV: right ventricle; RWMA: regional wall motion abnormality; TR: tricuspid regurgitation.

Causative factor	TEE finding	Treatment
1. Spurious reading	Normal examination	Correct transducer
Incorrectly positioned or zeroed transducers		
Peripheral-central gradient	Normal examination	Measure pressure from more central artery
2. Peripheral resistance (afterload)		
Vasodilatation	⬦ LVEDA, ⬦ FAC%	α_1 agonists
Structural disruption e.g. aortic dissection	Intimal flap	Surgical repair
Pulmonary hypertension	RV and RA overload, TR	NO, PGI_2
3. Rate and rhythm	Abnormal transmital and pulmonary venous Doppler flow patterns (lack of A-waves).	DC cardioversion to sinus rhythm Chronotropic agents: epinephrine, isoprenaline Pacing
4. Volume status		
Hypovolaemia	⬦ LVEDA, ⬦ FAC%	IV colloid, blood
Hypervolaemia	Bulging atrial septum, ⬦ Chamber dimensions	Vasodilators, diuretics, volume removal
5. Decreased contractility		
Systolic failure	⬦ FAC%	Inotropes, IABP, LVAD
• *Myocardial ischaemia*	RWMA	Nitrates, revascularise
Diastolic failure	E/A reversal, poor relaxation	Inodilators, nitrates, IABP
• *Myocardial ischaemia*	RWMA	
• *LVH*	⬦ LVED septal diameter	
6. Structural disorder		
Valve disruption, Incomplete correction	Regugitation, paravalvular leak	Surgery
Tamponade	Extracardiac fluid collection	Surgery
Dynamic obstruction	LVOT turbulence, MR	Volume, ⬦ inotropes
RV–LV interaction	⬦ RA and RV dimensions, TR, leftward septal shift	Inodilators, nitrates, Mechanical support
• *RV failure*		
• *Pulmonary hypertension*		
• *High PEEP*		

Myocardial ischemia

Myocardial ischemia represents a common cause of hypotension/low cardiac output state following cardiac surgery. Contributing factors include: pre-existing ischemic heart disease; inadequate coronary artery revascularization; poor myocardial preservation during coronary or valvular surgery; and coronary embolism.

Acute cessation of coronary blood flow results in impaired myocardial function in the area supplied by the vessel and re-establishment of flow is associated with normalization of these changes.[11] Battler *et al* demonstrated that these regional changes occurred *before* ECG changes in dogs,[12] a finding confirmed in humans by Hauser *et al*.[13] Wohlgelernter *et al*, using transthoracic echocardiography (TTE) to monitor regional wall motion changes during angioplasty, had a greater sensitivity than the 12-lead ECG for the detection of myocardial ischemia[14] leading to the development of TEE as a monitor of myocardial ischemia.

The most commonly used view for TEE monitoring of myocardial ischemia is the transgastric short axis cross-section of the left ventricle at the midpapillary level.[15,16] This view is usually chosen since it contains regions of the ventricular wall supplied by the three main coronary arteries. Identification of a dysfunctional region suggests which coronary vessel contributes to the ischemia. The typical regions perfused by the three main coronary arteries are shown in Figure 11.2. In routine clinical monitoring the transgastric short axis image is usually divided into six segments, and the motion at each segment, which together with systolic thickening are considered individually to give each segment a score ranging from normal to dyskinetic on a five-point scale. The segmental scores are then averaged to give an overall impression of ventricular function. The standards committee of the ASE has recommended that the left ventricle be divided into 16 segments imaged through five different planes.[17] Nevertheless during the vast majority of intraoperative studies a single transgastric short axis view has been used.

The onset of a new persistent regional wall motion abnormality (RWMA) is widely assumed to be ischemic in origin.[15, 18] The report by Koolen[19] that dysfunctional myocardium often improves immediately after coronary artery bypass graft (CABG) surgery, was the first to

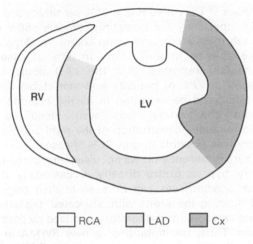

RCA   LAD   Cx

Figure 11.2

The transgastric short axis view at the level of the papillary muscles demonstrating the typical regions of myocardium perfused by each of the three main coronary arteries. RCA: right coronary artery; LAD: left anterior descending artery; Cx: circumflex artery.

describe the abolition of RWMA by revascularization. Leung and colleagues have shown that RWMAs are common in patients undergoing CABG,[16] and several groups have now demonstrated a relationship between the development of new persistent RWMA and an adverse cardiac outcome.[20, 21] More recently Shah examined the use of biplane monitoring to detect RWMA.[22] Of the 21% patients found to have a new RWMA, 30% were subsequently determined to have had an acute myocardial infarction. Of particular importance in this study is that new RWMAs were visible in both the transverse and vertical planes in only 45% of cases, 20% were only visible in the transverse plane and 35% only visible in the vertical plane. This finding lends further weight to the ASE recommendation to use multiple planes for assessing regional left ventricular function.[17] It must be stressed that adequate image quality and avoidance of an oblique cross section are vital in order to avoid erroneous diagnosis of RWMA.

Having determined which coronary artery is likely to be responsible for the myocardial ischemia it is worth considering the ability of TEE to directly image the coronary artery in question. Yoshida and colleagues were able to image the left main stem from its origin in the left coronary sinus to its bifurcation into the left anterior descending (LAD) and circumflex arteries in 90%

of cases.[23] They also had a 91% sensitivity and a 100% specificity for detecting stenosis >50% of the left main stem, and using color-flow Doppler were able to quantify flow in 85% of cases. Yamagishi reported that the LAD could be imaged in 77% of patients and that stable flow signals could be recorded in all the patients in whom the artery was well visualized.[24] Unfortunately, visualization of the right coronary artery was possible in only 26% of cases.

There is currently no way of visualizing coronary artery bypass grafts directly. Occasionally the aortic anastomoses can be seen at their origins and flushing the grafts with 'sonicated' (agitated) saline can confirm the territory perfused by patent grafts. Thus, the finding of a new RWMA in a grafted region is taken as an indication of graft dysfunction.

Valvular dysfunction

The anatomical and functional images produced by TEE provide information that would otherwise be impossible to achieve. The significance of this information in terms of planning the surgical procedure and evaluating its effects, including deciding whether further surgery is necessary, has led to valvular surgery being considered a category I indication for intraoperative TEE in its own right.[7]

Nowhere is this more important than in the evaluation of the effects of valvular repair procedures. These are continuing to increase in popularity owing to their reduced short-term and long-term mortality compared to valve replacement. At the Mayo Clinic more than 95% of patients with regurgitant mitral lesions are undergoing repair procedures, with 7% requiring reinstitution of CPB and a further repair.[25] The most frequent repair procedures are leaflet or chordal resections and mitral annuloplasty, with two or more distinct abnormalities occurring in over 90% of cases.[26] Following a resection procedure two-dimensional (2-D) echocardiography is used to image the mitral leaflets to assess the degree of coaptation as well as checking for residual prolapse. Normal closure is associated with considerable overlap of the leaflet tips producing a line of closure with appreciable depth. However, 2-D echocardiography may fail to reveal severe

functional inadequacy and color-flow Doppler mapping is used to assess the functional result. It is vital that at the time that functional regurgitation is assessed the hemodynamic loading of the left ventricle is normal since the mitral regurgitation (MR) may be absent in the setting of decreased left ventricular afterload. This risk of misinterpretation has led to many authorities recommending pharmacological manipulation (e.g. vasoconstriction) if necessary.[25, 27] Failure of a mitral repair procedure may also result in systolic anterior motion of the anterior mitral leaflet (SAM) resulting in MR as well as dynamic obstruction of the left ventricular outflow tract (LVOTO). This is discussed further below. A posterior mitral leaflet that has undergone extensive resection may appear as an immobile structure against which the anterior leaflet closes.[27] If the color Doppler suggests adequate function then this appearance should not be considered abnormal. Insertion of a ring prosthesis can cause distortion of the valve annulus resulting in leaflet prolapse or rarely, functional stenosis. However, a more common complication consists of new onset SAM-related dynamic LVOTO.[28]

Because prosthetic valves are designed to allow a continuous flow of blood to prevent blood clot formation on the exposed surfaces, 'physiological' regurgitation is a routine finding following valve replacement. The origins of these regurgitant, so-called 'wash jets' always lie *within* the sewing ring (see Figure 10.1); and different valves have differing patterns of 'normal' regurgitation. Even bioprosthetic valves may have a small central regurgitant jet. When only a limited number of imaging planes are used to it is possible to confuse the origin of these wash jets and to believe that they lie outside the sewing ring. Imaging in both transverse and long axis planes will usually confirm their origin within the sewing ring. A major problem with mechanical valves is their echogenic nature and the problems of echo drop-out (acoustic shadowing) behind a valve (see Figure 10.1). Individual valves can be recognized not only by their morphological features but also by their characteristic drop-out patterns. Some authorities have recommended that prosthetic valves are imaged using low gain settings in order to enhance image clarity accepting that surrounding native tissues will be less well seen.[27]

A major problem with all prosthetic valves is that of 'pathological' as opposed to 'physiological' regurgitation. TEE is exquisitely sensitive to detecting tiny amounts of regurgitation with color-flow Doppler. Assessment of the severity of regurgitation is based upon the normal echocardiographic standards for the valve in question. It must be remembered that what appears to be minimal regurgitation in one plane may appear to be very severe in another. Differentiating valvular from paravalvular regurgitation (see Figure 10.2) is often challenging, especially if the sewing ring is not well visualized. The technique of freezing the color-flow Doppler image superimposed on a 2-D image and then electronically subtracting and replacing the colour flow image often helps in identifying the origin of regurgitation.[29]

The final part of a TEE examination following valve surgery is inspection of neighbouring structures. Tears in the atrial septum caused by surgical retractors occasionally occur during mitral surgery giving rise to an atrial septal defect. It must also be remembered that a transatrial approach to the mitral valve might have be used. Other valves may also occasionally be damaged; catching one of the aortic valve cusps during insertion of a Carpentier mitral ring has been reported giving rise to florid aortic regurgitation.

Aortic dissection

A rare cause of the low cardiac output state that may manifest for the first time at separation from

CPB is aortic dissection. The most likely scenario is an intimal flap that has dissected more proximally to involve either the aortic valve or the coronary ostia. Although dissections due to aortic cannulation and aortic clamping have been reported they are fortunately rare. It is widely accepted that TEE is a superb tool for diagnosing aortic dissection.[27, 29] Given the close proximity of the aorta to the esophagus very detailed images are usually produced even using a single imaging plane. Regardless of the number of imaging planes used it is usually impossible to image the ascending aorta from about 5-cm distal to the aortic valve until well beyond the proximal aortic arch owing to the interposition of the air filled trachea between the aorta and esophagus.[30] Fortunately it is extremely rare for dissections to be confined to this region alone.[27] Data from the European Cooperative Study Group demonstrates a 99% sensitivity and 98% specificity for single transverse plane imaging,[31] although detection of the entry site is facilitated by the use of multiple windows afforded by multiplane systems.[27]

An aortic dissection is the result of a tear in the intima, which provides a site of entry for blood to dissect the intima away from the underlying media, and creates a second lumen for blood flow. Thus the diagnosis is made by finding two aortic lumens separated by an intimal flap and is shown in Figure 11.3. The intimal flap usually moves towards the false lumen, which is usually larger than the true lumen, during systole.

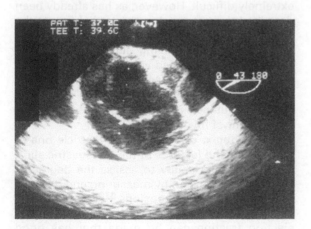

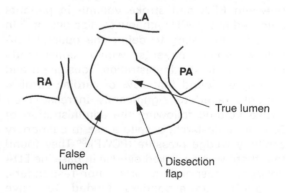

Figure 11.3

Transverse short axis view of the aorta in a patient with a type I dissection. The true lumen lies below, and separated from, the false lumen by an intimal flap. RA: right atrium; LA: left atrium; PA: pulmonary artery.

When hemodynamic problems are encountered at the time of separation from CPB these usually relate either to a recognized or acute intraoperative dissection or to complications related to the dissection such as proximal dissection to involve the aortic valve or coronary arteries,[32] or to aortic rupture. Retrograde dissection with rupture below the pericardial reflection will be immediately obvious intraoperatively since the rupture will occur into the pericardium. More distal rupture may be less obvious producing a hemothorax or hemoperitoneum, the patient presenting as hypotensive and hypovolemic despite volume expansion. However, these complications are usually detectable by TEE.

Hypovolemia

Intravenous fluids are frequently administered to patients following cardiac surgery to improve cardiovascular function by the Frank–Starling mechanism. Assessing preload in these patients can represent a challenge, the values obtained from both central venous and pulmonary artery catheters can, in some circumstances, be misleading and this has led to the exploration of the use of TEE for assessing preload.[33, 34] Assessment of left ventricular preload is carried out by measuring the end diastolic area (EDA) in the transgastric short axis view at the level of the papillary muscles, taking EDA as a surrogate for left ventricular end diastolic volume (LVEDV). Greim and colleagues found a good correlation between EDA and stroke volume in patients admitted to the ICU with low cardiac output.[35] In a study attempting to define the optimal EDA below which patients would consistently respond to fluid administration, Tousignant and colleagues found that 40% of cardiac surgical patients failed to significantly increase their stroke volume following the administration of 500 ml pentastarch, despite a rise in pulmonary capillary wedge pressure (PCWP).[36] They found that there was a marked overlap in baseline EDA between responders and non-responders, although non-responders tended to have reduced ventricular compliance.

Leung has shown that recognizing marked hypovolemia is simpler than assessing preload. She found that in hypovolemic patients there is obliteration of the left ventricular cavity during systole in the transgastric short axis view;[34] subsequently termed the 'kissing papillary muscles' sign. This is a simple screening test to apply, but needs to be used with care. It has been recognized for some time that in the setting of left ventricle hypertrophy, secondary to aortic stenosis or hypertension for example, using TEE estimates of ventricular filling tends to lead to overfilling the ventricle whilst using PCWP tends to lead to underfilling. It is also recognized that the hypertrophied left ventricle tends to have a reduced compliance.

The failing ventricle

One of the commonest causes for the low cardiac output state following cardiac surgery is a failing left and/or right ventricle. The underlying cause is most commonly ischemia or inadequate myocardial preservation during the operative period, although valvular dysfunction may also play a part. Even if the valves functioned normally before the operative event, as the heart undergoes progressive distension as it fails it undergoes progressive distension resulting in new mitral and tricuspid regurgitation (TR). This development of TR may make placement of a pulmonary artery flotation catheter difficult, if not impossible, without which assessment of left ventricular filling and cardiac output becomes extremely difficult. However, as has already been described the transgastric short axis view at the level of the papillary muscles provides a useful guide to ventricular filling although the caveat about the hypertrophied ventricle must be borne in mind. The same transgastric short axis view can also provide information about RWMA as has been outlined in the section describing the assessment of myocardial ischemia.

In the context of a failing left ventricle one of the most useful features of the transgastric short axis view is the ability to assess the degree of ventricular distension by measuring end diastolic and end systolic dimensions.[37] By measuring end systolic and diastolic areas, an estimate of ejection fraction can be made that has good agreement with ejection fraction estimated from ventriculography[38] and radionuclide angiography.[39] Using a truncated ellipsoidal model, Thys and colleagues have shown that it is possible to derive an approximation for changes in left ventricular volume and hence calculate cardiac output.[40] Cardiac output calculated using this technique shows a high correlation with cardiac output measured by thermodilution. Alternatively, cardiac output can be estimated by multiplying the cross-sectional area of one of the valves with the velocity time integral (VTI) of the blood flowing through it.

A major advantage of TEE is its ability to provide an anatomical real time picture. In the context of a failing ventricle this ability can be crucial in recognizing that the right ventricle has failed, and that the left side is actually hypovolemic. This scenario is most likely to be encountered postoperatively in patients with pre-existing pulmonary hypertension where, as well as supporting the failing right ventricle, treatment of the pulmonary hypertension will be required as well.

The mainstay of treatment for ventricular failure, once volume status has been optimized, is inotrope and inodilator therapy. TEE through its ability to assess ventricular volume status, ejection fraction and cardiac output has a major role to play in these patients in the absence of more invasive hemodynamic monitoring. In the setting of ventricular failure secondary to myocardial ischemia or inadequate myocardial preservation, or in patients with poor pre-existing ventricular function, off-loading the left ventricle while at the same time augmenting diastolic coronary perfusion with an intra-aortic balloon pump (IABP) maybe worth considering. TEE can be used to confirm correct intraluminal placement of the IABP, the tip of which should lie in the descending aorta just below the origin of the left subclavian artery; that is, just distal to the aortic arch.

Cardiac tamponade

Cardiac tamponade following cardiothoracic surgery is a life-threatening condition that requires prompt diagnosis and treatment and yet can be clinically challenging from a diagnostic standpoint. Based on the experience of the Mayo Clinic over a 19-year period, cardiac tamponade occurs in approximately 1% of cardiac surgical cases although the incidence varies dramatically with the surgical procedure.[41] An important finding in this report was that 30% of large (>400 ml) pericardial effusions were not associated with cardiac tamponade. Historically, the diagnosis of cardiac tamponade has been made on clinical findings. The classic triad of hypotension, elevated venous pressure and quiet heart sounds lacks specificity particularly in patients who develop cardiac tamponade following cardiac surgery;[42] in this group the same physical signs occur more commonly due to other conditions such as left ventricular dysfunction.[41] The detection of pericardial effusions has been greatly facilitated by the development of echocardiography which is now recognized as the gold standard diagnostic tool.[42, 43]

The volume of the pericardial effusion can be quantified by echocardiography and the hemodynamic effects assessed by looking for abnormal septal motion, right atrial[44] or right ventricular[45] diastolic collapse and a reduction in the changing diameter of the inferior vena cava during the respiratory cycle. When the volume of fluid in the pericardial space exceeds 25 ml an echo-free space around the heart persists throughout the cardiac cycle as shown in Figure 11.4. Smaller effusions may only be detected as an echo-free space posterior to the heart (i.e. between the TEE probe and the heart) during systole. With very large effusions the heart may have a swinging motion within the pericardial cavity and this may explain the observation of electrical alternans in the electrocardiogram.[43]

More recently it has been reported that Doppler echocardiograpic features are more sensitive than traditional echocardiography or clinical signs.[41, 46, 47] In the absence of pericardial tamponade, intrapericardial pressure, left ventricular diastolic pressure and intrathoracic pressure decrease to the same extent during the inspiratory phase of spontaneous respiration, and thus maintain the left ventricular filling pressure gradient. In cardiac tamponade, however, intrapericardial pressure decreases substantially less than intrathoracic pressure leading to a reduction in left ventricular filling during a spontaneous inspiration. A consequence of this reduction in left ventricular filling is that mitral valve opening is delayed, the isovolumic relaxation time is prolonged and the velocity of blood crossing the mitral valve during the

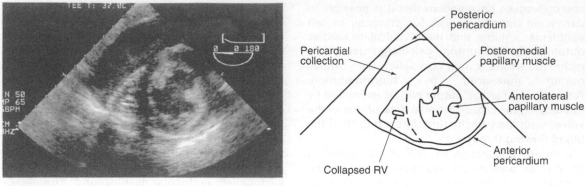

Figure 11.4

Transgastric short axis view during diastole demonstrating cardiac tamponade. There is an extracardiac collection of blood around the heart and marked collapse of the right ventricle (RV). LV: left ventricle.

early phase of left ventricular filling is reduced. On the other hand, during spontaneous exhalation the left ventricular filling pressure gradient is increased. Due to ventricular coupling in pericardial tamponade, with a relatively fixed cardiac volume, reciprocal changes occur in the right-sided chambers.[43]

Whilst it is widely recognized that echocardiography has a major role in the diagnosis of pericardial effusions what is much less well recognized is its utility in their treatment. Historically, treatment of pericardial effusions has been by blind, usually sub-xiphoid, aspiration or by surgery. Tsang and colleagues[41] have conclusively demonstrated the safety and effectiveness of echocardiographically guided pericardiocentesis, and this has led to recommendations that blind aspiration should be abandoned.[42] It is interesting to note that in this series from the Mayo Clinic two-thirds of the emergency evacuations of a pericardial tamponade were managed under echocardiographic control rather than with surgery.

Left ventricular outflow tract obstruction

Dynamic left ventricular outflow tract obstruction (LVOTO) can be one of the most difficult diagnoses to make without echocardiography,

requiring a high index of suspicion, particularly in the immediate post-CPB period. Unlike most other causes of the low cardiac output state, inotropes will tend to make the dynamic obstruction worse and treatment consists of volume loading and reduction of inotropic support. In severe cases, depression of the left ventricle with beta-blockers may be required. Dynamic LVOTO is most likely to occur in patients with hypertrophic obstructive cardiomyopathy or SAM.

The boundaries of the left ventricular outflow tract (LVOT) are superiorly the aortic valve, medially the interventricular septum and laterally the anterior leaflet of the mitral valve. The relations of the LVOT are readily seen in the five-chamber view. Other views that clearly demonstrate the LVOT include the midesophageal long axis view through the aortic valve and the transgastric and deep transgastric long axis views. These last two views are especially useful for quantifying the hemodynamic significance of the LVOTO by use of Doppler techniques to assess the degree of functional stenosis; normal LVOT flow velocity is less than 1.5 m s^{-1} and LVOT flow velocities in excess of this suggest significant obstruction.

Correction of a mitral leaflet prolapse may allow the previously prolapsing leaflet to exhibit SAM-related LVOTO (see Figure 10.4).[48] This anterior motion of the leaflet may also impair coaptation of the mitral leaflets resulting in MR and is a well-recognized complication of mitral valvular repair. SAM has also been reported to occur following aortic valve replacement in critical aortic stenosis.[49]

The immediate post-CPB period often features several factors that would be expected to exacerbate any predisposition to SAM. These factors include the presence of a low systemic vascular resistance in patients with preserved ventricular function, as well as a tendency to avoid any risk of left ventricular overdistension by maintaining a degree of hypovolemia.

Conclusions

Transesophageal echocardiography is a relatively non-invasive technique that produces both anatomical images and functional data in real time and has a major role to play in the management of the patient in the 'low cardiac output state'. Without the anatomical images provided by TEE some of the diagnoses would be impossible to reach and inappropriate therapies might be used.

References

1. Daniel WG, Erbel R, Kasper W et al. Safety of transesophageal echocardiography. A multicenter survey of 10,419 examinations. *Circulation* 1991;**83**:817–21.

2. Savino JS, Hanson CW 3rd, Bigelow DC et al. Oropharyngeal injury after transesophageal echocardiography. *J Cardiothorac Vasc Anesth* 1994;**8**:76–8.

3. Latham P, Hodgins LR. A gastric laceration after transesophageal echocardiography in a patient undergoing aortic valve replacement. *Anesth Analg* 1995;**81**:641–2.

4. Kharasch ED, Sivarajan M. Gastroesophageal perforation after intraoperative transesophageal echocardiography. *Anesthesiology* 1996;**85**:426–8.

5. Shanewise JS, Cheung AT, Aronson S et al. ASE/SCA guidelines for performing a comprehensive intraoperative multiplane transesophageal echocardiography examination: recommendations of the American Society of Echocardiography Council for Intraoperative Echocardiography and the Society of Cardiovascular Anesthesiologists Task Force for Certification in Perioperative Transesophageal Echocardiography. *Anesth Analg* 1999;**89**:870–84.

6. Frazin L, Talano JV, Stephanides L et al. Esophageal echocardiography. *Circulation* 1976;**54**:102–8.

7. Practice guidelines for perioperative transesophageal echocardiography. A report by the American Society of Anesthesiologists and the Society of Cardiovascular Anesthesiologists Task Force on Transesophageal Echocardiography. *Anesthesiology* 1996;**84**:986–1006.

8. Bennett S, Oduro A, Wright G, Younger J. *Cardiothoracic perioperative transoesophageal echocardiography.* Cambridge, UK: Association of Cardiothoracic Anaesthetists, 1999.

9. Reichert CL, Visser CA, Koolen JJ et al. Transesophageal echocardiography in hypotensive patients after cardiac operations. Comparison with hemodynamic parameters. *J Thorac Cardiovasc Surg* 1992;**104**:321–6.

10. Heidenreich PA, Stainback RF, Redberg RF et al. Transesophageal echocardiography predicts mortality in critically ill patients with unexplained hypotension. *J Am Coll Cardiol* 1995;**26**:152–8.

11. Tennant R, Wiggers CJ. The effect of coronary occlusion on myocardial contraction. *Am J Physiol* 1935;**112**:351–61.

12. Battler A, Froelicher VF, Gallagher KP et al. Dissociation between regional myocardial dysfunction and ECG changes during ischemia in the conscious dog. *Circulation* 1980;**62**:735–44.

13. Hauser AM, Gangadharan V, Ramos et al. Sequence of mechanical, electrocardiographic and clinical effects of repeated coronary artery occlusion in human beings: echocardiographic observations during coronary angioplasty. *J Am Coll Cardiol* 1985;**5**:193–7.

14. Wohlgelernter D, Cleman M, Highman HA et al. Regional myocardial dysfunction during coronary angioplasty: evaluation by two-dimensional echocardiography and 12 lead electrocardiography. *J Am Coll Cardiol* 1986;**7**:1245–54.

15. Rafferty TD. Left ventricular regional wall motion abnormalities as indicators of myocardial ischemia. *Basics of transesophageal echocardiography.* New York: Churchill Livingstone, 1995;111–6.

16. Leung JM, O'Kelly BF, Mangano DT. Relationship of regional wall motion abnormalities to hemodynamic indices of myocardial oxygen supply and demand in patients undergoing CABG surgery. *Anesthesiology* 1990;**73**:802–14.

17. Schiller NB, Shah PM, Crawford M *et al.* Recommendations for quantitation of the left ventricle by two-dimensional echocardiography. American Society of Echocardiography Committee on Standards, Subcommittee on Quantitation of Two-Dimensional Echocardiograms. *J Am Soc Echocardiogr* 1989;**2**:358–67.

18. Thys DM. The intraoperative assessment of regional myocardial performance. *J Cardiothorac Anesth* 1987;**1**:273–5.

19. Koolen JJ, Visser CA, van Wezel HB *et al.* Influence of coronary artery bypass surgery on regional wall motion: an intraoperative two-dimensional transesophageal echocardiographic study. *J Cardiothorac Anesth* 1987;**1**:276–84.

20. Leung JM, O'Kelly B, Browner WS *et al.* Prognostic importance of postbypass regional wall-motion abnormalities in patients undergoing coronary artery bypass graft surgery. SPI Research Group. *Anesthesiology* 1989;**71**:16–25.

21. Smith JS, Cahalan MK, Benefiel DJ *et al.* Intraoperative detection of myocardial ischemia in high-risk patients: electrocardiography versus two-dimensional transesophageal echocardiography. *Circulation* 1985;**72**:1015–21.

22. Shah PM, Kyo S, Matsumura M, Omoto R. Utility of biplane transesophageal echocardiography in left ventricular wall motion analysis. *J Cardiothorac Vasc Anesth* 1991;**5**:316–9.

23. Yoshida K, Yoshikawa J, Hozumi T *et al.* Detection of left main coronary artery stenosis by transesophageal color Doppler and two-dimensional echocardiography. *Circulation* 1990;**81**:1271–6.

24. Yamagishi M, Miyatake K, Beppu S *et al.* Assessment of coronary blood flow by transesophageal two-dimensional pulsed Doppler echocardiography. *Am J Cardiol* 1988;**62**:641–4.

25. Oh JK, Seward JB, Tajik AJ. Intraoperative echocardiography. In: *The echo manual*. Boston: Little Brown, 1994;221–8.

26. Galloway AC, Colvin SB, Baumann FG *et al.* Current concepts of mitral valve reconstruction for mitral insufficiency. *Circulation* 1988;**78**:1087–98.

27. Rafferty TD. Selected topics. *Basics of transesophageal echocardiography*. New York: Churchill Livingstone, 1995;147–71.

28. Lee KS, Stewart WJ, Lever HM *et al.* Mechanism of outflow tract obstruction causing failed mitral valve repair. Anterior displacement of leaflet coaptation. *Circulation* 1993;**88**:II24–9.

29. Blanchard DG, Dittrich HC, Mitchell M, McCann HA. Diagnostic pitfalls in transesophageal echocardiography. *J Am Soc Echocardiogr* 1992;**5**:525–40.

30. Konstadt SN, Reich DL, Quintana C, Levy M. The ascending aorta: how much does transesophageal echocardiography see? *Anesth Analg* 1994;**78**:240–4.

31. Erbel R, Engberding R, Daniel W *et al.* Echocardiography in diagnosis of aortic dissection. *Lancet* 1989;**1**:457–61.

32. Ballal RS, Nanda NC, Gatewood R *et al.* Usefulness of transesophageal echocardiography in assessment of aortic dissection. *Circulation* 1991;**84**:1903–14.

33. Cheung AT, Savino JS, Weiss SJ *et al.* Echocardiographic and hemodynamic indexes of left ventricular preload in patients with normal and abnormal ventricular function. *Anesthesiology* 1994;**81**:376–87.

34. Leung JM, Levine EH. Left ventricular end-systolic cavity obliteration as an estimate of intraoperative hypovolemia. *Anesthesiology* 1994;**81**:1102–9.

35. Greim CA, Roewer N, Apfel C *et al.* Relation of echocardiographic preload indices to stroke volume in critically ill patients with normal and low cardiac index. *Intensive Care Med* 1997;**23**:411–6.

36. Tousignant CP, Walsh F, Mazer CD. The use of transesophageal echocardiography for preload assessment in critically ill patients. *Anesth Analg* 2000;**90**:351–5.

37. Oh JK, Seward JB, Tajik AJ. Assessment of ventricular function. In: *The echo manual*. Boston: Little Brown, 1994;39–50.

38. Ren JF, Panidis IP, Kotler MN *et al.* Effect of coronary bypass surgery and valve replacement on left ventricular function: assessment by intraoperative two-dimensional echocardiography. *Am Heart J* 1985;**109**:281–9.

39. Clements FM, Harpole DH, Quill TJ *et al.* Simultaneous measurement of cardiac volumes, areas and ejection fractions by transesophageal

echocardiography and first pass radionuclide angiography. *Anesthesiology* 1988;**69**:A4.

40. Thys DM, Hillel Z, Goldman ME *et al*. A comparison of hemodynamic indices derived by invasive monitoring and two-dimensional echocardiography. *Anesthesiology* 1987;**67**:630–4.

41. Tsang TS, Barnes ME, Hayes SN *et al*. Clinical and echocardiographic characteristics of significant pericardial effusions following cardiothoracic surgery and outcomes of echo-guided pericardiocentesis for management: Mayo Clinic experience, 1979–1998. *Chest* 1999;**116**:322–31.

42. Fagan SM, Chan KL. Pericardiocentesis: blind no more! *Chest* 1999;**116**:275-6.

43. Oh JK, Seward JB, Tajik AJ. Pericardial diseases. In: *The echo manual*. Boston: Little Brown, 1994;165–76.

44. Gillam LD, Guyer DE, Gibson TC *et al*. Hydrodynamic compression of the right atrium: a new echocardiographic sign of cardiac tamponade. *Circulation* 1983;**68**:294–301.

45. Armstrong WF, Schilt BF, Helper DJ *et al*. Diastolic collapse of the right ventricle with cardiac tamponade: an echocardiographic study. *Circulation* 1982;**65**:1491–6.

46. Appleton CP, Hatle LK, Popp RL. Cardiac tamponade and pericardial effusion: respiratory variation in transvalvular flow velocities studied by Doppler echocardiography. *J Am Coll Cardiol* 1988;**11**:1020–30.

47. Burstow DJ, Oh JK, Bailey KR *et al*. Cardiac tamponade: characteristic Doppler observations. *Mayo Clin Proc* 1989;**64**:312–24.

48. Kupferschmid JP, Carr T, Connelly GP, Shemin RJ. Systolic anterior motion of the mitral valve after valve repair without an annular ring. *Ann Thorac Surg* 1994;**57**:484–6.

49. Cutrone F, Coyle JP, Novoa R *et al*. Severe dynamic left ventricular outflow tract obstruction following aortic valve replacement diagnosed by intraoperative echocardiography. *Anesthesiology* 1990;**72**:563–6.

12
Adult congenital heart disease

Matthew J Barnard

Introduction

Adult congenital heart disease is a relatively new medical specialty, which has developed as a direct result of improved medical and surgical management of pediatric congenital heart conditions.[1] Prior to 1960 less than 15% of neonates with congenital heart disease survived into adolescence. Presently over 90% of patients reach young adult life, including those with complex anomalies. This has created a new population of adults with both operated and unoperated congenital heart disease. It is estimated that this population is increasing by 2000 annually in the United Kingdom. These patients present complex medical, surgical and psychosocial problems.[2, 3]

Case report 1

A 26-year-old male presented with severe pulmonary regurgitation. His underlying cardiac pathology comprised transposition of the great arteries (TGA), ventricular septal defect (VSD) and left ventricular outflow tract (LVOT) obstruction. At age 5 years he underwent a Rastelli correction comprising patch closure of the VSD, thereby tunneling left ventricle to aorta, and insertion of a homograft conduit between the right ventricle and pulmonary artery. He had one episode of infective endocarditis 3 years before this admission. Homograft degeneration resulted in pulmonary regurgitation and increased right heart size and he was scheduled for elective replacement.

Past medical history	Rastelli procedure for TGA, VSD and LVOT obstruction 21 years ago. Infective endocarditis 3 years ago. Pulmonary regurgitation secondary to homograft degeneration.
Regular medications	Aspirin 75 mg OD. No allergies.
Examination	Weight 75 kg. Sternotomy scar noted. BP 110/70 mmHg. Palpable second heart sound and palpable thrill at left upper sternal edge. Single second heart sound. Grade 3/6 ejection systolic murmur, soft diastolic murmur.
Investigations	Hb 11.4 g dl^{-1}, WBC 3.1×10^9 l^{-1}, platelets 142×10^9 l^{-1}, creatinine 0.9 mg dl^{-1} (84 µmol l^{-1}). **CXR:** Cardiomegaly with calcification within conduit. **ECG:** Right bundle branch block. **Cardiac catheter:** RV 71/1 mmHg, RVEDP 16 mmHg, LV 104/4 mmHg, LVEDP 19 mmHg, PA (mean) 27/6 (19) mmHg. Proximal conduit narrowing with 44 mmHg gradient between RV and PA. No LVOT obstruction or aortic regurgitation. Good biventricular function. Pulmonary regurgitation

Elective femorofemoral cardiopulmonary bypass (CPB) was instituted due to the close proximity of the conduit to the sternum. Sternotomy was performed without incident and the conduit was then opened in preparation for removal, at which time transesophageal echocardiographic (TEE) monitoring demonstrated a significant amount of air in the systemic circulation. It was evident that a small and previously undetected residual VSD was present. The patient was placed head down, thiopental 1 g IV was administered and ice packs were placed around the head. One minute of circulatory arrest was required to control and close the defect. Significant ST segment elevation was evident on ECG for 30 minutes following this incident. Resection of muscular right ventricular outflow tract obstruction was then performed and a pulmonary homograft inserted. Following uneventful separation from CPB, the patient was transferred to intensive care receiving only an infusion of glyceryl trinitrate 2.6 µg kg^{-1} min^{-1}. The postoperative course was complicated by persistent pyrexia and bilateral pleural effusions. The patient was eventually discharged from hospital 25 days later, with no clinical evidence of neurological sequelae.

Case report 2

A 48-year-old woman presented with severe mitral regurgitation. She had a complex, unpalliated cyanotic heart defect comprising tricuspid atresia, with no connection between right atrium and right ventricle. There was a large naturally occurring secundum atrial septal defect (ASD) and a non-restrictive VSD. The pulmonary vasculature was protected from systemic pressures by significant pulmonary valve stenosis. Her past medical history included a transient ischemic attack (TIA) 9 years before admission, a cerebrovascular accident (CVA) resulting in right hemiparesis, 5 years before admission, and an episode of infective endocarditis and pulmonary edema necessitating an admission 1 year before this admission. She was receiving treatment for paroxysmal supraventricular tachycardias (SVT).

She underwent replacement of the mitral valve with a 33-mm Carbomedics (Sulzer Carbomedics; Austin, TX, USA) bileaflet mechanical prosthesis and further enlargement of the ASD. The procedure was conducted using CPB with cross-clamping of the aorta and antegrade cold blood cardioplegia. High-dose aprotinin (2 Mkiu bolus, 2 Mkiu prime and 0.5 Mkiu h^{-1}) was administered perioperatively. Monitoring included intraoperative TEE. Cardiopulmonary bypass was discontinued without difficulty and she was weaned from mechanical ventilation 6 hours after admission to the intensive care unit.

The first 6 days after surgery were uneventful. A pyrexia was observed on day 7 and she developed right chest pain, a right pleural effusion, and weight gain, while her urea rose from 5.8 to 13.8 mmol l^{-1}. Over the following 21 days her clinical progress was poor and she continued to complain of chest and abdominal discomfort. Clinical signs of pulmonary collapse/consolidation were accompanied by persistent pyrexia, leukocytosis (WBC 14.9×10^9 l^{-1}) and elevation of C-reactive protein (CRP >180 iu l^{-1}). Two episodes of fast atrial fibrillation (ventricular rate 150 beats min^{-1}) required DC cardioversion. She required overnight mechanical ventilation following one

Past medical history	Tricuspid atresia, ASD and VSD. TIA 9 years ago. CVA — right hemiparesis 5 years ago. Infective endocarditis 1 year ago. Paroxysmal SVTs.
Regular medications	Warfarin 3 mg OD, frusemide 40 mg OD, amiloride 5 mg OD, amiodarone 200 mg OD, metolazone 5 mg OD. No allergies.
Examination	Weight 80 kg. BP 110/70 mmHg.
Investigations	Hb 17.8 g dl^{-1}. SaO$_2$ (air) 80%. **TEE:** Situs solitus, absent right atrioventricular connection, ventricular disconcordance, severe subpulmonary and pulmonary stenosis, non-restrictive VSD, left atrioventricular regurgitation.

of these episodes due to inadequate spontaneous respiration. On postoperative day 28 ultrasound examination of the abdomen demonstrated an empyema of the gall bladder which was drained percutaneously. Multiple gallstones in the distal common bile duct necessitated endoscopic cholangiography and sphincterotomy 1 week later. Following this she again required several hours mechanical ventilation due to her general debilitation. Significant gastrointestinal hemorrhage followed reinstitution of heparin therapy. The source of this hemorrhage was assumed to be the sphincterotomy site.

Over the following 2 weeks the patient's condition gradually improved, although the clinical course was complicated by further episodes of fever and cholecystitis, a widespread vascular rash (attributed to drug reaction), chest pain and hemoptysis, bilateral tinnitus and left maxillary sinusitis. She was eventually discharged after 55 days in hospital.

Discussion

Surgical procedures

Adults with congenital heart disease who require surgery may present having had no previous surgery or for reoperations.[4] The former group comprises a small number of patients in whom a minor defect — such as secundum ASD — has not been detected, and patients with known lesions which have not previously required intervention. The majority of patients, however, have already undergone surgery. Currently 80% of surgical procedures in the author's unit are reoperations, including over 40% who have undergone two or more previous cardiothoracic procedures.

Table 12.1 lists the categories which define the indications for reoperation. A large number is described as inevitable on the basis that the categories constitute either completion of surgical repair, or deal with complications, which are an accepted fate of the original procedure.[5] Replacement of conduits connecting the right ventricle to pulmonary artery fall into this category. Residual abnormalities of an underlying lesion form another category, an example

Table 12.1 Indications for surgery in adults with congenital heart disease

- Inevitable reoperations
- Residual abnormalities
- Recurrence of original lesions
- Further palliation
- Unexpected complications
- Transplantation

being atrioventricular valve regurgitation in patients with atrioventricular septal defects. Recurrence of previous abnormalities such as aortic recoarctation or aortic valve restenosis forms a third group. Palliative procedures are a fourth group and are often aimed at optimizing pulmonary blood flow. Palliation may be permanent (for example systemic to pulmonary artery shunt formation for inadequate pulmonary blood flow), or may form part of a staged repair in high-risk patients who are deemed unsuitable for complete or radical repair at the time at which intervention is necessary. Unexpected developments such as infective endocarditis necessitate surgery in a small number of patients. Finally transplantation is the final fallback for some patients with end stage heart failure or pulmonary vascular disease.

The indications for the majority of procedures conducted are valve dysfunction, conduit failure, or recoarctation. Insertion or replacement of right heart conduits for pulmonary stenosis, pulmonary regurgitation or right ventricular aneurysm — as in the first case report — constitutes the single largest indication for surgery in the author's institution. A variety of biological and prosthetic substrates have been used. The timing of surgery is difficult and in general is best performed prior to the onset of symptoms, as up to 50% of patients with severe obstruction are symptom free.

Associated problems

Table 12.2 lists the important issues that must be considered in adults with congenital heart disease. Resternotomy represents a significant risk in patients who have undergone previous surgery for congenital heart disease.[6] The risk of major hemorrhage is substantially higher than in

Table 12.2 Important medical and surgical problems in adults with congenital heart disease

- Resternotomy in the presence of right ventricle to pulmonary artery conduits
- Cyanosis, hematological abnormalities and aortopulmonary collateral vessels
- Ventricular dysfunction and restrictive right ventricular physiology
- Arrhythmias
- Pulmonary vascular disease
- Comorbidity : congenital syndromes, scoliosis and respiratory compromise, acquired heart disease

patients undergoing reoperation for acquired heart disease and is attributable to the fact that right heart conduits almost inevitably require replacement — they lie directly behind the sternum and in some cases they actually erode the sternum. Careful preoperative assessment of the retrosternal space is therefore, essential. Although the position of the conduit may best be determined by magnetic resonance imaging[6] a lateral chest radiograph will often adequately demonstrate the position of a calcified conduit in many patients. Exposure of the femoral vessels is usually undertaken before resternotomy, and if preoperative investigation indicates that the conduit is at risk, femorofemoral CPB is instituted before sternotomy. In the absence of other lesions such as septal defects the operation can usually be performed on a beating heart, without the need for aortic cross-clamping. A VSD carries the additional risk of air entering the systemic circulation if the conduit is ruptured. In addition, systemic to pulmonary collateral arteries or shunts will decrease systemic perfusion, and aortic regurgitation can lead to severe ventricular distension. In these cases induction of hypothermia and circulatory arrest prior to sternotomy may be necessary. There is a risk of ventricular distension if ventricular fibrillation occurs and one solution is to vent the left heart through the chest wall. Alternatively, external cardiac massage prior to sternotomy is both simple and effective.

Ventricular dysfunction is common.[7] These patients manifest contractile failure, diastolic dysfunction and abnormalities of ventricular interaction. Ventricular impairment may be a result of delayed surgery, poor myocardial protection in an earlier era of cardiac surgery, pulmonary vascular disease, chronic pressure and volume overload, or inadequate previous repair. Right ventricular failure is common and important. The complex anatomy and loading conditions dictate that simple indices of ventricular function (ejection fraction) are often inadequate. Although myocardial protection may be more difficult in these patients, abnormal ventricular function, together with increased non-coronary collateral blood flow as well as the possibility of acquired coronary artery disease underlie its importance.

Hypertrophy results in reduced ventricular compliance, and the potential for low postoperative cardiac output. Loss of sinus rhythm and arrhythmias are poorly tolerated in this situation. Additionally residual hemodynamic lesions are also poorly tolerated and must be excluded with the aid of intraoperative TEE. Restrictive right ventricular physiology can arise postoperatively[8] and may be diagnosed by echocardiographic demonstration of diastolic antegrade flow through the pulmonary valve. It appears to be related to perioperative myocardial injury, as it correlates with troponin release and indicators of oxidative stress.[9]

Chronic cyanosis/hypoxemia indicates the possibility of aortopulmonary collateral arteries, hematological abnormalities, renal impairment and myocardial injury or fibrosis.[10] Collateral arteries may be acquired or congenital (e.g. complex pulmonary atresia). It is important to assess their presence and anatomy prior to operation with selective angiography. If appropriate (in terms of pulmonary blood supply) they may be embolized prior to surgery. Otherwise they are controlled or ligated before CPB to avoid systemic 'steal' and shunting of blood to the pulmonary arteries with ventricular distension. Visualization may be difficult, and hypothermic circulatory arrest or low-flow bypass together with appropriate ventricular venting may be required. Hematological abnormalities mandate meticulous surgical hemostasis, appropriate use of blood products and the use of aprotinin. Preoperative venesection is performed when the haematocrit is very high, although this is rare.[11] As a guide, venesection should be considered if the hemotocrit is greater than 65%. It is important to detect the syndrome of decompensated erythrocytosis which comprises polycythemia in association with headache, fatigue, dizziness, visual disturbances, paresthesiae, irritability, mylagia and anorexia.

Pulmonary vascular disease is common, but is often anatomical and asymmetric. While the pulmonary hypertensive crises often seen in infants are rare, right ventricular failure and low output are common. Elevated pulmonary vascular resistance is often the determining factor in whether a lesion is suitable for repair, and is associated with significantly elevated perioperative risk.

Specific anesthetic considerations

An understanding of the pathophysiology of the cardiac defect as well as the implications of previous interventions is essential.[12] Eight questions to consider during preoperative assessment are listed in Table 12.3.

Vascular access may present difficulties.[13] Arterial access can be problematic in recoarctation and previous Blalock Taussig shunts. Bilateral Blalock Taussig shunts mandate lower limb arterial pressure monitoring. Femoral vein thrombosis following previous catheterization can prevent access or the inferior vena cava may be interrupted, with hemiazygous continuation. It is best to avoid superior vena cava (SVC) catheters in Glenn (SVC to pulmonary artery) shunts and perhaps in other Fontan circulations, in order to avoid SVC thrombosis. Meticulous care must be taken to avoid intravenous air entry in patients with shunt lesions as systemic embolization can occur, even when shunting is predominantly left to right.

Table 12.3 Preoperative assessment of patients with congenital heart disease

- What is the anatomy of any previous repair?
- Are there any residual structural defects?
- Is ventricular function normal?
- Are there anatomical or physiological abnormalities of the pulmonary vasculature?
- Normal venous anatomy — connections, drainage and monitoring sites?
- Are there residual ECG abnormalities?
- What antibiotic prophylaxis is necessary?
- Is anticoagulation therapy employed and when should it be withdrawn and reinstituted?

External defibrillator pads are placed on patients undergoing reoperations, as access for internal paddles is usually impossible during chest opening. Conduit replacement is associated with a significant number of arrhythmias during conduit dissection.

Intraoperative nitric oxide is used during 5% of procedures in the author's unit. It is typically required for patients with Fontan circulations in whom weaning from CPB is problematic. Facilities for administration of nitric oxide into the inspiratory gases and appropriate monitoring should be available. Measurement of nitric oxide and nitrogen dioxide concentrations is most easily accomplished with electrochemical monitors. Infective endocarditis guidelines must be followed.[14]

Conclusions and learning points

- Adult congenital heart disease comprises a complex but increasing problem.
- Patients deserve a continuation of the excellence of care that they have received during their pediatric era.
- A multidisciplinary team in a specialized unit dedicated to their care best manages those with anything other than straightforward simple lesions.[15]

References

1. Somerville J. Management of adults with congenital heart disease: an increasing problem. *Annu Rev Med* 1997;**48**:283–93.

2. Baum VC, Perloff JK. Anesthetic implications of adults with congenital heart disease. *Anesth Analg* 1993;**76**:1342–58.

3. Webb GD, Harrison DA, Connelly MS. Challenges posed by the adult patient with congenital heart disease. *Adv Intern Med* 1996;**41**:437–95.

4. Laks H, Pearl JM. The surgeon's responsibility: operation and reoperation: the UCLA experience. *J Am Coll Cardiol* 1991;**18**:327–9.

5. Rosenthal A. Adults with tetralogy of Fallot—repaired, yes; cured, no. *N Engl J Med* 1993;**329**:655–6.

6. Surgery for congenital defects. In: Redington A, Shore D, Oldershaw P (eds) *Congenital heart disease in adults*. London: WB Saunders, 1994;171–8.

7. Perloff JK. Congenital heart disease in adults. A new cardiovascular subspecialty. *Circulation* 1991;**84**:1881–90.

8. Cullen S, Shore D, Redington A. Characterization of right ventricular diastolic performance after complete repair of tetralogy of Fallot. Restrictive physiology predicts slow postoperative recovery. *Circulation* 1995;**91**:1782–9.

9. Chaturvedi RR, Shore DF, Lincoln C *et al*. Acute right ventricular restrictive physiology after repair of tetralogy of Fallot: association with myocardial injury and oxidative stress. *Circulation* 1999;**100**:1540–7.

10. Perloff JK, Rosove MH, Child JS, Wright GB. Adults with cyanotic congenital heart disease: hematologic management. *Ann Intern Med* 1988;**109**:406–13.

11. Jones P, Patel A. Eisenmenger's syndrome and problems with anaesthesia. *Br J Hosp Med* 1995;**54**:214.

12. Findlow D, Doyle E. Congenital heart disease in adults. *Br J Anaesth* 1997;**78**:416–30.

13. Burrows FA. Anaesthetic management of the child with congenital heart disease for non-cardiac surgery. *Can J Anaesth* 1992;**39**:R60–70.

14. Child JS. Infective endocarditis: risks and prophylaxis. *J Am Coll Cardiol* 1991;**18**:337–8.

15. Connelly MS, Webb GD, Somerville J *et al*. Canadian Consensus Conference on Adult Congenital Heart Disease 1996. *Can J Cardiol* 1998;**14**:395–452.

13
The Fontan circulation

Matthew J Barnard

Introduction

The Fontan operation, as originally described,[1] refers to a specific procedure (atriopulmonary connection) whereas *Fontan circulation* is a term widely used to generically describe the final result of palliative procedures for patients who will ultimately be limited to a univentricular circulation. The new physiology involves diversion of all or part of the systemic venous return to the pulmonary circulation, usually without a subpulmonary ventricle.[2] The aim of these procedures is to separate the systemic and pulmonary circulations, but with systemic venous blood flowing to the lungs without the assistance of a right ventricle. This results in the normal arrangement of a series rather than parallel circulation. Flow across the lungs to the left atrium becomes entirely dependent on the pressure gradient between the venae cavae and the left atrium.

Case report

A 20-year-old male presented with recurrent atrial tachyarrhythmias and diminished exercise tolerance. The patient's underlying anatomy comprised a double inlet right ventricle, hypoplastic left ventricle, single ventricular septal defect (VSD), ventriculoarterial discor-

Past medical history	Univentricular type heart. Blalock Hanlon atrial septectomy and left modified Blalock Taussig shunt. Atriopulmonary (Fontan) connection. Recurrent atrial tachyarrhythmias and diminished exercise tolerance
Regular medications	Amiodarone 200 mg OD, warfarin as per INR
Examination	Weight 43 kg. Sternotomy scar noted. BP 115/60, HR 50. JVP elevated. RV heave. Single second heart sound. Soft systolic murmur at left sternal edge.
Investigations	Hb 14 g dl^{-1}, INR 1 1, creatinine 1.0 mg dl^{-1} (91 µmol l^{-1}). **CXR:** Mild cardiomegaly. **ECG:** Sinus rhythm and right atrial hypertrophy. **TEE:** Enlarged right atrium with spontaneous echo contrast. Impaired ventricular function. Large ventricular septal defect. **Angiography:** Obstructed atriopulmonary connection. Markedly enlarged right atrium wrapped over pulmonary artery. Ventricular function moderate (pressure-volume loops). SpO$_2$ 98%. Pulmonary arterial SO$_2$ 75%. **Intracardiac pressures:** Mean RA 12 mmHg, mean SVC 13 mmHg, PA 13/11 mmHg, mean IVC 11 mmHg, LV 85/13 mmHg.

dance with anterior aorta and common atrioventricular valve. Thus, he essentially had a univentricular type heart. Previous surgery included a Blalock Hanlon atrial septectomy and left modified Blalock Taussig shunt. Six years previously an atriopulmonary (Fontan) connection had been performed. He initially did well, but recently had developed problems with systemic ventricular impairment, atrial distension and persistent arrhythmias. He was scheduled for elective conversion of atriopulmonary connection to total cavopulmonary connection.

The operation was lengthy (720 minutes) due to attempted intraoperative radiofrequency ablation of arrhythmia pathways. Femoral arterial cannulation was performed before sternotomy and cardiopulmonary bypass (CPB) was instituted following bicaval cannulation. The aorta was cross-clamped but coronary perfusion was maintained via direct coronary cannulation. A single short right internal jugular catheter was inserted, as well as a triple lumen catheter in a femoral vein. Intraoperative monitoring included transesophageal echocardiography.

Separation from CPB was problematic. This was attributed to pre-existing ventricular dysfunction together with the consequences of a long CPB duration on pulmonary vascular resistance (PVR). Acceptable hemodynamics were eventually achieved with a combination of intravenous epinephrine 0.1 µg kg^{-1} min^{-1}, enoximone 5 mg/kg^{-1} min^{-1} and 10 ppm inhaled nitric oxide. Mechanical ventilation incorporated a long expiratory time (I:E ratio 1:3 to 1:4) and no positive end expiratory pressure. A high FiO$_2$ was administered and PaCO$_2$ was maintained below 34 mmHg (4.5 kPa). He made initial progress postoperatively and the trachea was extubated on the second postoperative day in line with the desire to minimize positive intrathoracic pressure. However progressive respiratory insufficiency supervened, and he sustained a sudden cardiac arrest on day 3 while preparations were being made to reinstitute mechanical ventilation. He was resuscitated following 35 minutes of electromechanical dissociation and ventricular fibrillation; but never subsequently regained consciousness. Investigations confirmed severe diffuse cerebral injury. He died 3 weeks later.

Discussion

Indications and types of operations

Essentially any condition resulting in absence or hypoplasia of a ventricular chamber, or the impossibility of biventricular repair may be considered for these procedures. This type of operation was originally described for tricuspid atresia but has now been extended to a wide variety of complex lesions, particularly double inlet ventricle.[3,4] Single ventricle type circulations with mixing of venous blood are inherently inefficient due to recirculation of blood through the pulmonary vasculature. Additionally they confer cyanosis, which in combination with volume overload, results in impaired ventricular function. Suitable candidates for surgery require a normal or low PVR, and normal left ventricular filling pressures.

Glenn operations are usually staging procedures performed as part of a sequence that culminates in a Fontan-type procedure. The bidirectional Glenn shunt comprises connection of the superior vena cava (SVC) to the pulmonary artery. Inferior vena caval blood usually continues to reach the heart and maintains a right to left shunt with resultant hypoxemia. The palliative effect diminishes over time, and between 5 and 15 years over 40% require conversion to Fontan.[5, 6] 'Glenn patients' can develop venous collaterals that communicate between the SVC and the inferior vena cava (and provide natural decompression of the high SVC pressures). Glenn procedures are infrequently performed as a primary procedure in adults due to the lower proportion of cardiac output returning via the SVC. Cases have been reported of attempted Glenn procedures in adults with postoperative emergency conversion to complete Fontan connections.[7]

The Fontan procedure involves an atriopulmonary anastomosis[1] which originally incorporated a valved conduit. This was superseded by direct connection between the right atrial appendage and main pulmonary artery. Sophisticated physiological models demonstrated that the right atrium provided an insignificant contribution to forward flow through the lungs, and could actually be detrimental in terms of energy losses.[8] As a result the total cavopulmonary connection (TCPC) was developed. This involves connecting the distal end of the SVC to the side of the right pulmonary artery, together with a conduit (e.g. a Goretex baffle along the free wall of the right atrium) connecting the inferior vena cava to the inferior aspect of the right pulmonary artery. The operation involves less right atrial dissection than a Fontan procedure and hence potentially less damage to the sino-atrial node. Exclusion of the right atrium results in less distension, and diminished turbulence. This ought to improve forward flow, and the hope is that this will result in fewer arrhythmias and a lower incidence of right atrial thrombosis.[2] More recently extracardiac inferior vena cava to pulmonary artery conduits have been reported.

Partial or fenestrated intra-atrial conduits incorporate a fenestration that allows right to left shunting of blood at atrial level. These were developed in response to the high mortality (up to 30%) and morbidity in high-risk candidates (e.g. those with borderline PVR).[9] The fenestration allows decompression of the systemic venous system and maintains or augments cardiac output, at the expense of increased cyanosis consequent upon the right to left shunt. Fenestrations may be subsequently closed or enlarged using minimally invasive transvenous techniques.

Risk determinants

Success depends on both low PVR and left atrial pressure. Pulmonary blood flow will diminish in the presence of elevated systemic ventricular end diastolic pressure, elevations of PVR, atrioventricular valve dysfunction, and loss of sinus rhythm. Systemic atrioventricular valve regurgitation — whether anatomical or functional in origin — may cause serious hemodynamic disturbance. Valve replacement in this setting is a high risk procedure.[10] Additional problems are pulmonary vein stenosis, pulmonary artery stenosis and cavopulmonary anastomotic obstruction.

Three preoperative risk factors are associated with definite poor outcome. These are a PVR in excess of 4 Wood units (320 dyne s cm^{-5}) or an increased pulmonary artery pressure (mean greater than 15 mmHg), age less than 2 or greater than 14 years, and systemic ventricular hypertrophy.[2]

Physiology

These patients have diminished reserve in terms of ability to increase cardiac output in response to exercise or stress. Minor hemodynamic changes can lead to severe deterioration. Cardiac index is decreased both at rest and during exercise[11] and ventilation perfusion abnormalities are common. A patient with a completed Fontan circulation should have a peripheral arterial saturation of approximately 95%. These patients are extremely sensitive to changes in PVR. Factors that influence PVR include pCO_2, pO_2, arterial pH, mean airway pressure, PEEP and extrinsic compression (at surgery). In practical terms therefore it is important to maintain central venous pressure, utilize positive pressure ventilation with caution and to be aware that reduced contractility and loss of sinus rhythm are poorly tolerated. Systemic ventricular function is often reduced,[12] particularly when it is morphologically a right ventricle. Diastolic function can be particularly affected.[13] Ventricular relaxation is incoordinate, with prolonged isovolumic relaxation, diminished early rapid filling and dominant atrial systolic filling. Systolic performance can be within normal limits in the presence of markedly abnormal diastolic function.[2]

Complications

These patients demonstrate high central, hepatic, mesenteric and renal venous pressures. These high pressures are important in the aetiology of late problems and complications including arteriovenous fistulae, arrhythmias, thrombosis, peripheral edema, protein-losing enteropathy (PLE) and pathway obstruction. Between 10 and 20% of patients who have had Glenn procedures develop pulmonary arteriovenous malformations.[14] They may be multiple and diffuse, and result in progressive cyanosis.

Arrhythmias are a major concern in the Fontan patient. All arrhythmias should provoke a search for underlying hemodynamic disturbances, such as pathway obstruction, decreased ventricular function and valve regurgitation.[15] Supraventricular tachycardia occurs in 20–40% of patients between 5 and 15 years from operation[16] and may be attributable to increased right atrial pressure and atrial distension. There seems to be a lower incidence with TCPC patients, although they still occur.[17]

Thrombosis and embolic stroke are particular risks, especially when there are low flow areas within the heart. The echocardiographic appearance of the right atrium is often large and dilated with marked 'spontaneous contrast'. An intrinsic thrombotic tendency exists in over 60% of patients which may be due to protein C deficiency.[18]

Within 10 years of operation, 10–15% of patients develop PLE and secondary hypoproteinemia.[10] Clinical features include hepatomegaly, ascites, cirrhosis, peripheral edema, and pleural and pericardial effusions. It carries a grim prognosis, with 50% of those affected dead at 5 years.[2]

Venous pathway or conduit obstruction can occur and is a serious complication. It may result in atrial arrhythmias, decreased functional capacity, fluid retention and PLE.[10]

Prognosis

Mortality from the early procedure is less than 5%. The 'ideal' survival at 15 years has been advocated as 73–90%,[19] but survival of 60% has been reported.[16] Reoperation carries a high mortality — in the presence of PLE it approaches 75%, although it is somewhat less than this if the problem is solely mechanical obstruction. Clinically a progressive deterioration in functional cardiac capacity occurs. Of 90% of patients whose activity postoperatively is class 1 NYHA, only 50% will remain so at 15 years.[19]

Management/treatment

As previously stated, adult patients very rarely present for Fontan procedures as a primary

Table 13.1 Assessment of the Fontan patient

- Ventricular function
- Pathway obstruction
- Residual shunts/baffle leaks
- Systemic atrioventricular valve regurgitation
- Right atrial thrombosis
- Arrhythmias
- Pulmonary arteriovenous malformations
- Protein/albumin levels
- Hepatic function

operation. Indications for cardiac surgery in adult life include relief of venous pathway obstruction, repair or replacement of atrioventricular valves and repair of residual shunts. Venous collateral channels may be closed by transcatheter coil occlusion, or altered with the introduction of an axillary arteriovenous fistula. The place of converting the Fontan connection to a TCPC or extracardiac conduit (as in the case report) is currently being evaluated. Table 13.1 lists factors that should be considered in preoperative assessment of patients presenting for surgery who have previously undergone a Fontan operation. Guiding principles in the approach to patients undergoing such operations include accurate preoperative diagnosis, selection of the correct procedure, excellent myocardial protection and elimination of residual anatomical defects.

Postoperative cardiac output

Low postoperative cardiac output may be due to left ventricular outflow tract obstruction, systemic atrioventricular valve regurgitation, impaired myocardial function, elevated PVR, residual defects, arrhythmias, tamponade, hypovolemia or inappropriate inotrope use. Escalating inotrope administration can be associated with acute ventricular hypertrophy and spiraling cardiac dysfunction. Cardiac performance may be evaluated with clinical measures, systemic venous oxygen saturation, serum lactate determination, urine output and echocardiography. Early return to the cardiac catheterization laboratory during the postoperative period is advisable to exclude or intervene in case of residual anatomical defects. Superior vena caval and left atrial (LA) catheters will allow calculation of the transpulmonary gradient. Hypovolemia will result in low SVC and LA pressures and low transpulmonary gradient. Venous pathway obstruction or high PVR will result in high right-sided pressure with low LA pressure and increased transpulmonary gradient. Left ventricular outflow obstruction, myocardial dysfunction or atrioventricular valve regurgitation will result in both pressures being high.

Cardiovascular therapy should be tailored to the underlying problem. Management includes volume loading, pacing, and optimization of mechanical ventilation. Vasodilators and inotropes may be necessary. Atrioventricular sequential pacing is greatly preferred for hemodynamic benefit, and epicardial leads are often used in order to minimize thrombotic risk. It should be emphasized that tachyarrhythmias can result in profound hemodynamic deterioration and are potentially life threatening in these patients. Attempts should be made to restore sinus rhythm as soon as possible, employing DC cardioversion as necessary.[9] Pharmacological correction of acid–base disturbances, negative pressure ventilation (cuirass) and extracorporeal membrane oxygenation can be considered. Continuous drainage of ascites and pleural effusions, opening the sternum and consideration of taking down the repair may be necessary to aid the failing heart. Inhaled nitric oxide can be a useful pulmonary vasodilator, but it is important that its use does not mask other (anatomical) reasons for failure.

Conclusions and learning points

- The Fontan circulation poses unique physiological challenges.
- Successful management of the patient with a Fontan circulation undergoing cardiac surgery requires complete understanding of the underlying anatomy, physiology and pathophysiology.
- Pharmacological and physiological manipulation of PVR is frequently necessary.
- These patients have minimal cardiac reserve and are at significant risk from any surgical intervention. They require careful and very close attention to detail.

References

1. Fontan F, Baudet E. Surgical repair of tricuspid atresia. *Thorax* 1971;**26**:240–8.

2. Univentricular atrioventricular connection and the Fontan procedure. In: Redington A, Shore D, Oldershaw P (eds) *Congenital heart disease in adults*. London: WB Saunders, 1994;89–100.

3. Yacoub MH, Radley-Smith R. Use of a valved conduit from right atrium to pulmonary artery for 'correction' of single ventricle. *Circulation* 1976;**54**:III63–70.

4. Franklin RC, Spiegelhalter DJ, Rossi Filho RI et al. Double-inlet ventricle presenting in infancy. III. Outcome and potential for definitive repair. *J Thorac Cardiovasc Surg* 1991;**101**:924–34.

5. di Carlo D, Williams WG, Freedom RM et al. The role of cava-pulmonary (Glenn) anastomosis in the palliative treatment of congenital heart disease. *J Thorac Cardiovasc Surg* 1982;**83**:437–42.

6. Kopf GS, Laks H, Stansel HC et al. Thirty-year follow-up of superior vena cava-pulmonary artery (Glenn) shunts. *J Thorac Cardiovasc Surg* 1990;**100**:662–70.

7. Surgery. In: Redington A, Shore D, Oldershaw P (eds) *Congenital heart disease in adults*. London: WB Saunders, 1994;179–90.

8. de Leval MR, Kilner P, Gewillig M, Bull C. Total cavopulmonary connection: a logical alternative to atriopulmonary connection for complex Fontan operations. Experimental studies and early clinical experience. *J Thorac Cardiovasc Surg* 1988;**96**:682–95.

9. Connelly MS, Webb GD, Somerville J et al. Canadian Consensus Conference on Adult Congenital Heart Disease 1996. *Can J Cardiol* 1998;**14**:395–452.

10. Webb GD, Harrison DA, Connelly MS. Challenges posed by the adult patient with congenital heart disease. *Adv Intern Med* 1996;**41**:437–95.

11. Gewillig MH, Lundstrom UR, Bull C et al. Exercise responses in patients with congenital heart disease after Fontan repair: patterns and determinants of performance. *J Am Coll Cardiol* 1990;**15**:1424–32.

12. Akagi T, Benson LN, Green M et al. Ventricular performance before and after Fontan repair for

univentricular atrioventricular connection: angiographic and radionuclide assessment. *J Am Coll Cardiol* 1992;**20**:920–6.

13. Penny DJ, Rigby ML, Redington AN. Abnormal patterns of intraventricular flow and diastolic filling after the Fontan operation: evidence for incoordinate ventricular wall motion. *Br Heart J* 1991;**66**:375–8.

14. Lamberti JJ, Spicer RL, Waldman JD *et al*. The bidirectional cavopulmonary shunt. *J Thorac Cardiovasc Surg* 1990;**100**:22–9.

15. Peters NS, Somerville J. Arrhythmias after the Fontan procedure. *Br Heart J* 1992;**68**:199–204.

16. Driscoll DJ, Offord KP, Feldt RH *et al*. Five- to fifteen-year follow-up after Fontan operation. *Circulation* 1992;**85**:469–96.

17. Gelatt M, Hamilton RM, McCrindle BW *et al*. Risk factors for atrial tachyarrhythmias after the Fontan operation. *J Am Coll Cardiol* 1994;**24**:1735–41.

18. Cromme-Dijkhuis AH, Henkens CM, Bijleveld CM *et al*. Coagulation factor abnormalities as possible thrombotic risk factors after Fontan operations. *Lancet* 1990;**336**:1087–90.

19. Fontan F, Kirklin JW, Fernandez G *et al*. Outcome after a 'perfect' Fontan operation. *Circulation* 1990;**81**:1520–36.

14
Heparin resistance in a patient requiring cardiopulmonary bypass

Rosalind J Mills and Helena M McKeague

Introduction

Several factors have been suggested to contribute to reduced heparin sensitivity in cardiac patients. The incidence of heparin resistance has been estimated to be as high as 20%. Preoperative therapy with heparin,[1, 2] intravenous glyceryl trinitrate (GTN),[3] aortic balloon pumps,[1] ventricular aneurysm with thrombus, autotransfusion[4] and infective endocarditis[5, 6] have all been implicated as causative factors. Heparin treatment in the preoperative period, which can lead to low plasma levels of the coagulation inhibitor antithrombin III (AT-III) is thought to be the most common cause.[2, 5]

Knowledge of the factors that affect patient sensitivity to heparin, and the appropriate management of these patients is vital in the context of cardiac surgery with cardiopulmonary bypass (CPB). Inadequate anticoagulation during CPB can lead to activation of hemostatic mechanisms with the consequent risk of intravascular thrombosis, thrombosis of the extracorporeal circuit, and increased postoperative bleeding.[7] Supplementation of low endogenous AT-III levels is the logical approach for the treatment of heparin resistant patients requiring surgery.

Case history

An 81-year-old female Caucasian presented for urgent CABG. The patient had a 2-year history of angina, with recurrent admissions for unstable angina. Previous coronary angiography had revealed diffuse triple vessel disease, with well-preserved left ventricular function. Two weeks

Past medical history	Hypertension. DVT of left calf 2 years earlier. Oesophageal reflux. Hypothyroidism. No known drug allergies.
Regular medications	Aspirin 75 mg OD, diltiazem 60 mg TDS, isosorbide mononitrate SR 120 mg OD, omeprazole 20 mg OD, simvastatin 10 mg OD, thyroxine 50 µg OD, glyceryl trinitrate 5–10 mg h^{-1} IV, heparin 5000 iu TDS SC
Examination	Weight 65 kg. BMI 26.3 kg m^{-2}. BP 140/70. Reduced air entry at left base. Bilateral varicose leg veins. Bilateral ankle edema. Clinically euthyroid.
Investigations	Hb 12.0 g dl^{-1}, WBC 9.14 × 10^9 l^{-1}, platelets 334 × 10^9 l^{-1}, PT 11 s, APTT 26 s [Na$^+$] 136 mmol l^{-1}, [K$^+$] 3.6 mmol l^{-1}, urea 4.7 mmol l^{-1}, creatinine 0.9 mg.dl-1 (83 µmol l^{-1}). **CXR**: Heart size normal, lungs clear, large fixed hiatus hernia in chest. **ECG**: Sinus rhythm 75 min^{-1}. No acute ischemic changes. **Cardiac catheter**: Good overall left ventricular function. Triple vessel disease.

prior to surgery the patient was admitted to a referring hospital with chest pain at rest which was treated with intravenous GTN and subcutaneous heparin. Transfer to a cardiac surgery unit was arranged for urgent coronary revascularization.

One hour prior to transfer to the anesthetic room the patient was premedicated with intramuscular morphine 10 mg and hyoscine 0.2 mg. The right radial artery and a right forearm vein were cannulated under local anesthesia. Following preoxygenation, anesthesia was induced with diazepam 7 mg, fentanyl citrate 0.5 mg, and suxamethonium 100 mg. A rapid sequence induction technique with application of cricoid pressure was performed as the patient had reported symptoms of gastroesophageal reflux, and the chest X-ray (CXR) suggested an intrathoracic stomach. Following tracheal intubation, the lungs were ventilated with an air/oxygen mixture. Anesthesia was maintained with an infusion of propofol 4mg kg^{-1} min^{-1} and a further 0.5 mg of fentanyl. Neuromuscular blockade was prolonged with pancuronium 12 mg. Before transfer to the operating theatre, the right internal jugular vein was cannulated and a urinary catheter was sited under antibiotic cover — flucloxacillin 1 g and gentamicin 120 mg.

At the start of surgery a baseline Celite activated clotting time (ACT) of 116 seconds was determined using the Automated Coagulation Timer II system (Medtronic Inc., Minneapolis, MA, USA) In addition, a heparin dose response (HDR) slope was calculated using the Hepcon Hemostasis Management System (Medtronic Inc.). This system carries out three dual-channel clotting tests simultaneously by comparing a patient's blood with no heparin in two channels, heparin 1.5 units ml^{-1} in another two channels and heparin 2.5 units ml^{-1} in the last two channels. As the response to heparin is linear up to 8 units ml^{-1}, the three clotting times can be plotted on a graph to produce an HDR curve. The HDR slope (in seconds per unit heparin per milliliter of blood) is the value that the ACT will increase by, for each unit of heparin given per milliliter of blood. This value, 66 s iu^{-1} ml^{-1} (normal HDR slope >80 s iu^{-1} ml^{-1}), indicated a reduced sensitivity to heparin in our patient.

Saphenous vein, the left internal mammary artery, and the left radial artery were harvested for use as revascularization conduits. After median sternotomy, just prior to the placement of the aortic purse string, anticoagulation was initiated with heparin 20 000 iu (300 iu kg^{-1}). Five minutes after heparin administration, the ACT had only reached 331 seconds — an inadequate response — so a further dose of heparin 100 iu kg^{-1} was given. The next ACT (402 seconds) was also below the target value of 480 s, so the patient was treated with recombinant human antithrombin III (rhAT-III) 75 u kg^{-1}, as dictated by a research protocol. Five minutes after the administration of rhAT-III adequate anticoagulation was demonstrated (ACT 654 seconds) allowing CPB to be established between the right atrium and the ascending aorta.

Three coronary bypasses were performed with antegrade cold blood cardioplegia for myocardial protection during 30 minutes of aortic cross-clamping. Throughout CPB (duration 74 minutes) the ACT remained >600 seconds. With the exception of heparin 5 000 iu, which was added to the CPB prime routinely, no additional heparin was administered.

Once ventilation had been re-established the patient was weaned from CPB with sequential (DDD) pacing. Residual heparin was reversed by the administration of protamine 300 mg. The postprotamine ACT was 136 seconds.

At the end of surgery the patient was transferred to the ICU. One adult dose (4 units = 4 individual donations) of platelets (237 ml) was given to the patient because aspirin therapy had been continued until the time of surgery. The patient was successfully weaned from mechanical ventilation and extubated 6 hours after arrival in the ICU. The left pleural drain and both pericardial drains were removed the following morning, and the patient was discharged from the ICU. The remainder of the postoperative course was uncomplicated, and the patient was transferred to a convalescence home 7 days after surgery.

Discussion

Patients undergoing cardiac surgery with CPB require full anticoagulation with heparin to prevent clotting. Coagulation can be initiated by contact of blood with the artificial surfaces of the heart–lung machine circuitry.[8, 9] A degree of heparin resistance is common in patients who have received preoperative heparin therapy. [1, 4–6] Low levels of AT-III are important in the etiology of heparin resistance, since heparin requires AT-III to exert its anticoagulant effect (Figure 14.1).[10] The primary function of heparin is to inhibit the activity of thrombin which is responsible for fibrin production.[11,12]

AT-III is a naturally occurring enzyme inhibitor formed from activated factor X. AT-III inhibits and destroys thrombin, as well as decreasing the activity of factors IX, X, XI, and XII. Deficiency of AT-III can be hereditary or acquired. The acquired form usually results from chronic heparin administration (intravenous or subcutaneous) when demand for AT-III outstrips supply producing a relative resistance to heparin. Therefore, in the presence of low AT-III levels, a normal dose of heparin will not achieve full anticoagulation.

Low intrinsic levels of AT-III can be boosted, by administering exogenous AT-III, to enhance the therapeutic effect of heparin in resistant patients. [7, 13, 14] The most obvious reason for avoiding incomplete anticoagulation during CPB is to prevent coagulation within the circulation and consequent thromboembolic phenomena. There are also more subtle reasons. If the coagulation cascade is not 'switched off' during CPB, coagulation factors are consumed, resulting in a deficiency in the postCPB period.[7] This can exacerbate postoperative bleeding and increase transfusion requirements. The use of exogenous

AT-III to facilitate complete anticoagulation during CPB has also been shown to produce less platelet activation, and better preservation of platelet function.[10] AT-III therapy, by decreasing heparin requirements in resistant patients, avoids the need for excessive doses of protamine to be administered.[14]

The use of fresh frozen plasma (FFP) or blood, which both contain AT-III, is one way to overcome heparin resistance.[15, 16] Specific AT-III preparations are now commercially available and provide a more logical choice to augment the efficacy of heparin, and have the advantage of immediate availability. Currently marketed preparations consist of dried human plasma fraction enriched with AT-III, which are reconstituted with water for injection. The preparation is derived from the plasma of multiple donors, and as for all blood-derived products, there is a possible risk of transmission of infective agents. The production process includes pasteurization which is effective in removing or inactivating both enveloped and non-enveloped viruses, including HIV.

The newest, and not yet commercially available, form of AT-III is a transgenically produced recombinant human AT-III (rhAT-III) which is currently undergoing phase III clinical trials to assess the effectiveness of rhAT-III in reducing FFP administration to restore heparin sensitivity in resistant patients undergoing elective heart surgery with CPB. Initial results indicate a statistically significant decrease in the dose of FFP required to achieve adequate anticoagulation for CPB. In addition, blood levels of AT-III were found to be increased to normal throughout CPB in patients receiving rhAT-III, unlike the patients who received placebo and FFP, in whom AT-III levels only reached 40% of normal values. A further finding was that fibrinolysis was inhibited to a significantly greater degree in patients receiving rhAT-III, although there appeared to be no difference in demonstrated thrombin activity between the two groups.

Recombinant human AT-III may in time prove to be the ideal therapy for managing heparin resistant patients. It appears to be both safe and effective in clinical trials, and has the potential for unlimited availability combined with the avoidance of use of donor blood products (Table 14.1). Where an excessive dose of heparin has been administered in an attempt to achieve safe prolon-

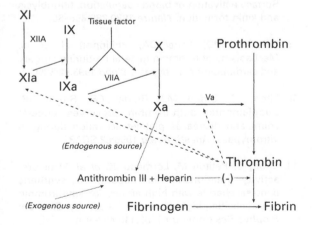

Figure 14.1

Interaction of heparin with antithrombin III on coagulation

Table 14.1 Advantages and disadvantages of the different sources of exogenous ATIII

ATIII Source	Efficacy	Cost	Infection risk	Immediate Availability	Unlimited Availability
Fresh frozen plasma	++	+	+	+	–
Blood	+	+	+	+	–
Dried human plasma fraction	+++	++	+++	++++	–
rhAT III	++++	++++	?/–	++++	++++

gation of the ACT for CPB, it is advisable to titrate the post-CPB protamine dose according to the residual heparin activity remaining after discontinuation of extracorporeal circulation. Providing that heparin activity is adequately reversed with protamine, administration of AT-III has not been shown to cause rebound anticoagulation.

Conclusions and learning points

- Heparin resistance is relatively common, particularly in patients receiving heparin for treatment of unstable angina.
- Heparin resistance can be usefully predicted on the grounds of clinical suspicion and calculating a heparin-dose response curve.
- A low blood level of AT-III is the commonest cause of heparin resistance.
- Exogenous AT-III can restore efficacy of heparin, manifested by an increase in ACT values.
- Detection and treatment of AT-III-mediated heparin resistance may be important with respect to preservation of coagulation factors and platelets, which may in turn reduce blood loss and limit transfusion requirements.
- Transgenically produced recombinant human AT-III may provide an unlimited, donor-free supply of AT-III.

References

1. Staples MH, Dunton RF, Karlson KJ et al. Heparin resistance after preoperative heparin therapy or intraaortic balloon pumping. Ann Thorac Surg 1994;**57**:1211–6.

2. Dietrich W, Spannagl M, Schramm W et al. The influence of preoperative anticoagulation on heparin response during cardiopulmonary bypass. J Thorac Cardiovasc Surg 1991;**102**:505–14.

3. Habbab MA, Haft JI. Heparin resistance induced by intravenous nitroglycerin. A word of caution when both drugs are used concomitantly. Arch Intern Med 1987;**147**:857–60.

4. Mummaneni N, Istanbouli M, Pifarre R, El-Etr AA. Increased heparin requirements with autotransfusion. J Thorac Cardiovasc Surg 1983;**86**:446–7.

5. Ranucci M, Isgro G, Cazzaniga A et al. Predictors for heparin resistance in patients undergoing coronary artery bypass grafting. Perfusion 1999;**14**:437–42.

6. Anderson EF. Heparin resistance prior to cardiopulmonary bypass. Anesthesiology 1986;**64**:504–7.

7. Despotis GJ, Levine V, Joist JH et al. Antithrombin III during cardiac surgery: effect on response of activated clotting time to heparin and relationship to markers of hemostatic activation. Anesth Analg 1997;**85**:498–506.

8. Heimark RL, Kurachi K, Fujikawa K, Davie EW. Surface activation of blood coagulation, fibrinolysis and kinin formation. Nature 1980;**286**:456–60.

9. Boisclair MD, Lane DA, Philippou H et al. Mechanisms of thrombin generation during surgery and cardiopulmonary bypass. Blood 1993;**82**:3350–7.

10. Fitch JC, Smith MJ, Rinder CS, Smith BR. Supplemental antithrombin preserves platelet count and decreases platelet activation during in vitro bypass. Anesth Analg 1996;**82**:SCA3.

11. Choay J, Petitou M, Lormeau JC et al. Structure-activity relationship in heparin: a synthetic pentasaccharide with high affinity for antithrombin III and eliciting high anti-factor Xa activity. Biochem Biophys Res Commun 1983;**116**:492–9.

12. Hirsch J, Raschke R, Warkentin TE et al. Heparin: mechanism of action, pharmacokinetics, dosing

considerations, monitoring, efficacy, and safety. *Chest* 1995;**108**:258S–60S.

13. Montes FR, Levy JH. Can we alter heparin dose-responses with antithrombin III? *Anesth Analg* 1996;**82**:SCA94.

14. Kanbak M. The treatment of heparin resistance with Antithrombin III in cardiac surgery. *Can J Anaesth* 1999;**46**:581–5.

15. Sabbagh AH, Chung GK, Shuttleworth P *et al.* Fresh frozen plasma: a solution to heparin resistance during cardiopulmonary bypass. *Ann Thorac Surg* 1984;**37**:466–8.

16. Barnette RE, Shupak RC, Pontius J, Rao AK. In vitro effect of fresh frozen plasma on the activated coagulation time in patients undergoing cardiopulmonary bypass. *Anesth Analg* 1988;**67**:57–60.

15
Heparin-associated thrombocytopenia and thrombosis

Gautam Sreeram, Ajeet D Sharma and Thomas F Slaughter

Introduction

Heparin-associated thrombocytopenia (HAT) comprises an immune-mediated syndrome of thrombocytopenia and/or thrombosis in a subset of patients exposed to heparin. Although the incidence of HAT in the general population is low, patients requiring cardiac surgery and cardiopulmonary bypass (CPB) may be at particular risk because of prior heparin exposure and the requirement for anticoagulation during the period of extracorporeal circulation.[1]

Case history

A 68-year-old male with a history of coronary artery disease presented with exertional angina and dyspnea. Two months earlier he had undergone percutaneous transluminal coronary angioplasty (PTCA) of the right coronary artery (RCA).

At that time, thrombocytopenia (platelet count 52×10^9 l^{-1}) developed 6 days after beginning heparin administration. Testing for heparin/platelet factor 4 (PF_4) antibodies by enzyme-linked immunosorbent assay (ELISA) was positive supporting a diagnosis of HAT. The thrombocytopenia resolved with heparin discontinuation, and the remainder of the patient's hospital course was unremarkable. The patient remained healthy until this current hospital admission for unstable angina.

Because of the recent history of HAT, repeat testing for heparin/PF_4 antibodies was performed after hospital admission. Both heparin/PF_4 ELISA and serotonin release assay (SRA) testing confirmed the presence of heparin-associated antibodies. Platelet aggregation testing with the heparinoid, danaparoid (Orgaran, Organon Inc; West Orange, NJ, USA), failed to induce platelet aggregation. Electrocardiogram (ECG) signs of ischemia resolved with administration of aspirin, atenolol, nitroglycerin, and oxygen. However, the patient continued to experience exertional

Past medical history	Hypertension. Hypercholesterolemia. Esophageal reflux. Ischemic heart disease. Previous PTCA of RCA. Heparin-associated thrombocytopenia.
Regular medications	Isosorbide mononitrate SR 120 mg OD, glyceryl trinitrate 0.5 mg PRN, omeprazole 20 mg OD, metoprolol 25 mg OD. No known drug allergies.
Examination	Weight 90 kg. Height 1.7 m. BMI 31 kg.m^{-2}. Alert and orientated. Pulse 70 regular. BP 114/64. Chest clear to auscultation. No murmurs, rubs or gallops.
Investigations	Hb 14 g dl^{-1}, platelets 220×10^9 l^{-1}, creatinine 0.8 mg dl^{-1} (71 µmol l^{-1}). **CXR:** Unremarkable. **ECG:** Sinus rhythm with ST elevation in leads II, III and aVF. **Coronary angiography:** 75% stenosis of left main and right coronary arteries with 95% stenosis of proximal circumflex and obtuse marginal coronary arteries.

angina. Following coronary angiography and surgical consultation, the patient was scheduled for coronary artery bypass graft (CABG) surgery.

In addition to routine monitoring, both an arterial and pulmonary artery catheter were inserted under local anesthesia prior to the induction of anesthesia. No heparin was added to the vascular catheter flush solutions, and a pulmonary artery catheter with no heparin bonding was selected.

Because of the presence of heparin-associated antibodies, danaparoid was selected as the alternative anticoagulant for CPB. A bolus dose of danaparoid 11 250 units (125 u kg^{-1}) prior to CPB resulted in an anti-Xa concentration of 0.80 u ml^{-1}. Danaparoid was added to the CPB prime to a final concentration of 2 u ml^{-1}. A danaparoid infusion of 630 u hour^{-1} (7 u kg^{-1} hour^{-1}) was maintained during CPB. Anti-Xa concentration achieved during CPB approximated 1.2 u ml^{-1}. After initiating CPB, no overt clot formation was evident. Surgery proceeded uneventfully and three coronary artery bypass grafts were completed. Approximately 45 minutes before completion of surgical revascularization, the danaparoid infusion was discontinued. The patient was separated uneventfully from CPB after a total time of 90 minutes. Clot formation was apparent in the surgical field approximately 20 minutes after completion of CPB. Laboratory investigation of blood drawn immediately after CPB revealed a hemoglobin concentration of 9 g dl^{-1} and a platelet count of 140 × 10^9 l^{-1}.

Chest tube drainage postoperatively necessitated the transfusion of packed red blood cells. The patient remained in the ICU overnight and was transferred to the floor the following day.

On the first postoperative day, aspirin therapy was begun at a dose of 325 mg day^{-1}. Daily platelet counts were performed. On the fifth postoperative day, the platelet count remained stable with no symptoms or signs suggestive of a thrombotic complication. The patient was discharged home on the eighth postoperative day.

Discussion

Heparin-associated thrombocytopenia has been reported in approximately 3% of patients after heparin exposure. The prevalence of heparin-associated antibodies may be even greater in patients requiring cardiac surgery.[2] Two 'types' of HAT have been reported in the literature. Type I HAT, which generally resolves spontaneously, is typically associated with an early onset (1–2 days after heparin administration) and mild thrombocytopenia (platelet counts >100 × 10^9 l^{-1}). In contrast, type II HAT, which generally persists until heparin discontinuation, is typically associated with a delayed onset (5–15 days after heparin administration), severe thrombocytopenia (platelet counts <100 × 10^9 l^{-1}), and the potential for thrombotic complications. Whether types I and II HAT represent different pathophysiologic processes or merely gradations of the same process remains unclear.

Substantial evidence suggests that type II HAT results from an immune-mediated process. Recent findings suggest that autoantibodies generated against heparin/PF$_4$ complexes mediate the pathophysiologic effects of HAT. Heparin/PF$_4$ complexes bind to and activate platelets by way of platelet FcγRII receptors.[3] These antibodies also may bind to complexes on the vascular endothelium, composed of heparin-like proteins and PF$_4$, resulting in 'activation' of endothelial cells and expression of tissue factor.[4]

The diagnosis of HAT is usually first entertained after the appearance of thrombocytopenia during heparin therapy. Although thrombocytopenia typically develops 5–8 days after initiation of heparin therapy, patients with prior heparin exposure may develop thrombocytopenia within 1–2 days of heparin re-exposure.[5] Occasionally, thrombosis occurs concurrently with the onset of thrombocytopenia. Thrombosis of both arterial and venous systems have been described in the setting of HAT.

The laboratory diagnosis of HAT has traditionally relied on platelet aggregation-based assays; however, immunoassays may provide a simpler alternative. Platelet aggregation-based assays include the ^{14}C-SRA and a heparin-induced platelet-aggregation (HIPA) assay. The ^{14}C-SRA has been considered the 'gold standard' diagnostic test for HAT. In the SRA, serum from a suspect patient is incubated with platelets containing [14]C. Known concentrations of heparin are added to the reaction mixture. In the presence of heparin-associated antibodies, the platelets are activated releasing radioactive ^{14}C into the supernatant, which can be measured.

The specialized skills necessary to perform this assay, limit its use to research settings. Although somewhat less sensitive, the HIPA assay offers a non-radioactive and less technically demanding method for diagnosis of heparin-associated antibodies. In this technique, platelet aggregatory response is measured using donor platelets incubated with a patient's serum and known concentrations of heparin. The HIPA method offers acceptable sensitivity and specificity for detection of heparin-associated antibodies, but requires extremely careful attention to selection of donor platelets and assay conditions. Most recently, ELISA-based assays for the quantification of heparin/PF_4 complexes have demonstrated substantial sensitivity and specificity, exceeding 90%, to detect heparin-associated antibodies.[3] Given that no single assay is 100% sensitive and specific, both aggregation and ELISA-based methods may be needed to definitively exclude the diagnosis of HAT.[3]

The patient with pre-existing HAT requiring cardiac surgery presents a particular challenge for perioperative management of anticoagulation. Administration of heparin, in the setting of HAT, may pose a substantial risk for the patient. Several alternative strategies have been successfully employed to manage these patients during cardiac surgery with CPB. These include: (1) delay surgery until the heparin-associated antibodies are no longer present in serum concentrations adequate to induce platelet aggregation in response to heparin; (2) administer platelet inhibitors (i.e. aspirin or prostacyclin) in addition to heparin; or (3) replace heparin with an alternative anticoagulant.[1] Each of these alternatives has inherent risks and limitations. Regardless of the approach chosen, it is critical to eliminate or minimize any perioperative heparin exposure.

In vitro testing of patient serum has demonstrated heparin-induced platelet aggregation months, and even years, after an episode of HAT.[6] Consequently, many patients cannot delay surgery until heparin-associated antibodies are cleared from the circulation. While plasmapheresis may accelerate elimination of heparin-associated antibodies, the need for exchange transfusions with fresh frozen plasma make this option less than ideal. Furthermore, the response of patients to recurrent heparin exposure after plasmapheresis remains unknown.[1]

Successful administration of heparin to patients with HAT after pretreatment with platelet-inhibiting drugs has been described. Antiplatelet drugs used in this setting include aspirin, dipyridamole, and the prostanoid inhibitor iloprost. Unfortunately, neither aspirin nor dipyridamole reliably inhibit platelet aggregation in the setting of heparin-associated antibodies. Iloprost has been administered successfully as a continuous infusion in patients receiving a full dose of unfractionated heparin prior to CPB. However, vasodilatory effects of iloprost may require a vasoconstrictor infusion to alleviate systemic hypotension.

Alternative anticoagulants offer a third approach to management of the patient requiring anticoagulation for CPB. Direct thrombin inhibitors administered in the setting of HAT include recombinant hirudin and argatroban. In addition, the heparinoid, danaparoid, has been successfully administered in this setting. To date, the majority of clinical experience with alternative anticoagulants during CPB has been attributable to recombinant hirudin and danaparoid.

Hirudin, derived from leech salivary gland extract, specifically binds and inhibits thrombin's proteolytic activity. Advantages of this drug include the lack of cross-reactivity with heparin-associated antibodies and a relatively short elimination half-life of 30–60 minutes.[7] Disadvantages of hirudin include dependence on renal function for elimination. Point-of-care monitoring of hirudin concentration with the ecarin clotting time (ECT) has been reported; however, this test is not yet widely available. An ECT >400 s has been reported to correspond with recombinant hirudin concentrations, in citrate-containing whole blood, greater than 4 µg ml^{-1}.[7] Successful anticoagulation during CPB has been reported by maintaining recombinant hirudin concentrations of 3-4 µg ml^{-1} (ECT: 350–400 s).[8]

Another alternative to heparin is danaparoid. This drug is a porcine mucosal extract — a heparinoid comprised of heparan, dermatan, and chondroitin sulfates.[9] The anticoagulant effect of danaparoid is primarily mediated by factor Xa inhibition with a lesser inhibitory effect on thrombin. The optimal dosing regimen for danaparoid in the setting of CPB remains unclear. One strategy, successfully used in adults, has been reported to include an initial

125 u kg^{-1} bolus with an additional 2 u ml^{-1} added to the CPB priming solution. Once CPB begins, a continuous infusion of 7 u kg^{-1} hr^{-1} is maintained until approximately 45 minutes before termination of CPB.[10] Disadvantages of danaparoid include a 10% cross-reactivity with heparin/ PF$_4$ antibodies, although this compares favorably with low molecular weight heparins which have 90% cross-reactivity. The potential for danaparoid to induce platelet aggregation in HAT must be tested in vitro before administration of the drug in a clinical setting. In addition, because of anti-Xa activity, traditional methods for measurement of surgical anticoagulation, such as the activated clotting time (ACT) and activated partial thromboplastin time (APTT), are unreliable. Anti-factor Xa measurements are necessary to monitor danaparoid therapy during CPB.[11] Unfortunately, at present, the time to obtain laboratory-based anti-Xa measurements may exceed 1 hour in many institutions — making intraoperative dosing adjustments difficult. As with hirudin, no effective means of reversing the activity of danaparoid is available.

Regardless of the method chosen to provide anticoagulation for cardiac surgery, all unnecessary perioperative heparin exposure should be avoided (i.e. heparin-bonded catheters and heparin in flush solutions), antiplatelet therapies should be reinstituted as soon as possible after surgery, and daily platelet counts should be monitored until resolution of the thrombocytopenia.

Conclusions and learning points

- Heparin-associated thrombocytopenia occurs in 1–3% of patients after heparin exposure but may be more prevalent in cardiac surgical patients.
- Heparin-associated thrombocytopenia (HAT), an immune-mediated process, typically causes severe thrombocytopenia which persists until heparin is discontinued.
- HAT may be accompanied by thrombotic complications.
- Alternative anticoagulants for patients with HAT undergoing CPB include either direct thrombin inhibitors (i.e. hirudin or argatroban) or a heparinoid (i.e. danaparoid).

- Treatment failures during CPB may result in intraoperative thromboses and/or excessive postoperative bleeding.

References

1. Slaughter TF, Greenberg CS. Heparin-associated thrombocytopenia and thrombosis: implications for perioperative management. *Anesthesiology* 1997;**87**:667–75.

2. Bauer TL, Arepally G, Konkle BA *et al.* Prevalence of heparin-associated antibodies without thrombosis in patients undergoing cardiopulmonary bypass surgery. *Circulation* 1997;**95**:1242–6.

3. Chong BH, Eisbacher M. Pathophysiology and laboratory testing of heparin-induced thrombocytopenia. *Semin Hematol* 1998;**35**:3–8.

4. Cines DB, Tomaski A, Tannenbaum S. Immune endothelial-cell injury in heparin-associated thrombocytopenia. *N Engl J Med* 1987;**316**:581–9.

5. Warkentin TE. Clinical presentation of heparin-induced thrombocytopenia. *Semin Hematol* 1998;**35**:9–16.

6. Kapsch DN, Adelstein EH, Rhodes GR, Silver D. Heparin-induced thrombocytopenia, thrombosis, and hemorrhage. *Surgery* 1979;**86**:148–55.

7. Koster A, Kuppe H, Hetzer R *et al.* Emergent cardiopulmonary bypass in five patients with heparin-induced thrombocytopenia type II employing recombinant hirudin. *Anesthesiology* 1998;**89**:777–80.

8. Bauer M, Koster A, Pasic M *et al.* Recombinant hirudin for extended aortic surgery in patients with heparin-induced thrombocytopenia. *J Thorac Cardiovasc Surg* 1999;**118**:191–2.

9. Meuleman DG. Orgaran (Org 10172): its pharmacological profile in experimental models. *Haemostasis* 1992;**22**:58–65.

10. Ortel TL, Chong BH. New treatment options for heparin-induced thrombocytopenia. *Semin Hematol* 1998;**35**:26–34.

11. Gitlin SD, Deeb GM, Yann C, Schmaier AH. Intraoperative monitoring of danaparoid sodium anticoagulation during cardiovascular operations. *J Vasc Surg* 1998;**27**:568–75.

16
Management of bleeding following cardiac surgery: the thrombelastographic approach

Alan M Cohen and Sally Tomkins

Introduction

Postoperative bleeding is a major cause of morbidity following cardiac surgery. Preoperative medication, intraoperative anticoagulation and reversal, cardiotomy suction, and not least cardiopulmonary bypass (CPB) can all cause derangements of haemostasis, most commonly platelet dysfunction, although inadequate reversal of heparin and, less frequently, fibrinolysis may also be important.[1] These effects are rarely detectable using commonly available laboratory tests, so that the traditional approach to the patient who is bleeding following cardiac surgery involves the use of empirically administered blood products. Such an approach is inappropriate in many patients resulting not only in unnecessary exposure to the undesirable effects of blood component therapy but also delayed management of the other main cause of bleeding, namely inadequate surgical haemostasis. The use of thrombelastography (TEG) offers a rational means of avoiding such an empirical approach.

Case history 1

A 66-year-old Caucasian female with a history of two myocardial infarctions 10 years previously, followed by stable (CCS class II/III) angina, presented with unstable (CCS class IV) angina and dyspnoea (NYHA class IV). Coronary angio-graphy and ventriculography revealed severe coronary artery disease and impaired left ventricular function. Shortly after angiography the patient's symptoms deteriorated further and she was therefore treated with enoxaparin pending urgent coronary artery bypass surgery.

Surgery was carried out 9 days after admission. The patient was premedicated with oral lorazepam 3 mg. Intravenous access and invasive arterial monitoring were established under local anaesthesia and the patient was subsequently anaesthetized using fentanyl 0.5 mg, etomidate 14 mg and midazolam 4 mg, with pancuronium 10 mg to obtain neuromuscular blockade. Following tracheal intubation, the lungs were ventilated with a mixture of oxygen (FiO_2 0.5), air and isoflurane 0.5%. Anesthesia was supplemented with propofol 4 mg kg^{-1} h^{-1} and incremental doses of fentanyl. A quadruple-lumen catheter was inserted into the right internal jugular vein for measurement of central venous pressure and administration of vasoactive drugs. During the period before CPB, tranexamic acid 2 g was given, as well as a glucose–insulin–potassium infusion. The left internal mammary artery, left radial artery and left long saphenous vein were harvested and anticoagulation was subsequently obtained using heparin 300 iu kg^{-1}, resulting in a celite activated clotting time (ACT) of 574 seconds.

Cardiopulmonary bypass was instituted between the right atrium and aortic root using a roller pump and membrane oxygenator, with a crystalloid prime that included heparin 5 000 iu

Past medical history	Myocardial infarctions (×2) 10 years earlier, hypertension, ex-smoker.
Regular medications	Aspirin 75 mg BD, enoxaparin 20 mg (SC) BD (both stopped 1 day prior to surgery), atenolol 25 mg OD, lisinopril 10 mg OD, atorvastatin 10 mg OD, isosorbide dinitrate SR 60 mg BD, bumetanide 1 mg OD, amlodipine 5 mg OD.
Examination	Weight 62 kg. BP 130/70. Bilateral basal inspiratory crackles. Otherwise unremarkable.
Investigations	Hb 12.3 g dl^{-1}, WBC 5.3 × 10^9 l^{-1}, platelets 204 × 10^9 l^{-1}. PT 13 s (INR 1.0), APTT 25.2 s (APTT ratio 0.78), fibrinogen 5.09 g l^{-1}. [Na$^+$] 130 mmol l^{-1}, [K$^+$] 5.6 mmol l^{-1}, urea 14.7 mmol l^{-1}, creatinine 1.8 mg dl^{-1} (162 μmol l^{-1}), glucose 99 mg dl^{-1} (5.5 mmol l^{-1}), bilirubin 0.6 mg dl^{-1} (11 μmol l^{-1}), aspartate transaminase 14 u.l^{-1}, alkaline phosphatase 72 u l^{-1}, total protein 71 g l^{-1}, albumin 46 g l^{-1}, globulin 25 g l^{-1}. **ECG:** Sinus rhythm, T wave inversion in lead V$_1$ to V$_4$. **Cardiac catheterization:** Severe triple vessel coronary artery disease. Anterior hypokinesia. LVEF 40%.

and tranexamic acid 2 g. Nasopharyngeal temperature was maintained at 34°C until the latter stages of the CPB period. Warm, blood-based antegrade cardioplegia was used for myocardial protection during the period of aortic cross-clamping while bypass grafts were anastomosed to the left anterior descending, first obtuse marginal, and the posterior descending coronary arteries. Following aortic declamping, enoximone 25 mg and triiodothyronine (T$_3$) 40 μg were administered in preparation for separation from CPB and dopamine 4 μg.kg^{-1} min^{-1} and noradrenaline 0.05 μg.kg^{-1} min^{-1} infusions commenced. Subsequent weaning from CPB was uneventful. Total CPB duration was 82 minutes. No additional heparin was given during CPB and the ACT prior to separation from CPB was 615 seconds. Protamine 200 mg was administered and, following routine surgical attention to haemostasis, the chest was closed uneventfully and no problems in relation to bleeding were noted at this stage. The extracorporeal circuit was drained of blood, which was reinfused to the patient. No further protamine was administered.

On arrival in the intensive care unit the patient was haemodynamically stable (BP 100/60) and normothermic. The haematocrit was 28.4%. Drainage from the chest tubes over the next 3 hours was 125 ml, 150 ml and 200 ml. Thrombelastography was performed at this stage and the trace is shown in Figure 16.1. The drainage over the next hour was 275 ml and it was therefore

decided to transfer the patient back to the operating theatre for re-exploration. At this stage, having received 4% succinylated gelatin (Gelofusine®, Braun; Melsungen, Germany) 1000 ml and 2 units of packed red cells, the haematocrit had fallen to 21.4%.

On re-exploration, profuse bleeding was noted from the right atrial cannulation site, though the remainder of the operative field was dry in appearance. The bleeding source was oversewn and the patient was returned to the ICU. Her further course was uneventful with no further significant chest tube drainage. Neither platelets nor fresh frozen plasma were given at any stage.

Case history 2

A 72-year-old female presented with chest pain. She had a long history of stable angina that had deteriorated suddenly, requiring admission to hospital. She was treated with streptokinase, but nevertheless sustained a full thickness inferior myocardial infarction and continued to suffer occasional chest pain with ST depression. Coronary angiography and ventriculography revealed significant left main stem stenosis, severe triple vessel coronary artery disease and moderately impaired left ventricular function. She was therefore scheduled for urgent coronary artery bypass surgery, which she underwent 16 days following angiography.

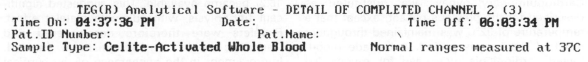

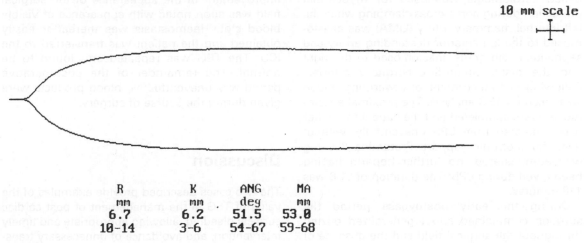

Figure 16.1

TEG from patient 1. See text and Figure 16.4 for explanation of the various TEG parameters. The normal ranges are shown below each individual parameter. Although the MA is less than the lower limit of the 'normal' range seen in non-surgical patients, this is acceptable coagulation following cardiac surgery.

Past medical history	Hypertension. Non-smoker.
Regular medications	Aspirin 75 mg OD (stopped 1 day before surgery), lansoprazole 30 mg OD, frusemide 40 mg BD, isosorbide mononitrate 20 mg BD, perindopril 2 mg OD, atenolol 12.5 mg OD.
Examination	Weight 67 kg. BP 100/60. Dependent ankle oedema.
Investigations	Hb 10.6 g dl^{-1}, WBC 4.7 × 10^9 l^{-1}, platelets 241 × 10^9 l^{-1}. INR 1.0, APTT ratio 1.2, fibrinogen 4.1 g l^{-1}. [Na$^+$] 132 mmol l^{-1}, [K$^+$] 3.1 mmol l^{-1}, urea 6.1 mmol l^{-1}, creatinine 0.9 mg dl^{-1} (85 μmol l^{-1}). Liver function tests — normal. **ECG:** Sinus rhythm, Q-waves and-T wave inversion in inferior leads. **Cardiac catheterization:** Left main stenosis. Severe triple vessel coronary artery disease. Inferior hypokinesia. LVEF 40%.

The patient was premedicated with oral lorazepam 3 mg. Intravenous access and invasive arterial monitoring were established under local anaesthesia and the patient was subsequently anaesthetized with fentanyl 1 mg and propofol 40 mg. Neuromuscular blockade was obtained with pancuronium 10 mg. Following tracheal intubation, the lungs were ventilated with a mixture of oxygen (FiO$_2$ 0.5), nitrous oxide and isoflurane 0.3%. Anaesthesia was maintained with propofol 3 mg kg^{-1} hour^{-1}. Administration of heparin 300 iu kg^{-1} resulted in an ACT of 441 seconds.

Cardiopulmonary bypass was instituted as described for the previous patient, except that a temperature of 32°C was maintained throughout most of the bypass period. Antegrade blood-based cardioplegia was used for myocardial protection during aortic cross-clamping while the left internal mammary artery (LIMA) was anastomosed to the left anterior descending artery and saphenous vein grafts anastomosed to the right and the distal circumflex coronary arteries. Following commencement of rewarming, blood was taken for TEG analysis. The proximal anastomoses were completed and the patient thereafter was separated from CPB uneventfully, without need for inotropic support. Protamine 200 mg was administered, no further heparin having been given during CPB. The duration of CPB was 118 minutes.

During the early postbypass period the surgeon complained about generalized oozing throughout the surgical field and the absence of visible blood clot and requested further protamine to be given and, in view of the recent aspirin therapy, platelets to be ordered. However, at this stage the completed TEG trace (Figure 16.2) became available. This suggested significant fibrinolysis, with adequate platelet effect. Platelets were therefore not ordered and traneamic acid 2 g administered instead. Improvement in the appearance of the surgical field was soon noted with appearance of visible blood clot. Haemostasis was thereafter easily obtained and the patient was transferred to the ICU. The TEG was repeated and found to be normal. The remainder of the postoperative period was uneventful. No blood products were given during the course of surgery.

Discussion

The two cases described provide examples of the value of TEG in the management of post cardiac surgical bleeding, allowing appropriate and timely intervention, and avoidance of unnecessary transfusion of blood products. Thrombelastography is not, however, a new test, having been developed over 50 years ago.[2] For 35 years it remained primarily a research tool, until the development of

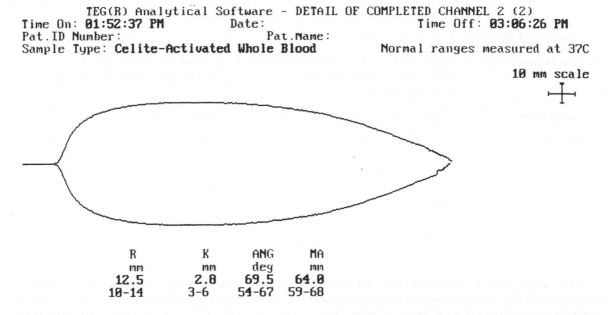

TEG(R) Analytical Software – DETAIL OF COMPLETED CHANNEL 2 (2)

Time On: **01:52:37 PM**   Date: Time Off: **03:06:26 PM**
Pat.ID Number: Pat.Name:
Sample Type: **Celite-Activated Whole Blood**   Normal ranges measured at 37C

10 mm scale

R mm	K mm	ANG deg	MA mm
12.5	2.8	69.5	64.0
10–14	3–6	54–67	59–68

Figure 16.2

TEG from patient 2. Significant fibrinolysis is clearly evident. The relevant TEG parameter, the LY30 was 9.5% (upper limit of normal 7.5%).

liver transplantation in the early 1980s provided the need for a test that could provide rapid, 'point of care' information about the major and complex hemostatic changes occurring during such surgery.[3] Spiess and co-workers subsequently assessed the applicability of TEG to the less severe perturbations of hemostasis found in cardiac surgical patients and showed that TEG predicted postoperative bleeding with considerably greater sensitivity and specificity than commonly available laboratory tests of coagulation.[4] Subsequent increase in use of the TEG was aided by development of the currently used computerized display (with automated measurement of TEG parameters), which replaced the pen recorder output system and simplified interpretation. Further refinements in the mid-1990s included the celite activated TEG and the heparinase TEG (see below).

In 1999, Shore-Lesserson and co-workers reported the first prospective randomized comparison of TEG-based management versus management based on traditional coagulation tests, in cardiac surgical patients assessed as being at moderate to high risk of transfusion.[5] In the traditional group, 30% of patients received platelets and 32% received fresh frozen plasma (FFP), whereas in the TEG group 14% received platelets and 8% received FFP, with no difference between the groups in chest tube drainage. Similar results were reported from the UK by von Kier and Royston.[6] Throughout this period of TEG development, concerns with transfusion-related viral transmission — retroviruses in particular — provided further stimulus to the uptake of the technique, especially in the United States. In the United Kingdom, concern about the possibility of transmission of new variant Creutzfeld–Jacob disease[7] led to the requirement for all blood products to be leucodepleted. The significant increase in the cost of the blood supply that this has caused has prompted a surge of interest in TEG as a means of reducing transfusion-related expenses.

The principles of TEG (Haemoscope Corp; Skokie, Illinois, USA) are shown in Figure 16.3.

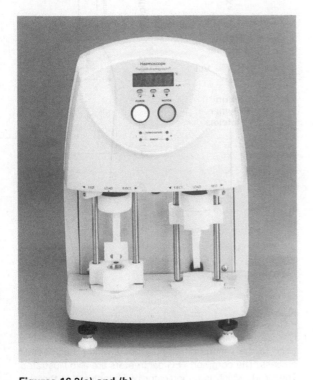

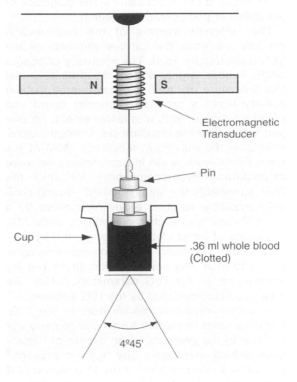

Figures 16.3(a) and (b)

(a) Photo of the TEG machine
(b) Diagram of the cup, pin and transducer

Whole blood is placed in a cuvette into which a piston is suspended and the cuvette is rotated back and forth, the temperature of the cuvette being maintained at 37°C. At first the piston remains motionless, until blood clot starts to form allowing the rotational movement of the cuvette to be transferred to the piston. As the clot strengthens the rotation of the piston increases and the resulting changes in torsion of the suspending wire are transduced and displayed graphically against time that, in the normal state, results in a characteristic 'cigar' shaped trace. In this way the TEG measures the kinetics of clot formation, as well as the strength and stability of the final clot.[8] The test, as currently performed, uses the addition of celite as an activating substance enhancing the rate of reaction. Although a completed TEG takes about an hour to perform, the majority of useful information is actually available within the first 15 minutes. The results of TEG are therefore, more rapidly available than those of traditional tests of coagulation, apart from the ACT, which although more rapid, is of limited value in the diagnosis of the cause of postoperative bleeding.

The different aspects of the haemostatic process influence the various elements of the TEG trace (Figure 16.4). The adequacy of coagulation factors largely affects the time to initial clot formation (R time), whereas overall platelet activity (itself a product of platelet count and platelet function) and, to a lesser extent, fibrinogen level affect the resultant clot strength, represented as the maximum amplitude (MA) of the trace. Fibrinolysis results in a subsequent decrease in amplitude. Hypercoagulability, for which the TEG is probably the 'gold standard' among clinically available tests, is easily recognised by a short R time and a characteristically wide MA. Diagnosis of gross clotting derangements therefore is largely a matter of simple pattern recognition, although less severe disturbances require assessment of the TEG parameters, which are measured automatically by the TEG software.

A further important modification of the TEG, routinely used in cardiac surgery, is to carry out the test in the presence of an excess of heparinase, which inactivates any heparin present.[9] This allows interpretation of the TEG during CPB or any other periods of intended heparinization, so that any problems with haemostasis, separate from heparin effect, can be identified well in advance of reversal with protamine and, if necessary, the need for additional therapy to be anticipated. Furthermore, following protamine administration, a 'plain' TEG and a heparinase TEG can be run concurrently from the same sample. Abnormalities seen in the 'plain' TEG (most notably prolongation of the R time) and not the heparinase-TEG, indicate the presence of unneutralised heparin and the need for further protamine. This is particularly useful in cases of heparin resistance — where calculation of the protamine dose required may be difficult — and when heparin 'rebound' is suspected.

An important principle of TEG interpretation is that a normal trace virtually eliminates the possibility of significant haemostatic abnormality.[10]

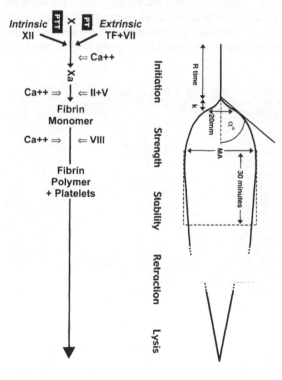

Figure 16.4

Diagram showing relationship of the elements of the TEG trace to the various different aspects of the haemostatic process. The common TEG parameters are also illustrated. The LY30, which is an indicator of fibrinolysis, is the area (shaded) outside the TEG trace in the 30 minutes following the MA, expressed as a percentage of the total area bounded by the dotted lines.

Under such circumstances, any clinically significant bleeding must, as demonstrated in the first case, be due to surgical causes. Without the aid of TEG it is likely that preoperative enoxaparin and aspirin, and the presence of heparin in the blood salvaged from the extracorporeal circuit, would have been implicated as the cause of postoperative bleeding. This would have undoubtedly prompted initial treatment with additional protamine, platelets and possibly FFP, with surgical re-exploration being considered only once these measures had been implemented (unless haemodynamic instability had developed in the interim). The hazards of such unnecessary transfusion are worth considering. The risks of viral transmission[11] or immunological reactions[12] are well known. Other hazards such as volume overload, haemodilution, hypothermia, and possibly increased risk of postoperative wound infection[13] and pulmonary infection[14] are less widely publicized, but may be no less important, particularly in higher risk patients. To these must be added the expense and scarcity of blood products, as well as the advantages of more expedient management, benefiting the patient, their family and, not least, the organization of the surgical service.

In patients with non-surgical bleeding, the abnormal TEG result allows appropriately targeted intervention, which results in avoidance of the transfusion related hazards described above. TEG abnormalities associated with cardiac surgery include; presence of heparin effect, seen as prolongation of the R time in the plain TEG compared to a concurrent heparinase TEG; and platelet dysfunction, represented by a low MA (less than 50 mm for a celite activated sample). Excessive fibrinolysis, as seen in the second case, is less commonly seen, but is an important cause of bleeding when it occurs. Interestingly, the patient described had received prior thrombolytic therapy, although the interval between thrombolysis and surgery would suggest that this was probably coincidental. In this patient, as in the previous case, the administration of aspirin up until the day of surgery would probably have been considered more relevant, prompting the administration of a platelet transfusion. Likewise, the request to administer additional protamine would also have been inappropriate. Although the use of additional doses of protamine appears to be commonplace and, in most cases, fairly innocuous, its adverse effects on platelet function are becoming more greatly appreciated[15] and it is preferable to avoid significant excesses of the drug. The abnormal TEG trace can therefore be used to guide appropriate therapy, although the general principle of treating the patient and not the test is as relevant to the TEG as to any laboratory investigation. Thus, transfusion should be withheld in a patient who is not bleeding, despite an abnormal TEG.

Although a TEG service has the potential for a unit to make significant savings in its blood product budget, the introduction of the test requires investment in several areas. In addition to the capital investment in the TEG hardware, there are organizational issues relating to training, operation and maintenance of the service, which must include a rigorous quality control programme. Most important however, is the change in attitude required of clinicians who may have used the empirical approach for many years. Some may find it difficult, at first, to put their faith in a test that is both new (to them) and different. For example, in the case of a patient with moderate postoperative haemorrhage and a normal TEG, they may wish to resort to the empirical approach, with reliance on the 'tried and trusted' INR and APTT. However, both the INR and APTT are known to be poor predictors of post-bypass bleeding, with a false positive rate of about 50%.[4] Since these tests are plasma based, they cannot possibly take into account the effect of the platelet surface, which is important in modulating reactions of the coagulation cascade in vivo. It is not surprising therefore that such tests give results which are both at variance with the clinical situation and a whole blood test such as the TEG, in which the platelet surface is present. Compliance with TEG-based management is aided by the use of guidelines, both for deciding when to use the test and in the resultant choice of treatment (Table 16.1). Guidelines allow the new user to become comfortable with the test and to accept its superiority over the empirical approach. Such guidelines will vary according to local factors, such as the delay or otherwise of obtaining blood products.

Future developments in TEG include the extension of the test to other perioperative areas. Addition of the powerful anti-platelet drug

Table 16.1 Treatment guidelines used at the Bristol Royal Infirmary, for Celite activated TEGs (modified from similar guidelines used by Harefield Hospital, UK)

Systematic TEG interpretation requires assessment of **R time** (compared between heparinase and non-heparinase traces) and **MA**. Fibrinolysis is assessed using the **LY30**, though is usually clear from inspection of the trace.

TEG values	Clinical cause	Treatment
Normal TEG	Any excess bleeding is 'surgical'	Re-exploration if necessary
Abnormal TEG		
R time (non-heparinase) greater than 1.5 × R time (heparinase)	Heparin present	Protamine (50 –100mg)
R time (heparinase) greater than 20mm?	↓ ↓ Clotting factors	R time 21 – 28: 2 units FFP
		R time > 28: 4 units FFP
MA less than 48mm?	↓ Platelet activity, or hypofibrinogenemia	Platelets (Cryoprecipitate, if low fibrinogen)
LY30 greater than 7.5%	Fibrinolysis	Tranexamic acid, 2g IV (over 2 min)

abciximab allows separate assessments of platelet and fibrinogen activities, and may become more frequently performed.[16] Addition of tissue factor is a particularly important development as it permits the assessment of fibrinolysis within minutes. This may have a great impact on the provision of a TEG service.[17] Finally, the use of TEG as a tool to assess hypercoagulability may allow an assessment of the importance of postoperative hypercoagulability in the development of postoperative thrombotic complications.

Learning points

- The TEG is a whole blood test, which simply measures the strength of the developing blood clot.
- Advantages of the TEG are that it is quick, can be carried out at the 'point of care' and assesses multiple aspects of haemostasis, including interactions between the various haemostatic components.
- The TEG provides information on fibrinolysis, residual heparinization, and hypercoagulability, which are not usually available from commonly available laboratory tests.
- The most important parameters of the TEG trace are the reaction (R) time, which is primarily dependent on the adequacy of the coagulation cascade, and the maximum amplitude (MA), which is mainly dependent

on overall platelet activity (including function).
- Modification of the TEG with added heparinase is extremely sensitive for the detection of residual heparinization.
- TEG-based management in cardiac surgery has been shown to reduce transfusion of blood products, compared to the empirical approach using commonly available laboratory based test, thereby reducing the multiple potential side effects of exposure.

Thromboelastograph and TEG are registered trademarks of Haemoscope Corporation, Skokie, Illinois, USA.

References

1. Body SC, Morse DS. Coagulation, transfusion and cardiac surgery. In: Spiess BD, Counts RB, Gould SA (eds) *Perioperative transfusion medicine*. Baltimore: Williams & Wilkins, 1998;419–460.

2. Hartert H. Blutgerinnungstudien mit der Thrombelastographic, einen neuen Untersuchungsverfahren. *Klin Wochenschr* 1948;**26**:577–83.

3. Kang YG, Martin DJ, Marquez J *et al*. Intraoperative changes in blood coagulation and thrombelastographic monitoring in liver transplantation. *Anesth Analg* 1985;**64**:888–96.

4. Spiess BD, Tuman KJ, McCarthy RJ *et al*. Thromboelastography as an indicator of post-

cardiopulmonary bypass coagulopathies. *J Clin Monit* 1987;**3**:25–30.

5. Shore-Lesserson L, Manspeizer HE, DePerio M *et al.* Thromboelastography-guided transfusion algorithm reduces transfusions in complex cardiac surgery. *Anesth Analg* 1999;**88**:312–9.

6. Von Kier S, Royston D. Reduced hemostatic factor transfusion using heparinase-modified thrombelastography (TEG) during cardiopulmonary bypass (CPB). *Anesthesiology* 1998;**89**:A911.

7. Seghatchian J. nvCJD and leucodepletion: an overview. *Transfus Sci* 2000;**22**:47-8.

8. Mallett SV, Cox DJ. Thrombelastography. *Br J Anaesth* 1992;**69**:307–13.

9. Tuman KJ, McCarthy RJ, Djuric M *et al.* Evaluation of coagulation during cardiopulmonary bypass with a heparinase-modified thromboelastographic assay. *J Cardiothorac Vasc Anesth* 1994;**8**:144–9.

10. Whalen J, Tuman KJ. Monitoring hemostasis. *Int Anesthesiol Clin* 1996;**34**:195–213.

11. Warner MA. Infectious risks of transfusion. In: Spiess BD, Counts RB, Gould SA (eds) *Perioperative transfusion medicine*. Baltimore: Williams & Wilkins, 1998; 97–110.

12. Petz LD. The surgeon and the transfusion service: essentials of compatibility testing, surgical blood ordering, emergency blood needs, and adverse reactions. In: Spiess BD, Counts RB, Gould SA (eds) *Perioperative transfusion medicine*. Baltimore: Williams & Wilkins, 1998;45–60.

13. Carson JL, Altman DG, Duff A *et al.* Risk of bacterial infection associated with allogeneic blood transfusion among patients undergoing hip fracture repair. *Transfusion* 1999;**39**:694–700.

14. Vamvakas EC, Carven JH. Transfusion and postoperative pneumonia in coronary artery bypass graft surgery: effect of the length of storage of transfused red cells. *Transfusion* 1999;**39**:701–10.

15. Ammar T, Fisher CF. The effects of heparinase 1 and protamine on platelet reactivity. *Anesthesiology* 1997;**86**:1382–6.

16. Kettner SC, Panzer OP, Kozek SA *et al.* Use of abciximab-modified thrombelastography in patients undergoing cardiac surgery. *Anesth Analg* 1999;**89**:580–4.

17. McCarthy RJ, Pharm D, Stancic Z *et al.* Use of recombinant human tissue factor (RTF) thromboplastin as an adjunct to whole blood thromboelastograph (TEG) coagulation monitoring. *Anesth Analg* 1996;**82**:S306.

17
Renal failure following cardiopulmonary bypass

William T McBride

Introduction

Although relatively uncommon, clinically significant renal problems following cardiac surgery constitute a significant prolongation of postoperative recovery time with increased morbidity and mortality.

Case history

A 71-year-old Caucasian male was transferred to the cardiac surgical unit for urgent coronary revascularization. One month earlier he presented at a referring hospital with a 48-hour history of severe central chest pain. There was no cardiac enzyme rise but an electrocardiogram (ECG) showed acute anteroseptal infarction. Treadmill testing 5 days later was strongly positive for myocardial ischemia. Although he did not develop chest pain, the patient exercised for just 3 minutes of a modified Bruce protocol before developing marked hypotension with significant ST-segment elevation in the inferolateral leads. Coronary angiography revealed severe triple vessel disease and impaired left ventricular function. While awaiting surgery he was confined to bed due to minimal exertion angina and episodes of nocturnal angina.

On the day of surgery the patient was premedicated with oral lorazepam 2 mg (90 minutes before induction) and intramuscular morphine sulfate 5 mg and hyoscine 200 μg. Supplemental oxygen at 4 l min $^{-1}$ was administered by face-mask. The patient was comfortable and already well sedated

on arrival in the operating room. As is routine procedure in our unit, intravenous access was initially established under local anesthesia (LA) in the left forearm and left external jugular vein. Two 500 ml infusions of Hartmann's solution were commenced and the right radial artery cannulated for invasive arterial pressure monitoring. Under LA a triple-lumen catheter was placed in the right internal jugular vein together with a continuous cardiac output pulmonary artery flotation catheter (PAC). Methylprednisolone 1 g (15 mg kg^{-1}) was administered prior to induction of anesthesia.

Anesthesia was induced using fentanyl 1 mg and target controlled infusion (TCI) of propofol of 0.5 μg l^{-1}. Muscle relaxation was achieved with pancuronium 8 mg. Following tracheal intubation, anesthesia was maintained with TCI propofol and incremental doses of fentanyl and pancuronium. The lungs were ventilated with an air–oxygen mixture (FiO$_2$ 50%). No volatile anesthetic agent was used. At this stage the patient was hemodynamically stable and ST-segment analysis was normal in all ECG leads. However, during sternotomy he developed ST-segment elevation in leads II, aVF and V$_5$, accompanied by a dramatic deterioration in hemodynamics. The heart rate increased to 140 beats min^{-1}, systolic arterial pressure fell to 80 mmHg and the pulmonary artery diastolic pressure (PAD) rapidly rose from a post induction level of 12 to 26 mmHg. Mixed venous oxygen saturation (SvO$_2$) fell from 78 to 40%. It was decided to fully heparinize the patient and proceed to emergency cardiopulmonary bypass (CPB). For 10 minutes before the institution of CPB it was only possible to maintain a systolic arterial pressure of between 50 and 70 mmHg with epinephrine 800 μg in divided

Past medical history	Hypertension and hypercholesterolemia. Asbestos exposure but no shortness of breath. Previous cholecystectomy (20 years earlier) and bilateral inguinal hernia repair (4 years earlier). Scarlet fever in childhood.
Regular medications	Metoprolol 25 mg QID, trandolopril 1 mg OD, pravastatin 20 mg OD, amlodipine 5 mg OD, isosorbide mononitrate LA 50 mg OD, diazepam 2 mg BD, GTN spray PRN, aspirin 300mg OD (discontinued 5 days before surgery), enoxaparin 20 mg OD.
Examination	Weight 69.2 kg, BSA 1.7 m^2. Very anxious. Apyrexial. HR 54 bpm (sinus rhythm), BP 112/72 mmHg. Normal heart sounds, no murmurs. Chest clear.
Investigations	[Na$^+$] 139 mmol l^{-1}, [K$^+$] 4.5 mmol l^{-1}, urea 24 mg dl^{-1} (8.6 mmol l^{-1}), creatinine 1.5 mg dl^{-1} (131 (mol l^{-1}), total protein 67 g l^{-1}, [Mg^{2+}] 0.84 mmol l^{-1} Hb 12.7 g dl^{-1}, Hct 37%, WBC 5.26 × 10^9 l^{-1}, platelets 185 × 10^9 l^{-1}. **CXR:** Lungs clear. Normal heart size. **ECG:** Sinus bradycardia. Previous anteroseptal infarction. **Cardiac catherization:** Severe left main stem disease. Occlusion of proximal left anterior descending (LAD) coronary artery. Severe stenosis in the circumflex. Diffuse right coronary artery (RCA) disease with a high-grade stenosis at mid-level and at the crux. Impaired left ventricular function (ejection fraction 35%). Anterolateral akinesia with mural calcification consistent with healed infarction.

doses. At this point an infusion of dopamine 3 μg kg^{-1} min^{-1} was commenced. Following the institution of CPB, frusemide 20 mg was administered and an infusion of dopexamine 0.5 μg kg^{-1} min^{-1} commenced.

During CPB the patient was cooled to 28°C. The surgeon used antegrade cold crystalloid (St Thomas' I) cardioplegia and topical cooling for myocardial protection. The CPB time was 106 minutes and the ischemic time 59 minutes. Saphenous vein grafts were anastamosed to the LAD, the posterior descending and second obtuse marginal branch of the circumflex coronary arteries. The quality of the vessels was described by the surgeon as 'very poor'. Weaning from CPB was eventually achieved with epinephrine 0.075 μg kg^{-1} min^{-1}, noradrenaline 0.04 μg kg^{-1} min^{-1}, dopamine 6 μg kg^{-1} min^{-1} and dopexamine 0.3 μg kg^{-1} min^{-1}. Insertion of an intra-aortic balloon pump (IABP) via the left common femoral artery resulted in an improvement in hemodynamics allowing the rate of epinephrine and noradrenaline infusion to be reduced (epinephrine 0.0625 μg kg^{-1} min^{-1} and noradrenaline 0.0125 μg kg^{-1} min^{-1}). Intermittent positive pressure ventilation was continued and adequate sedation achieved with a propofol infusion 2–5 mg kg^{-1} hour^{-1}.

Overnight the patient developed a marked fall in systemic vascular resistance requiring an increase in noradrenaline infusion rate to 0.0625 μg kg^{-1} min^{-1} (Figure 17.1) in order to maintain arterial pressure. This was followed by oliguria

Inotropes used postoperatively

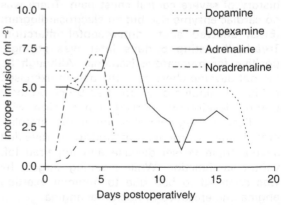

Figure 17.1

Inotropes (ml h^{-1}) over the first 17 days postoperatively. For dopamine and dopexamine 1ml h^{-1} = 1 μg kg^{-1}min^{-1}. For adrenaline and noradrenaline 4 ml h^{-1} = 0.05 μg kg^{-1} min^{-1}.

(Figure 17.2) and a markedly increasing metabolic acidosis (pH 7.26, serum lactate 83 mg dl^{-1} (9.23 mmol l^{-1}) — normal $\leq$ 18 mg dl^{-1} (2 mmol l^{-1})) and base excess –10.6 mmol l^{-1}). The dopexamine infusion rate was increased to 0.5 μg kg^{-1} min^{-1} (Figure 17.3) and an infusion of frusemide 2 mg $hour^{-1}$ commenced. Sodium bicarbonate 50 mmol was administered and repeated to achieve a base excess $\geq$ –5 mmol l^{-1}. Over the next 24 hours the acidosis and lactatemia resolved and urine output improved (Figure 17.2). Plasma concentrations of urea and creatinine began to rise precipitously (Figure

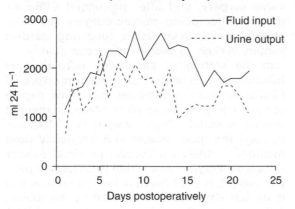

Figure 17.2

Fluid input and urinary output each 24 hours postoperatively.

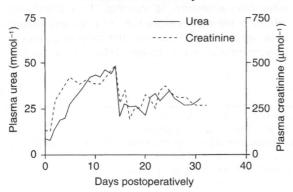

Figure 17.3

Plasma urea and creatinine concentrations postoperatively.

17.3) although the potassium concentration remained relatively stable. Measurement of urinary electrolytes suggested poor tubular concentration ability. At this stage the ECG and cardiac enzymes suggested an evolving large left ventricular infarction.

On the second day, the patient suffered an episode of ventricular fibrillation. Despite prompt resuscitation, arterial hypotension persisted for several hours. Intermittent episodes of sustained ventricular tachycardia were not effectively controlled with lignocaine 200 mg (in divided doses). Eventually arrythmia control was achieved with a combination of amiodarone (300 mg followed by an infusion of 48 mg h^{-1}) and mexilitene (250 mg over 10 minutes, 4 mg min^{-1} for 1 hour, 2 mg min^{-1} for 1 hour, followed by a gradually reducing maintenance dose commencing at 20 mg h^{-1}). These infusions continued for 2 weeks. Transesophageal echocardiography (TEE) revealed good right ventricular function and reasonable left ventricular function — albeit with anteroseptal akinesis and posterolateral hypokinesis. The IABP was removed at this point as the left foot was becoming critically ischemic. Following this perfusion of the left foot improved. On the third day, bowel sounds returned and nasogastric feeding was successfully introduced.

On the sixth postoperative day the patient was still mechanically ventilated. Fever and the development of bilateral pulmonary infiltrates on the chest radiograph were consistent with pulmonary infection. The leukocyte count rose from 5.26 to 17.4 $\times$ 10^9 l^{-1} and pulmonary function deteriorated (PaO_2 146 mmHg (19.5 kPa) with FiO_2 0.8 and PEEP 5 cmH_2O). The isolation of Gram-negative rods, from a sputum sample taken on the fourth day, prompted the introduction of piperacillin and tazobactam (Tazocin, Wyeth Laboratories; Maidenhead, Berks, UK) 2.25 g TDS. Propofol sedation was continued and, for the first time, the patient was noted to respond appropriately to commands. Over the next few days he became afebrile and his chest infection clinically improved. The leukocytosis, however, persisted and he remained in positive fluid balance (Figure 17.2) with very high urea and creatinine. The development of a systolic murmur over the precordium was thought likely to be due to Dressler's syndrome. A TEE examination revealed no valvular pathology.

By the thirteenth day, despite hemodynamic stability, there was no sign of recovery of renal function (Figures 17.2 and 17.3). Because of continued positive fluid balance, poor pulmonary function and uremia, a hemodialysis catheter was sited in the left subclavian vein and intermittent hemodialysis (3 hours daily) commenced (Filtral 20, Hospal AG; Lyon, France; [Na+] 140 mmol l⁻¹, [K+] 3.0 mmol l⁻¹). An episode of ventricular tachycardia during dialysis was thought to be due to an acute reduction in mexilitine levels. An increase in the rate of mexelitine infusion to 20 mg h⁻¹ during this and subsequent treatments prevented further dysrhythmia. A further deterioration in pulmonary function led to the antibiotic regimen being changed to netilmicin 2 mg kg⁻¹ (administered at the end of each dialysis treatment) and gentamicin (initially 80 mg after dialysis and subsequent doses dependent on plasma peak and trough monitoring). Hemodialysis was performed daily and, over the next 96 hours, respiratory function improved.

On the seventeenth day the propofol infusion was discontinued and the patient was weaned from mechanical ventilation and extubated. Hemodialysis was discontinued on the twentieth day and thereafter renal function gradually began to improve. It was felt that the failure to spontaneously recover from renal dysfunction after initial cardiovascular stabilization lay with a combination of ongoing renal 'insults' such as hypotension secondary to ventricular dysrhythmia and the use of nephrotoxic antibiotics in the face of sepsis.

Discussion

The definition of renal dysfunction varies from center to center. Nevertheless it is helpful to consider postoperative renal dysfunction as a spectrum ranging from subclinical renal dysfunction (i.e. dysfunction not detected by routine biochemical tests) to dialysis (in)dependent renal failure (Table 17.1).

Renal failure immediately after cardiac surgery is invariably oliguric. Acute dialysis dependent renal failure (ARF) occurs in approximately 1% patients following cardiac surgery and has an overall mortality of 30–60%.[1,2] Non-dialysis dependent clinical renal dysfunction occurs in approximately 8% of patients following cardiac surgery and has an overall mortality of less than 2%.[2] Acute postoperative renal failure is more likely in patients over 65 years of age, following valve surgery, and after prolonged CPB.[3] As patients undergoing cardiac surgery are more elderly, renal dysfunction following cardiac surgery is likely to become more common.[1]

In the setting of apparently normal renal function, the detection of urinary markers of tubular dysfunction indicates that some degree of renal injury has taken place.[4] Measurement of urinary N-acetyl-β-D-glucosaminidase (NAG) is perhaps the most reliable and frequently used method.[5–7] NAG is a specific proximal tubular lysosomal enzyme which, due to its large molecular weight, is not filtered at the glomerulus and is neither absorbed nor secreted by the tubule. Any increase in the urinary concentration of NAG may be considered a result of tubular damage. It is conventional to express urinary NAG as a function of urinary creatinine (the NAG:Cr ratio) in order to minimize error due to dilutional or concentrational effects. Urinary NAG is detectable in patients in whom the plasma creatinine concentration is normal. In patients in whom plasma concentrations of urea and creatinine are elevated however, the degree of elevation correlates with urinary NAG.[8] In a bovine

Table 17.1 The spectrum of renal dysfunction

Dialysis (in)dependent renal failure	Urine output < 0.3 ml kg⁻¹h⁻¹ (oliguric)
	OR urine output > 2.0 ml kg⁻¹ h⁻¹ (polyuric)
	AND a rise in plasma creatinine concentration >40 mmol l⁻¹ day⁻¹
Clinically detectable renal dysfunction	Urine output <1 ml kg⁻¹ hour⁻¹.
	AND plasma creatinine >1.25 mg dl⁻¹ (110 µmol l⁻¹)
	AND plasma urea >25 mg dl⁻¹ (9 mmol l⁻¹)
Subclinical renal dysfunction	Urine output normal
	Plasma urea and creatinine within normal range
	Creatinine clearance normal

model of renal dysfunction, urinary NAG levels have been shown to correlate with the histopathological severity of the renal lesions.[9] Other markers of subclinical tubular dysfunction include ß$_2$-microglobulin and α_1-microglobulin. As both are filtered at the glomerulus and 95% reabsorbed at the proximal tubule, any increase in urinary concentration would suggest proximal tubular dysfunction. Recent research suggests that subclinical renal dysfunction occurs in all patients following cardiac surgery conducted with CPB.[5, 8] A greater understanding of the mechanisms of subclinical renal dysfunction may lead to a greater understanding and subsequent prevention of clinically significant renal dysfunction.

Predisposing factors

In the case described, one can easily identify many perioperative factors, which no doubt contributed to postoperative renal problems. The plasma creatinine concentration was elevated before surgery. Although the reason for this was not clear, several factors may have contributed. Exposure to radiographic contrast media (e.g. during cardiac catheterization) is known to be associated with renal dysfunction. Whether this is due to renal vasoconstriction or direct tubulo-toxicity is unclear.[10] The risk of renal dysfunction increases with the volume of contrast used and is greater in patients with a pre-existing renal dysfunction and in diabetics.[10]

Other risk factors in the patient described include a long history of essential hypertension and administration of the angiotensin-converting enzyme inhibitor, trandolopril. This drug may be indirectly nephrotoxic by interfering with circulatory control within the glomerulus mediated by bradykinin. There may also be a direct toxic action on the distal tubule.

In a study of 2222 patients[11] undergoing myocardial revascularization with or without concurrent valvular surgery, 171 patients (7.7%) developed postoperative renal dysfunction. Of these, 30 (17.5%) had oliguric renal failure that required dialysis. Independent preoperative predictors of renal dysfunction included age at least 70 years; congestive heart failure; previous myocardial revascularization; insulin-dependent

diabetes mellitus or preoperative serum glucose level >300 mg dl^{-1} (16.6 mmol l^{-1}); and preoperative serum creatinine levels of 1.4–2.0 mg dl^{-1} (124–177 (mol l^{-1}). Perioperative factors that increased the risk of renal dysfunction were CPB duration of at least 3 hours and ventricular dysfunction. Davila-Roman and colleagues have demonstrated that the severity of atherosclerosis of the ascending aorta is also a predictor of renal dysfunction after cardiac operations.[12]

In the case presented, the most obvious intra-operative risk factor for renal dysfunction was the episode of arterial hypotension before the onset of CPB. Let us consider a simplified overview of the effect of hypotension on the kidney. Initially, as blood pressure falls, glomerular perfusion pressure (GPP) falls and there is a reduction in glomerular filtration rate (GFR) and urinary output. At first this is 'tubuloprotective' as the energy requirements and oxygen demand required for tubular sodium transport are reduced. As mean arteriolar pressure falls, renal and splanchnic vasoconstriction diverts blood to vital organs such as the brain and heart, thus GPP is further jeopardized. In the presence of persistent hypotension, however, angiotensin II (AgII) is produced via the renin–angiotensin–aldosterone axis. Stimulation of efferent arteriolar AgII receptors leads to some restoration of GPP, an improvement in GFR and, possibly, an increase in urine production. However, this does not mean that all is well because the efferent arteriolar vasoconstriction may jeopardize oxygen delivery to the energy-hungry regions of the nephron. Particularly vulnerable areas are the distal segments of the proximal tubule and thick ascending medullary segments of the loop of Henlé involved in sodium reabsorption and urine concentration. Initially the poor performance of these tubular cells is reflected in 'poor quality' urine — urine with a sodium concentration ≥10 mmol l^{-1} — even though the volume of urine produced may be satisfactory. This state of affairs may well be easily reversible if oxygen delivery to these cells is restored. If not there is a real risk of irreversible damage of these cells and acute tubular necrosis (ATN).

Clearly, in this situation, arterial hypotension must be rapidly corrected to avoid ATN. In this case, where a catastrophic left ventricular pump failure was evolving secondary to critical left main stem coronary artery disease, there was little option but to support the failing heart with substantial doses of epinephrine while the surgeon rapidly instituted CPB. During CPB renal perfusion would have been somewhat restored but there is little doubt than an initial insult had taken place. As previously mentioned, subclinical renal injury occurs in virtually all patients subjected to CPB.[5,8] In the case described CPB was used to 'rescue' the patient from cardiovascular collapse even though this would have a deleterious effect on renal function. The nature of CPB-mediated renal injury is far from clear. Decreased GPP during CPB may be a factor, but it is possible that the rapidly evolving inflammatory response during and after CPB may also play a role. In this connection it is interesting to note that in a hypotensive murine model of ATN, mice unable to express intercellular adhesion molecule-1 (ICAM-1 'knock out' mice) are less susceptible to develop ATN than normal mice.[13] It is also noteworthy that the proinflammatory cytokines interleukin 8 (IL-8), monomeric tumour necrosis factor alpha (TNF-α) and IL-1β, implicated in the CPB mediated inflammatory response, all have molecular weights less than 20 000 Daltons and thus, are readily filtered at the glomerulus. In contrast the larger, balancing anti-inflammatory cytokines (IL-10, IL-1ra and TNF soluble receptors) are larger and less readily filtered. It is tempting to suggest that during CPB, tubular cells may be particularly vulnerable to the actions of these inflammatory cytokines. This hypothesis is supported by the demonstration in vitro that proximal tubular cells respond to proinflammatory cytokine challenge via the induction of nitric oxide synthetase (NOS) and generation of cytotoxic concentrations of nitric oxide, suggesting a mechanism for direct proinflammatory cytokine-mediated proximal tubular cytotoxicity.[14, 15] This work suggests that the tubular cells, while important in disposing of proinflammatory cytokines,[16] may themselves be damaged in the process. Further support for this idea comes from the recent demonstration that the magnitude of the increase in plasma TNF-α and IL-8 following elective CABG surgery with CPB, correlates with the magnitude of proximal tubular injury as measured by urinary NAG/creatinine.[17] In this connection it is interesting that ulinistatin, which is known to reduce the IL-8 response to CPB,[18] is also known to *reduce* CPB-mediated subclinical renal dysfunction.[19]

What measures can be taken to minimize the tubular damage in such a situation? Four theoretical principles govern renal protective strategies.

1. Restore oxygen delivery and perfusion to the tubules.
2. Reduce the oxygen demand of the tubules.
3. Reduce the magnitude of the inflammatory response.
4. Avoid further nephrotoxic insults.

Restoration of oxygen delivery to the tubules

Since the underlying problem in this case was one of decreased mean arterial pressure the therapeutic response lay in correcting this. Following CPB, this involved inotropic support as well as use of the IABP. This approach required constant reassessment as some combinations of inotropes may have a deleterious effect on the kidney. Since a PAC was in place, inotropic support could be adjusted according to systemic vascular resistance (SVR) and stroke volume. Following CPB this patient had profoundly low SVR and required noradrenaline to effect vasoconstriction to maintain a satisfactory MAP. Although vascular indices may be improved, the overall outlook may be worsened if noradrenaline-mediated renal and splanchnic vasoconstriction exacerbates renal and splanchnic ischemia. This could lead to ATN and increased gut permeability with endotoxin translocation and development of a systemic inflammatory response. In routine clinical practice this should be suspected if there is elevated plasma lactate and negative base excess, especially if oxygen delivery remains stable. Ideally one should endeavor to reduce the noradrenaline, but the problem is that this may again lead to hypotension which could be life-threatening bearing in mind the pressure dependent coronary artery perfusion.

A frequently asked question is whether dopamine can improve renal and splanchnic perfusion in hypotensive states. At normal arterial pressures, dopamine improves RBF via its dopaminergic receptor effect and hence increases both GFR and urine output. However, as blood pressure falls this is not maintained, probably due to the inability of dopamine to overcome reflex α-adrenergic vasoconstriction or a direct α-adrenergic effect on afferent and efferent arterioles. Because efferent arteriolar vasoconstriction occurs in the face of hypotension, GPP may be adequate to maintain GFR. Although urine output may be preserved, ischemia of the nephron may be developing as a result of efferent arteriolar vasoconstriction. It is no surprise, therefore, that studies have not shown a renal protective effect of dopamine in either cardiac or vascular surgery.[20, 21]

Is it possible to retain the benefits of noradrenaline in maintaining a satisfactory arterial pressure to perfuse a critically ischemic myocardium and still overcome the problem of renal and splanchnic hypoperfusion? It is in this setting that dopexamine has a theoretical role to play. This is an inotropic agent with vasodilator properties mediated by both dopaminergic and β_2-adrenergic receptors. It lacks α-adrenergic activity and has been shown to enhance liver blood flow,[22] to reduce gastrointestinal permeability[23] following CPB and to improve splanchnic blood flow in the critically ill.[24] At low doses, it has been shown to improve creatinine clearance following cardiac surgery.[25] Low-dose dopexamine could, therefore, theoretically overcome renal and splanchnic hypoperfusion in conditions of low arterial pressure requiring noradrenaline infusion. Clinical studies are necessary to demonstrate this, although in the author's experience it is ethically difficult to withhold low-dose dopexamine in such situations. In the author's unit it is usual practice to introduce dopexamine in such situations starting at 0.5 µg kg^{-1} min^{-1} and increasing the dose (in increments of 0.5 µg kg^{-1} min^{-1} every 15 minutes) as necessary, to a maximum of 1.5 µg kg^{-1} min^{-1} (Figure 17.1). Usually, as in the case presented, elevated plasma lactate concentrations and negative base excess should normalize over several hours. If, however, following the administration of low-dose dopexamine, there is no significant improvement in lactatemia and base excess despite the presence of adequate oxygen delivery and blood glucose, then the rare but very real possibility of irreversible gut ischemia should be urgently considered. Dopexamine, by virtue of its β_2–adrenergic action, tends to prevent hyperkalemia which may delay or even help avoid the need for dialysis. Of interest, the patient discussed did not develop hyperkalemia (Figure 17.3).

Reducing oxygen demand by the tubules

The loop diuretic frusemide blocks active sodium potassium transport in the thick ascending limb of the loop of Henlé. In isolated kidney models of renal ischemia, frusemide has been shown to confer protection against ATN, but several clinical studies have been disappointing.[26] In the case presented, frusemide was administered as a bolus before the institution of CPB and by infusion thereafter. Further well-controlled clinical studies are needed to determine if the very clear theoretical benefits of this drug are reflected by clinical benefit.

Reducing the magnitude of the inflammatory response

The goal here is to reduce the magnitude of inflammatory mediators that the kidney filters and denatures during a period of renal hypoperfusion. Just as a combination of many factors contribute to the magnitude of the inflammatory response, a combination of many strategies is needed to minimize it.[27] Ulinastatin reduces IL-8 release and also reduces the severity of subclinical perioperative renal dysfunction. In the case presented, methylprednisolone was given preoperatively and this would be expected to reduce the proinflammatory (IL-8) response at cardiac surgery and magnify the anti-inflammatory (IL-10) response. In the author's unit all patients considered to be at high risk of developing a detrimental inflammatory response are routinely given methylprednisolone 15 mg kg^{-1} before the onset of CPB. This is half of the dose of methylprednisolone reported by Tabardel and colleagues[28] to significantly reduce the IL-8 response and increase the IL-10 response in patients undergoing coronary revascularization. The addition of a similar dose of methylprednisolone to an isolated extracorporeal circuit has been shown to significantly reduce the IL-8 response.[29] The effect of lower doses of methylprednisolone on cytokine responses has yet to be determined and further studies will be required to demonstrate any protective effect of methlylprednisolone on renal function.

Avoiding further nephrotoxic insults

Sepsis and the resulting inflammatory response is nephrotoxic. This situation is further complicated by the fact that many antibiotics are nephrotoxic. Nevertheless, in life threatening infections the required antibiotics need to be given and the kidneys supported as necessary. The use of piperacillin, tazobactam, netilmicin and gentamicin in this case was justified on clinical grounds despite their undoubtedly adverse impact on renal function and the requirement for dialysis. Where possible nephrotoxic drugs should be avoided. In this context it should be recalled that non-steroidal anti-inflammatory drugs are potentially nephrotoxic.

In most centers, renal replacement therapy falls into one of two categories: intermittent hemodialysis (IHD); and continuous renal replacement therapy (CRRT). The simplest form of CRRT is continuous arteriovenous hemofiltration (CAVHF). While this approach has the advantage of simplicity, it is unsuitable for use in the hemodynamically unstable patient. For this reason, continuous venovenous hemo(dia)filtration (CVVHF) is more commonly employed. Although CVVHF is more complex to institute and manage than CAVHF, it confers greater hemodynamic stability, avoids rapid fluid and electrolyte shifts, permits nutrition without restriction, and may be tailored to the changing needs of the patient. In addition, the technique allows the use of more biocompatible membranes and the necessity for uninterrupted anticoagulation. The relative merits of IHD versus CRRT in terms of mortality must await further study. However, there is already evidence of decreased morbidity in CRRT patients. Bellomo and colleagues[30] have shown that changing the form of renal replacement therapy from IHD to continuous hemofiltration was associated with improved control of azotemia and superior adequacy of small solute clearance. In addition, Ronco and colleagues[31] have demonstrated that patients treated with CVVHF had less intracerebral fluid shift (quantified by computed tomography) than patients treated with IHD. The authors suggested that IHD might lead to a postdialysis brain edematogenic state. This may be of relevance in the patient with multiorgan system failure following cardiac surgery when cerebral function may be impaired.

A unifying theme affecting our understanding of the etiology of renal failure, and our treatment thereof, is the perioperative inflammatory response. The production and release of both proinflammatory and anti-inflammatory cytokines is a normal, physiological response to surgery and CPB. Under normal conditions, these cytokines are rapidly cleared from the blood, and the kidney plays an important role in this process. However, in some situations proximal tubular cells may be vulnerable (at least in vitro) to proinflammatory cytokine-mediated cytotoxicity.[15] In situations of renal hypotension the smooth execution of proinflammatory cytokine disposal by the kidneys may be impaired. This may lead, not only to a reduction in proinflammatory cytokine clearance, but also reduced oxygen supply to the kidney when energy requiring mechanisms are required for the safe disposal of filtered proinflammatory cytokines. Proximal tubular damage may then be more likely. It is therefore, not surprising that factors likely to increase the inflammatory response — such as prolonged CPB time, poor splanchnic perfusion and sepsis — increase the likelihood of renal dysfunction.[11] In this case study, several examples of anti-inflammatory strategies have been alluded to. These included methylprednisolone (through reducing IL-8 and increasing IL-10), dopexamine (through improvement of splanchnic perfusion and reducing IL-6) and aggressive treatment of sepsis. Finally, until the inflammatory response is settled permanent renal dysfunction should not be diagnosed.

Conclusions and learning points

- Preoperative renal dysfunction should be anticipated in patients recently undergoing cardiac catheterization, who have had a recent episode of arterial hypotension or who are taking angiotensin-converting enzyme inhibitors.
- Perioperative hypotension, as well as the CPB insult itself, may contribute to the renal dysfunction.
- Strategies to prevent and treat developing ATN will involve; restoring oxygen delivery to the tubules, reducing tubular oxygen demand, reducing the inflammatory response and avoiding any subsequent nephrotoxic events, especially, where possible avoiding nephrotoxic drugs.

- When dialysis is needed there is now increasing evidence that continuous renal replacement therapy such as CVVHF may be superior to intermittent hemodialysis.

References

1. Chertow GM, Levy EM, Hammermeister KE et al. Independent association between acute renal failure and mortality following cardiac surgery. Am J Med 1998;**104**:343-8.

2. Conlon PJ, Stafford-Smith M, White WD et al. Acute renal failure following cardiac surgery. Nephrol Dial Transplant 1999;**14**:1158-62.

3. Mangos GJ, Brown MA, Chan WY et al. Acute renal failure following cardiac surgery: incidence, outcomes and risk factors. Aust N Z J Med 1995;**25**:284-9.

4. Kleinschmidt S, Bauer M, Grundmann U et al. Effect of gamma-hydroxybutyric acid and pentoxifylline on kidney function parameters in coronary surgery interventions. Anaesthesiol Reanim 1997;**22**:102-7.

5. Westhuyzen J, McGiffin DC, McCarthy J, Fleming SJ. Tubular nephrotoxicity after cardiac surgery utilising cardiopulmonary bypass. Clin Chim Acta 1994;**228**:123-32.

6. Price RG. The role of NAG (N-acetyl-beta-D-glucosaminidase) in the diagnosis of kidney disease including the monitoring of nephrotoxicity. Clin Nephrol 1992;**38 (Suppl 1)**:S14-9.

7. Price RG. Measurement of N-acetyl-beta-glucosaminidase and its isoenzymes in urine methods and clinical applications. Eur J Clin Chem Clin Biochem 1992;**30**:693-705.

8. Jorres A, Kordonouri O, Schiessler A et al. Urinary excretion of thromboxane and markers for renal injury in patients undergoing cardiopulmonary bypass. Artif Organs 1994;**18**:565-9.

9. Sato R, Sano Y, Sato J, Naito Y. N-acetyl-beta-D-glucosaminidase activity in urine of cows with renal parenchymal lesions. Am J Vet Res 1999;**60**:410-3.

10. McCullough PA, Wolyn R, Rocher LL et al. Acute renal failure after coronary intervention: incidence, risk factors and relationship to mortality. Am J Med 1997;**103**:368-75.

11. Mangano CM, Diamondstone LS, Ramsay JG et al. Renal dysfunction after myocardial revascularization: risk factors, adverse outcomes, and hospital resource utilization. The Multicenter Study of Perioperative Ischemia Research Group. Ann Intern Med 1998;**128**:194-203.

12. Davila-Roman VG, Kouchoukos NT, Schechtman KB, Barzilai B. Atherosclerosis of the ascending aorta is a predictor of renal dysfunction after cardiac operations. J Thorac Cardiovasc Surg 1999;**117**:111-6.

13. Kelly KJ, Williams WW Jr, Colvin RB et al. Intercellular adhesion molecule-1-deficient mice are protected against ischaemic renal injury. J Clin Invest 1996;**97**:1056-63.

14. Traylor LA, Proksch JW, Beanum VC, Mayeux PR. Nitric oxide generation by renal proximal tubules: role of nitric oxide in the cytotoxicity of Lipid A. J Pharmacol Exp Ther 1996;**279**:91-6.

15. Chatterjee PK, Hawksworth GM, McClay JS. Cytokine-stimulated nitric oxide production in the human proximal renal tubule and its modulation by natriuretic peptides: A novel immunomodulatory mechanism? Exp Nephrol 1999;**7**:438-48.

16. Bocci V, Paulesu L, Pessina GP. The renal catabolic pathways of cytokines. Contrib Nephrol 1993;**101**:55-60.

17. Gormley SM, McBride WT, Armstrong MA et al. Plasma and urinary cytokine homeostasis and renal dysfunction during cardiac surgery. Anesthesiology 2000;**93**:1210-6.

18. Kawamura T, Inada K, Akasaka N, Wakusawa R. Ulinastatin reduces elevation of cytokines and soluble adhesion molecules during cardiac surgery. Can J Anaesth 1996;**43**:456-60.

19. Ueki M, Yokono S, Nogaya J et al. Effects of ulinastatin on postoperative renal function after cardiopulmonary bypass. Masui 1995;**44**:691-7.

20. Myles PS, Buckland MR, Schenk NJ et al. Effect of 'renal dose' dopamine on renal function following cardiac surgery. Anaesth Intensive Care 1993;**21**:56-61.

21. Baldwin L, Henderson A, Hickman P. Effect of post operative low-dose dopamine on renal function

after elective major vascular surgery. *Ann Intern Med* 1994;**120**:744–7.

22. Sharpe DA, Mitchel IM, Kay EA *et al.* Enhancing liver blood flow after cardiopulmonary bypass: the effects of dopamine and dopexamine. *Perfusion* 1999;**14**:29–36.

23. Sinclair DG, Houldsworth PE, Keogh B *et al.* Gastrointestinal permeability following cardiopulmonary bypass: a randomised study comparing the effects of dopamine and dopexamine. *Intensive Care Med* 1997;**23**:510–6.

24. Maynard ND, Bihari DJ, Dalton RN *et al.* Increasing splanchnic blood flow in the critically III. *Chest* 1995;**108**:1648–54.

25. Berendes E, Mollhoff T, Van Aken H *et al.* Effects of dopexamine on creatinine clearance, systemic inflammation, and splanchnic oxygenation in patients undergoing coronary artery bypass grafting. *Anesth Analg* 1997;**84**:950–7.

26. Heyman SN. Furosemide and oxygen sparing. In: Galley H (ed) *Critical care focus. Renal failure.* London: BMJ Books, 1999; 45–59.

27. McBride WT, McBride SJ. The balance of pro and anti-inflammatory cytokines in cardiac surgery. *Curr Opin Anaesthesiol* 1998;**11**:15–22.

28. Tabardel Y, Duchateau J, Schmartz D *et al.* Corticosteroids increase blood interleukin-10 levels during cardiopulmonary bypass in men. *Surgery* 1996;**119**:76–80.

29. Gormley SMC, Armstrong MA, McMurray TJ, McBride WT. The effect of methylprednisolone on the immune response using an isolated cardiopulmonary bypass circuit. *Anesth Analg* 1999;**88**:SCA17.

30. Bellomo R, Farmer M, Bhonagiri S *et al.* Changing acute renal failure treatment from intermittent hemodialysis to continuous hemofiltration: impact on azotemic control. *Int J Artif Organs* 1999 **22**:145–50.

31. Ronco C, Bellomo R, Brendolan A *et al.* Brain density changes during renal replacement in critically ill patients with acute renal failure. Continuous hemofiltration versus intermittent hemodialysis. *J Nephrol* 1999;**12**:173–8

18

The inotropic action of glucose–insulin–potassium infusions

Christopher J Broomhead, Susan J Wright and M Peter Colvin

Introduction

We describe the case history of a patient who benefited from the inotropic effects of an infusion of glucose–insulin–potassium (GIK), and then discuss the physiological basis for its action and the clinical evidence supporting its use.

Case history

A 54-year-old merchant seaman presented to the casualty department with a short history of chest pain of sudden onset. The pain was typically cardiac in nature, described as central chest tightness, associated with nausea and tachycardia.

He had no past cardiac or other medical history, although he was a heavy smoker with a strong family history of cardiac disease, his father having died aged 58 of a myocardial infarction. He appeared distressed, was hypertensive and tachycardic. There was no evidence of cardiac failure. All investigations were normal, including the electrocardiogram (ECG), which showed sinus tachycardia but no acute changes. However, the troponin T level was elevated, and a diagnosis of unstable angina was made. He was admitted and treated with glyceryl trinitrate (GTN) and heparin infusions, and intermittent doses of diamorphine. His pain rapidly settled and the cardiac enzyme rise was minimal at 24 hours.

On day 2 he developed further chest pain, again without ECG changes, which quickly

Past medical history	None prior to admission. Prior to surgery aspirin 75 mg OD, clopidogrel 75 mg OD, GTN infusion at 3 mg h^{-1}.
Examination prior to surgery	Weight 84 kg. BP 110/50, HR 110 SR, JVP +4, fine bibasal crepitations.
Investigations prior to surgery	Hb 10.2 g dl^{-1}, WBC 14.2 × 10^9 l^{-1}, platelets 140 × 10^9 l^{-1}. creatinine 3.0 mg dl^{-1} (266 mmol l^{-1}), urea 22 mmol l^{-1}, glucose 162 mg dl^{-1} (9 mmol l^{-1}), LFTs mildly deranged. Troponin T raised **CXR:** Heart size normal, lung fields upper lobe blood diversion, fluid in the horizontal fissure and small bilateral pleural effusions. **ECG:** Sinus rhythm, 110 bpm, no acute changes. **TTE:** Hypertrophied left ventricle with moderate function, no structural abnormality. **Coronary angiogram:** Mild anterior hypokinesia, moderate overall left ventricular function, critical lesion in the proximal LAD treated by PTCA

resolved with further diamorphine. There was no further cardiac enzyme rise although the troponin T level remained significantly raised. Over the following 3 days, this pattern of recurrent angina without ECG changes continued, so he was transferred to the regional cardiac unit for further investigation. On arrival he was complaining of severe pain and breathlessness, and was obviously distressed. On examination he was hypotensive and tachycardic with a gallop rhythm. The peripheral oxygen saturation was 92% on oxygen 6 l min^{-1} administered via a facemask, he was tachypneic, and there were widespread crepitations in the mid and lower zones of his chest bilaterally. There were no ECG changes, and his cardiac enzymes were not further elevated. Blood gas analysis revealed a mild respiratory alkalosis with a PCO_2 of 25.5 mmHg (3.4 kPa), and a metabolic acidosis with a base deficit of 6 mmol l^{-1}. Transthoracic echocardiography revealed a hypertrophied left ventricle with moderate function and no structural abnormalities. The patient was treated with intravenous frusemide and an intra-aortic balloon pump (IABP) was inserted. Over the following 24 hours the pulmonary edema cleared, his blood pressure improved and the tachycardia resolved. Blood tests remained normal except for the renal function, which had deteriorated significantly, the creatinine rising to 3.2 mg dl^{-1} (287 µmol l^{-1}) having been normal at first presentation.

The patient continued to have short-lived episodes of angina despite intravenous heparin and GTN, the IABP, and maximal medical therapy. Nevertheless he remained clinically stable, and there was no further deterioration in renal function. On day 6 after admission, it was decided that he was stable enough to undergo coronary angiography with a plan to proceed to angioplasty (PTCA) if appropriate. The only demonstrable lesion was significant proximal disease in the left anterior descending coronary artery. Following PTCA, two stents were inserted into the LAD with a good radiological result, and the patient was commenced on abciximab and clopidogrel. However immediately following the procedure, the patient again developed hypotension with pulmonary edema and became anuric. A pulmonary artery catheter was inserted, which showed a raised pulmonary artery occlusion pressure, low cardiac index and raised systemic vascular resistance, consistent with a diagnosis of cardiogenic shock. Infusions of dopamine 2.5 µg kg^{-1} min^{-1} and epinephrine 10 µg min^{-1} (0.12 µg kg^{-1} min^{-1}) were commenced. Despite a dramatic increase in the dose of epinephrine to 25 µg min^{-1} (0.3 µg kg^{-1} min^{-1}) there was little improvement in cardiac index and the patient remained hypotensive and was unable to tolerate any increase in the rate of GTN administration.

At this stage the patient was transferred from coronary care unit (CCU) to the ICU with a view to commencing continuous venovenous hemofiltration (CVVHF) since he had been anuric since PTCA and was now developing a severe metabolic acidosis. On admission a GIK infusion was commenced. Glucose 50% (i.e. 500 mg ml^{-1}) and human soluble insulin 1 iu ml^{-1} was infused at a rate of 5–10 ml hour^{-1}. Serum concentrations of glucose and potassium were measured at 30 minute intervals. The GIK infusion rate was adjusted to maintain a serum glucose concentration between 140 and 216 mg dl^{-1} (8–12 mmol l^{-1}) and potassium chloride (5–10 mmol) was administered to maintain a serum [K$^+$] between 4.5 and 5.5 mmol l^{-1}. Within 60 minutes of starting GIK, the cardiac index had risen from 1.8 to 3.0 l min^{-1} m^{-2}, and the mixed venous saturation rose from 57 to 75%. Over the next 4 hours the epinephrine infusion was weaned from 25 to 5 µg min^{-1}, without any deterioration in cardiac index. The blood pressure increased to the patient's prePTCA level and the urine output was restored with the assistance of a low-dose frusemide infusion, and the need for hemofiltration was avoided. By 24 hours after PTCA, the patient was pain free, normotensive, had an acceptable urine output, no metabolic acidosis and the pulmonary edema had resolved. After a further 24 hours, all pharmacological support had been weaned off and the patient remained stable and pain-free.

Unfortunately 72 hours after the PTCA he again developed chest pain without ECG changes, which did not settle with diamorphine and GTN infusions. At this stage it was felt that coronary artery bypass grafting was a better option than a further PTCA. Surgery was undertaken within 2 hours of the onset of chest pain. Since the patient was surprisingly stable after induction of anesthesia, the left internal mammary artery was harvested and anastomosed to the LAD, and a saphenous vein graft was placed on the circumflex artery. In view of his previous ventricular dysfunction, he was weaned from cardiopulmonary bypass supported by the IABP and a low-dose epinephrine infusion. After routine chest closure he was transferred to the ICU, cardiovascularly stable on epinephrine 10 μg min[-1] and the IABP. There was significant loss into his chest drains over the first 4 hours, despite normal ACT, clotting screen and platelet count. This was attributed to the combined effects of aspirin, clopidogrel and abciximab, so platelets were administered with a good effect.

Twelve hours postoperatively, there was a sudden deterioration in gas exchange associated with marked hypotension, oliguria and a severe metabolic acidosis. A pulmonary artery catheter was inserted, confirming the diagnosis of postoperative cardiogenic shock. TTE demonstrated globally impaired left ventricular function but no significant cardiac effusion. The epinephrine infusion was increased to 30 μg min[-1] (0.36 μg kg[-1] min[-1]) with minimal increase in the cardiac index, and no improvement in the blood pressure. Dopamine was introduced as an alternative inotrope, with no success. However, just as previously, when a GIK infusion was commenced there was a dramatic and sustained improvement in cardiac index. Over the following 24 hours all the inotropic support was weaned, except for the GIK infusion. The patient was weaned from mechanical ventilation and the trachea extubated 36 hours after surgery. After a further 36 hours of stability, the IABP was removed; the GIK infusion stopped and the patient remained stable. The pulmonary artery catheter was removed, and the patient transferred back to CCU. Over the next 8 days the patient's renal function returned to normal, he remained pain-free and was discharged to cardiac rehabilitation. Six months after surgery he was making good progress and had remained pain-free.

Discussion

The effects of insulin on glucose metabolism have been known since its discovery, but the effects of insulin on the cardiovascular system were not described until 1927.[1] The use of glucose–insulin–potassium (GIK) infusions to ameliorate ischemic myocardial dysfunction, and

to a lesser degree, infarction and cardiac failure has been expounded for nearly 40 years, even though the mechanism of its complex actions in myocardial pathophysiology have only recently been revealed. Large-scale clinical studies are now beginning to reveal the true potential of GIK therapy. That such an inexpensive therapy may reduce the mortality rate in acute myocardial infarction by 30% seems astounding. In reality it is not surprising that manipulating metabolic controls during a long period of ischemia can produce beneficial effects, since ischemia in itself produces metabolic disruption, which leads to myocardial dysfunction and eventually cell death.

In the 1960s, when GIK first became popular, it was initially suggested that the beneficial effect had two components. Firstly, insulin stimulates myocardial sodium–potassium ATPase ($Na^+K^+ATPase$), leading to an increased reuptake of K^+, which was believed to stabilize the cell membrane so reducing the incidence of dysrhythmias.[2] Secondly, insulin stimulated the myocardial uptake of glucose, increasing the provision of intracellular substrate thus helping to maintain cellular integrity. Although this concept of balancing the energy provision with the cellular metabolic requirements seems attractive, it also appears to be rather simplistic.

GIK enhances anaerobic oxidation in hypoxic myocardium, but the evidence for attenuation of ischemia-induced reductions in ATP stores is scanty.[3] However, the positioning of the glycolytic enzymes within the cell may ensure that the little ATP that is produced is located in regions critical to the maintenance of cellular membrane functions such as calcium and sodium homeostasis.[4, 5] Provision of a high glucose substrate has been shown to protect myocytes from the toxic effects of the increase in intracellular calcium induced by ischemia.[6] Extraction of glucose by ischemic myocardium increases as coronary blood flow reduces due to up-regulation of glucose transporters, particularly GLUT-4,[7] the delivery of glucose being the rate limiting step.[8] Importantly, more recent studies of myocardial infarction have shown that the acute infarct area is a region of low flow, not zero flow, that is sufficient to deliver substrate and remove lactate.[9, 10] This provides a rationale for treatment in the setting of acute ischemia and infarction.[11]

Ischemia also has other important metabolic effects. Increased catecholamine production leads to glucose intolerance[12] and increased concentrations of free fatty acids (FFA).[13] Under the normal conditions of plentiful oxygen supply, FFA are preferentially metabolized by the myocardium and are the more efficient source of energy. FFA metabolism produces more ATP per carbon atom than glucose metabolism, but demands more oxygen in order to do so. However, the high level of FFA generated during ischemia can generate dysrhythmias,[14] and may endanger the recovery of ischemic but viable tissue.[13] Insulin has an antiFFA effect, which may be particularly important in situations of raised catecholamine production when the toxic effects of FFA are accentuated.[15]

Clinical studies in myocardial infarction

Clinical studies date back to 1962 when Sodi-Pollares et al demonstrated a beneficial effect of GIK infusions administered to patients with acute myocardial infarction.[2] A Medical Research Council-funded working party was unable to reproduce these results, and following a review in the *Lancet*,[16] the use of GIK was largely abandoned. It was not until the 1980s that interest was rekindled by the work of Rackley et al, who not only confirmed the improvement in infarct patients, but also defined the optimal dose of insulin as that required to suppress FFA levels.[17] A meta-analysis, published in 1997, of the prospective randomized trials in the prethrombolytic era, provided the first firm evidence in support of GIK.[18] An editorial published with this article, described the treatment as simple and safe, and called for a trial to be undertaken in patients undergoing thrombolysis.[19]

The following year, the Estudios Cardiologicos Latinoamerica (ECLA) Collaborative Group reported the results of a prospective, randomized examination of GIK in over 400 patients with myocardial infarction who were also reperfused.[20] Remarkably it showed a 66% reduction (from 15.2 to 5.2%) in hospital mortality, for reperfusion and GIK therapy compared to reperfusion alone. This survival benefit was still apparent at 1 year. The combined endpoint of death, severe heart failure and non-fatal ventricular fibrillation was reduced by 40%. This is all the more surprising considering the average time from onset of symptoms of acute myocardial infarction to initiating treatment was 10–11 hours. An accompanying review stated that ECLA provided 'strong clinical and scientific evidence to support the use of GIK in acute myocardial infarction'.[11] A repeat of the meta-analysis including the ECLA trial showed a reduction in mortality of 44% with a probability of 0.07 and an odds ratio of 0.56 with a confidence interval that reaches unity.[21] Although this tends to support the benefits of GIK, a large-scale trial is still required to confirm the encouraging results seen so far.

Clinical studies in cardiac surgery

By its very nature cardiac surgery produces a period of myocardial ischemia, followed by reperfusion. There are few trials of GIK use in cardiac surgery, and interpretation of their results is handicapped by the poor design, a small study population, the choice of GIK dose and the timing of administration in relation to the ischemic insult, and the outcomes studied. However, they do tend to show a similar pattern of benefit with increases in cardiac index, decreased requirement for inotropic and mechanical support and a reduction in dysrhythmias.

Three studies have used GIK in the preoperative period. In a randomized, prospective study of GIK in urgent CABG for unstable angina, GIK was commenced prior to CPB and continued for 12 hours afterwards. The GIK group had a markedly greater cardiac index with less inotropic support, and the incidence of perioperative atrial fibrillation was dramatically reduced.[22] Another blinded, controlled study showed GIK started before bypass produced a marked improvement in cardiac index, with the greatest effect in those patients with the worst left ventricular function.[23] The last study demonstrated that GIK reduced postoperative hypotension and arrhythmias in patients undergoing mitral valve replacement.[24]

Cardiogenic shock after cardiac surgery is associated with a mortality rate of 30%.[25] In 1991, Svedjeholm et al showed that GIK enhanced the inotropic effects of dopamine in the postoperative period whilst decreasing FFA levels.[26] Subsequently they demonstrated hemodynamic improvements in a small group of patients with post-CPB cardiac failure, compared to historical controls.[27] Taegtmeyer's group also demonstrated that GIK markedly decreased FFA levels whilst increasing cardiac index by approximately 40% without change in inotropic dosages. By contrast, in the control group cardiac index remained unchanged despite a doubling of inotropic support. In a larger follow-up study, 322 patients with pump failure post-CPB were treated with GIK, reducing in-hospital mortality by one-third and the length of both ICU and hospital stay.[25]

The case described demonstrates the inotropic actions of GIK in ischemic myocardial dysfunction. Although dramatic responses were seen in this patient, and evidence is accumulating to support its use, as yet it is not standard practice. It will not be long before clear evidence appears to support its use in myocardial infarction. Hopefully similar studies will follow clarifying its role in cardiac surgery.

References

1. Visscher M, Muller, E. The influence of insulin on the mammalian heart. *J Physiol* 1927;**62**:341–8.

2. Sodi Pollares D, Testelli, M. Fishleder B *et al*. Effects of an intravenous influsion of a potassium-glucose-insulin infusion on the electro-cardiographic signs of myocardian infarction. *Am J Cardiol* 1962;**9**:166–81.

3. Eberli FR, Weinberg EO, Grice WN *et al*. Protective effect of increased glycolytic substrate against systolic and diastolic dysfunction and increased coronary resistance from prolonged global under-perfusion and reperfusion in isolated rabbit hearts perfused with erthrocyte suspensions. *Circ Res* 1991;**68**:466–81.

4. Xu KY, Zweier JL, Becker LC. Functional coupling between glycolysis and sarcoplasmic reticulum Ca^{2+} transport. *Circ Res* 1995;**77**:88–97.

5. Weiss JN, Lamp ST. Glycolysis preferentially inhibits ATP-sensitive K^+ channels in isolated guinea pig cardiac myocytes. *Science* 1987;**238**:67–9.

6. Kondo RP, Apstein CS, Eberli FR *et al*. Increased calcium loading and inotropy without greater cell death in hypoxic rat cardiomyocytes. *Am J Physiol* 1998;**275**:H2272–82.

7. Young, LH, Renfu, Y, Russell R *et al*. Low-flow ischemia leads to translocation of canine heart GLUT-4 and GLUT-1 glucose transporters to the sarcolemma in vivo. *Circulation* 1997;**95**;415–22.

8. King LM, Opie LH. Glucose delivery is a major determinant of glucose utilisation in the ischemic myocardium with a residual coronary flow. *Cardiovasc Res* 1998;**39**:381–92.

9. Christian TF, O'Connor MK, Schwartz RS *et al*. Technetium-99m MIBI to assess coronary collateral flow during acute myocardial infarction in two closed-chest animal models. *J Nucl Med* 1997;**38**:1840–6.

10. Milavetz GG, Giebel DW, Christian TF *et al*. Time to therapy and salvage in myocardial infarction. *J Am Coll Cardiol* 1998;**31**:1246–51.

11. Apstein CS. Glucose–insulin–potassium for acute myocardial infarction: remarkable results from a new prospective, randomized trial. *Circulation* 1998;**98**:2223–6.

12. Sowton E. Cardiac infarction and the glucose-tolerance test. *BMJ* 1962;i:84–86.

13. Opie LH. Metabolic response during impending myocardial infarction. I. Relevance of studies of glucose and fatty acid metabolism in animals. *Circulation* 1972;**45**:483–90.

14. Oliver MF, Opie LH. Effects of glucose and fatty acids on myocardial ischaemia and arrhythmias. *Lancet* 1994;**343**:155–8.

15. Gal J, Smith A, Riedel B, Royston D. Preservation and protection of myocardial function. *J Cardiothorac Vasc Anesth* 2000;**14(Suppl 1)**:22–36.

16. Medical Research Council working party on the treatment of myocardial infarction. Potassium, glucose and insulin treatment for acute myocardial infarction. *Lancet* 1968;**2**:1355–60.

17. Rackley CE, Russell RO Jr, Rogers WJ *et al*. Clinical experience with glucose-insulin-potassium therapy in acute myocardial infarction. *Am Heart J* 1981;**102**:1038–49.

18. Fath-Ordoubadi F, Beatt KJ. Glucose-insulin-potassium therapy for treatment of acute myocardial

infarction: an overview of randomized placebo-controlled trials. *Circulation* 1997;**96**:1152–6.

19. Apstein CS, Taegtmeyer H. Glucose-insulin-potassium in acute myocardial infarction: the time has come for a large, prospective trial. *Circulation* 1997;**96**:1074–7.

20. Diaz R, Paolasso EA, Piegas LS *et al* for the ECLA (Estudios Cardiologicos Latinoamerica) Collaborative Group. Metabolic modulation of acute myocardial infarction. *Circulation* 1998;**98**:2227–34.

21. Fath-Ordoubadi F, Beatt KJ. Glucose-insulin-potassium in acute myocardial infarction. *Lancet* 1999;**353**:1968.

22. Lazar HL, Philippides G, Fitzgerald C *et al*. Glucose-insulin-potassium solutions enhance recovery after urgent coronary artery bypass grafting. *J Thorac Cardiovasc Surg* 1997;**113**:354–60.

23. Girard C, Quentin P, Bouvier H *et al*. Glucose and insulin supply before cardiopulmonary bypass in cardiac surgery: a double-blind study. *Ann Thorac Surg* 1992;**54**:259–63.

24. Oldfield GS, Commerford PJ, Opie LH. Effects of preoperative glucose-insulin-potassium on myocardial glycogen levels and on complications of mitral valve replacement. *J Thorac Cardiovasc Surg* 1986;**91**:874–8.

25. Taegtmeyer H, Goodwin GW, Doenst T, Frazier OH. Substrate metabolism as a determinant for postischemic functional recovery of the heart. *Am J Cardiol* 1997;**80**:3A–10A.

26. Svedjeholm R, Hallhagen S, Ekroth T *et al*. Dopamine and high-dose insulin infusion (glucose-insulin-potassium) after a cardiac operation: effects on myocardial metabolism. *Ann Thorac Surg* 1991;**51**:262–70.

27. Svedjeholm R, Huljebrant I, Hakanson E, Vanhanen I. Glutamate and high-dose glucose-insulin-potassium (GIK) in the treatment of severe cardial failure after cardiac operations. *Ann Thorac Surg* 1995;**59**:S23–30.

19
Severe bronchospasm following cardiopulmonary bypass

Joseph E Arrowsmith

Introduction

Severe bronchospasm occurring at the end of cardiopulmonary bypass (CPB) is a fortunately rare but potentially fatal complication of cardiac surgery. The patient must be subjected to extra-corporeal support for an extended duration while the problem is treated. Weaning from CPB cannot be undertaken until adequate mechanical ventilation is re-established.

Case history 1

A 68-year-old Caucasian male presented 15 years after coronary artery bypass graft (CABG) surgery with a 2 year history of gradually worsening exertional (NYHA class III) angina and dyspnea. On the basis of the findings at cardiac catheterization the patient was offered repeat coronary revascularization.

On admission to hospital the day before surgery the patient gave a history of dyspnea, fever and a cough productive of purulent sputum. Examination of the chest revealed coarse bilateral basal inspiratory crackles.

Past medical history	CABG (×3) 15 years earlier, hypertension, hypercholesterolemia, Adult onset asthma, varicose veins, esophageal reflux. No known drug allergies.
Regular medications	Diltiazem SR 90 mg BD, bendrofluazide 2.5 mg OD, simvastatin 10 mg OD, aspirin 150 mg OD, prednisolone 5 mg OD, isorbide mononitrate SR 120 mg OD, glyceryl trinitrate 0.5 mg PRN, omeprazole 20 mg OD
Examination	Obese — weight 99 kg, BMI 29.9 kg m^{-2}. BP 110/70 mmHg. Sternal and leg scars consistent with previous CABG and varicose vein surgery.
Investigations	Hb 15.4 g dl^{-1}, WBC 10.9 ×10^9 l^{-1}, platelets 206 × 10^9 l^{-1} [Na$^+$] 139 mmol l^{-1}, [K$^+$] 3.8 mmol l^{-1}, urea 9.8 mmol l^{-1}, creatinine 1.5 mg dl^{-1} (132 µmol l^{-1}) **CXR:** Consistent with previous cardiac surgery, heart size normal, lungs clear. **ECG:** Sinus bradycardia. **Cardiac catheterization:** Vigorous left ventricle. Severe native coronary artery disease. Vein graft to first diagonal branch of the left anterior descending (LAD) coronary artery patent. Vein grafts to distal right and mid LAD coronary arteries occluded.

Surgery was postponed and the patient discharged home on antibiotics.

Two months later the patient was readmitted for surgery. The patient again gave a history of recent upper respiratory tract infection for which he had been prescribed co-amoxiclav (amoxycillin and potassium clavulanate), prednisolone 30 mg daily and nebulized salbutamol and ipratropium bromide. Apart from a healed sternotomy scar, examination of the chest on this occasion was unremarkable and it was agreed that surgery should go ahead as planned.

On the day of surgery the patient was premedicated with morphine sulfate 15 mg and hyoscine hydrobromide 0.3 mg IM an hour before transfer to the operating theater. On arrival in the anesthetic room a forearm vein and the right radial artery were cannulated under local anesthesia and an intravenous infusion of crystalloid and invasive arterial monitoring were established. In view of the history of esophageal reflux the patient was preoxygenated and a rapid sequence induction performed using diazepam 10 mg, fentanyl citrate 500 µg and succinylcholine 100 mg with cricoid pressure. Following tracheal intubation, the lungs were ventilated with 100% oxygen and neuromuscular blockade was prolonged with pancuronium bromide 12 mg. Anesthesia was maintained with propofol 4 mg kg^{-1} hr^{-1} and incremental doses of fentanyl. Following catheterization of the urinary bladder and cannulation of the right internal jugular vein with a triple-lumen catheter the patient was transferred to the operating room.

Full anticoagulation (Celite activated clotting time; ACT >450 s) with heparin sodium was achieved prior to sternotomy. Saphenous vein and both the left and right internal mammary arteries were harvested and, following division of pericardial adhesions, normothermic CPB (>35°C) was established between the right atrium and ascending aorta. A total of five coronary artery bypasses were fashioned using both antegrade and retrograde cold crystalloid (St Thomas' I) cardioplegia for myocardial protection.

Following completion of the proximal (aortic) anastamoses the surgeon asked for the lungs to be manually ventilated prior to separation from extracorporeal support. Both lungs were seen to inflate but showed no signs of significant deflation. A second inflation caused the lungs to bulge further into the operative field. The right

atrial pressure was not elevated and arterial pressure remained unchanged. Further attempts at ventilation were immediately abandoned and the breathing circuit was disconnected from the endotracheal tube.

Fiberoptic tracheobronchoscopy was performed to exclude mechanical obstruction of the proximal airways. The tip of the endotracheal tube was found to be well above the carina and there was no cuff herniation. The endobronchial anatomy was unremarkable — specifically there was no evidence of bronchial edema, mucosal erythema or mucous plugging.

Having excluded proximal airway obstruction, the gross pulmonary air-trapping observed was assumed to be secondary to acute bronchospasm. Dilute (1:100 000) epinephrine 100 µg was instilled into each main bronchus via the bronchoscope. Intravenous aminophylline 500 mg (in divided doses), ketamine 3 mg.kg^{-1} (in divided doses), magnesium sulfate 20 mmol, chlorpheniramine 10 mg, pancuronium 4 mg, hydrocortisone 100 mg, and epinephrine 15 µg (in divided doses) were then administered. Dopamine 2.5 µg kg^{-1} min^{-1}, epinephrine 0.05 µg kg^{-1} min^{-1} and salbutamol 4 µg kg^{-1} min^{-1} were administered by continuous IV infusion. Additional heparin was administered to maintain adequate anticoagulation and full CPB was continued.

Over the following 15 minutes the lungs gradually began to deflate. After another 15 minutes manual, and later mechanical, ventilation was cautiously restarted. Pulmonary compliance continued to improve such that 20 minutes later the patient could be easily weaned from CPB. The rest of the surgery was uneventful.

Following surgery the patient was transferred to the intensive care unit (ICU). On arrival ventilation with tidal volumes up to 850 ml was possible with peak airway pressures of only 22–24 cmH$_2$O. Arterial blood gases on 60% oxygen were pH 7.244, PaO$_2$ 182 mmHg (24 kPa), PaO$_2$/FiO$_2$ 304 mmHg (40 kPa), and PaCO$_2$ 48 mmHg (6.3 kPa). Auscultation of the chest revealed good air entry bilaterally but no audible wheeze. The intravenous infusions of dopamine, epinephrine and salbutamol were continued.

The following morning the patient was successfully weaned from mechanical ventilation and the trachea was finally extubated 16 hours after the end of surgery. The intravenous infusions were gradually reduced over the following 24 hours and the patient was discharged from the ICU the next day.

The remainder of the postoperative course was complicated by a transient ileus, fast atrial fibrillation, and frank pulmonary infection. A sternal wound infection required surgical debridement under general anesthesia on postoperative day 19. The patient was finally discharged home 38 days after his coronary revascularization. At an outpatient clinic visit some 5 weeks later the patient was reported to be making a slow but steady recovery.

Case history 2

A 69-year-old Caucasian female was admitted to hospital with a 3 week history of worsening paroxysmal nocturnal dyspnea and angina at rest (NYHA class IV). She was treated with intravenous heparin and nitrates and, following coronary angiography, referred for urgent CABG. Eighteen months earlier she had presented with exertional and nocturnal dyspnea and was referred to a cardiologist for investigation. She declined coronary angiography and underwent transthoracic echocardiography which revealed normal left ventricular function and trivial mitral regurgitation. A subsequent exercise 'Cardiolite' test revealed mild inferior posterobasal ischemia.

On the day of surgery, the patient was premedicated with methadone 10 mg by mouth 1 hour before transfer to the operating theater. On arrival in the anesthetic room, a peripheral venous crystalloid infusion was commenced. The patient was sedated with midazolam 4 mg and oxygen 4 l min^{-1} administered via nasal cannulae. Radial arterial pressure monitoring was established and a pulmonary artery catheter sited under local anesthesia. Arterial blood gas analysis revealed: pH 7.43, PO_2 70 mmHg (9.3 kPa), PCO_2 40.4 mmHg (5.4 kPa). The baseline Celite ACT was 189 s, consistent with preoperative heparin administration.

Following transfer to the operating room the patient was preoxygenated and anesthesia was induced with thiopental 125 mg, fentanyl 500 µg, and pancuronium 10 mg. The trachea was intubated and the lungs ventilated with oxygen and air (FiO_2 0.6–1.0). Anesthesia was maintained throughout the procedure with isoflurane (0.4–1.5% inspired) and incremental doses of fentanyl, midazolam and pancuronium. Infusions of dopamine 2.7 µg kg^{-1} min^{-1} and glyceryl trinitrate 170 µg min^{-1} were commenced and a multiplane transesophageal echocardiography (TEE) probe was placed in the esophagus without difficulty. Routine, prophylactic doses of cefuroxime 1.5 g were administered following induction of anesthesia and after separation from CPB.

Past medical history	Moderate/severe chronic airflow obstruction. Smoking – 8 pack per year history. Hemorrhoidectomy. Repair of right patellar fracture. Hypercholesterolemia. No previous anesthetic complications.
Regular medications	Hydrochlorothiazide 25 mg OD, metoprolol 50 mg OD, beclomethasone inhaler, albuterol inhaler, benazepril 20mg OD, atorvastatin 10 mg OD, estrogen/progesterone (PremPro) 0.625 mg/2.5 mg OD. Allergic to 'Sulfa' antibiotics.
Examination	Weight 78.5 kg. Height 1.63 m. BP 158/82 mmHg. No jugular venous distension. RR 18 min^{-1}. Large ventral hernia.
Investigations	[Na$^+$] 141 mmol l^{-1}, [K$^+$] 3.8 mmol l^{-1}, [Cl$^-$]101 mmol l^{-1}, [HCO$_3^-$] 28 mmol l^{-1}, urea 9 mmol l^{-1}, creatinine 0.8 mg dl^{-1} (70 µmol l^{-1}), glucose 88 mg dl^{-1} (4.9 mmol l^{-1}). Hb 13.5 g dl^{-1}, Hct 41%. **Spirometry:** FEV$_1$ 1.31 liters (58% predicted) **Carotid Doppler:** 80% left and 40% right internal carotid artery stenoses. **Left heart catheter:** Good LV function (EF ≥ 55 %). Complete occlusion of mid RCA, 75% stenoses of mid LAD and first diagonal branch. 50% left circumflex stenosis.

Surgery proceeded without incident. Following saphenous vein harvest and dissection of the left internal mammary, heparin 25 000 units (320 u kg^{-1}) was administered resulting in an ACT of 413 s. A further 15 000 units were required to achieve an ACT >480 s. A 10 g bolus of the lysine analogue, ε-aminocaproic acid was then administered followed by an infusion of 200 mg h^{-1}. Hypothermic (32°C) CPB was established between the right atrium and ascending aorta and three coronary bypass grafts fashioned using a single aortic cross-clamp technique and cold antegrade blood cardioplegia. After rewarming and removal of the aortic cross-clamp (ischemic time: 51 minutes), normal sinus rhythm was restored with lidocaine 200 mg and a single DC shock.

In preparation for separation from CPB, the lungs were ventilated with 100% oxygen. The lungs could be readily inflated but showed no signs of deflation. Further attempts at ventilation were abandoned and full CPB continued. Fiberoptic bronchoscopy revealed no obvious endobronchial abnormality and dilute (1:1 000 000) epinephrine (80 ml in total) was administered into the main bronchi. Intravenous heparin 5 000 units, hydrocortisone 100 mg, aminophylline 250mg, diphenhydramine 50 mg, ketamine 450 mg (in divided doses), magnesium sulfate 32 mmol (in divided doses), midazolam 2 mg, pancuronium 8 mg were administered and an infusion of epinephrine 1.25 μg kg^{-1} min^{-1} commenced. After 30 minutes, when the lungs had begun to deflate, pressure limited ventilation (30 cmH$_2$O, FiO$_2$ 1.0) was cautiously started. Exhaled tidal volumes gradually increased from 300 ml to 690 ml over the following 25 minutes at which time the patient was easily separated from CPB (total CPB time; 141 minutes) and protamine 350 mg administered without incident. At the request of the surgeon, procainamide (500 mg bolus and 120 mg h^{-1} by infusion) was administered for prophylaxis against atrial fibrillation. Arterial blood gas analysis at the end of the procedure revealed: pH 7.39, PO$_2$ 237 mmHg (31.6 kPa), PCO$_2$ 37.8 mmHg (5.0 kPa).

On arrival in the ICU, pulmonary compliance had improved sufficiently to allow the use volume controlled ventilation. Auscultation of the chest revealed good air entry and minimal bilateral expiratory wheeze. On the morning after surgery the patient was successfully weaned from mechanical ventilation and the infusions of dopamine and epinephrine discontinued. The patient subsequently made an uncomplicated recovery and was discharged home on the fifth postoperative day on aspirin, procainamide, frusemide, inhaled salbutamol and salmeterol, and a tapering dose of prednisolone. Four months later she underwent elective repair of her ventral hernia without complication.

Discussion

Severe bronchospasm following CPB has been described in both adults and children;[1] in native and transplanted lungs[2] in the presence[3, 4] and in the absence of a history of asthma or atopy,[5] and in patients who have had previously uneventful CPB. Most reports consistently describe high initial pulmonary inflation pressures, hyperinflation and inability to deflate the lungs immediately prior to the termination of CPB. A single case report describes bronchospasm in an asthmatic patient associated with cooling during the onset of CPB.[6] Features suggestive of anaphylactic or anaphylactoid reactions, marked arterial hypotension and cutaneous manifestations such as urticaria, erythema and edema, are invariably absent.

The small number of published reports describing the condition suggests that this is a rare phenomenon. In a series of 3714 cardiac surgical procedures undertaken in Strasbourg between 1978 and 1983, severe bronchospasm following CPB was noted on six (0.16%) occasions.[7] Interestingly, one patient developed the condition twice within the same year.

Possible etiologies include: products of complement activation[5, 8] reflex bronchiolar muscle contraction secondary to inadequate or 'light' anesthesia,[8] prolonged CPB, the cold urticaria syndrome,[9] exacerbation of preoperative bronchospastic disease, mitral stenosis,[7, 10, 11] allergic reactions to drugs or blood products,[1, 8] and β-adrenergic blockade.[12] Given that the first patient, described above, had undergone CPB without incident 15 years earlier it was speculated that the history of recurrent respiratory tract infection was, at least in part, a contributory factor. In most cases however, the precise etiology is unknown.

An acute allergic reaction to an anesthetic drug, an antimicrobial agent, an intravenous colloid solution, a component of the priming and/or cardioplegia solution, a blood product or latex may cause severe bronchospasm. While protamine sulfate and commonly used antibiotics are the most likely causes of allergic reactions in this setting neither can be reasonably implicated. In most cases antibiotics were given without incident after induction of anesthesia and bronchospasm was noted *before* protamine administration. Severe bronchospasm in the absence of cutaneous manifestations, airway edema, stridor, hypotension or dysrhythmia in most reported cases would tend to suggest a mechanism other than allergy.

A further interesting case is that of a 64-year-old man who had received cimetidine 400 mg and labetalol 650 mg prior to coronary artery surgery.[12] Arterial hypotension, which proved unresponsive to phenylephrine (total dose 14 mg), persisted throughout the first hour of CPB. During rewarming however, mean arterial pressure gradually rose to 150 mmHg. At the termination of CPB, severe bronchospasm was observed. The authors concluded that the arterial hypotension observed was a result of reduced labetalol clearance secondary to the effects of hypothermia and cimetidine administration. The severe and protracted bronchospasm were attributed to the combination of labetalol induced β-adrenoceptor antagonism and phenylephrine-induced α-adrenoceptor agonism.

The hallmark of the cold urticaria syndrome is well-circumscribed wheals with raised, erythematous borders. The condition, which is usually innocuous, is caused by IgE-dependent mast cell degranulation triggered by cold exposure. In addition to skin wheals, life-threatening hypotension, bronchospasm and/or laryngeal edema may occur in some patients.[1, 9] The management of patients with the condition who require CPB has been previously reported.[13]

Most authors conclude that bronchospasm following CPB should be diagnosed only after other causes of failure to inflate and/or deflate the lungs have been excluded. Extracorporeal support should be continued until adequate mechanical ventilation can be re-established. Continued attempts to ventilate may cause pulmonary barotrauma or disrupt an internal mammary artery graft.[14] A mechanical cause of acute pulmonary venous congestion should be excluded: compression of the left atrium by a retained swab may result in raised airway pressures and arterial hypotension.[15] After excluding a malfunction of the ventilator and/or breathing system most authors report proceeding rapidly to bronchoscopy. The fiberoptic bronchoscope allows examination of the proximal airways, aspiration of secretions under direct vision and endobronchial administration of drugs.

The goals of therapy in this situation are to reverse the bronchospasm, re-establish mechanical ventilation and separate the patient from extracorporeal support. In most published reports a favorable clinical outcome has followed the near simultaneous administration of several bronchodilator drugs into the airway, subcutaneously and into the circulation. Specific mention of deepening of anesthesia and the administration of supplemental doses of opioids and neuromuscular blocking drugs is made by a few authors. In a review of 23 published cases, Ecoff and colleagues noted that reported therapies have included: inhalational anesthetic agents (sevoflurane, isoflurane, enflurane, and halothane); β-adrenoceptor agonists (epinephrine, dopamine, terbutaline, salbutamol and isoprenaline); corticosteroids; aminophylline; antihistamines (cimetidine, ranitidine and diphenhydramine); and other drugs such as atropine, frusemide, lidocaine, and ketamine.[1] The use of magnesium sulfate in the cases described is novel in this setting but by no means its first reported use in the treatment of acute bronchospasm.[16]

Conclusions and learning points

- Severe bronchospasm is a rare, but potentially life-threatening sequel of CPB.
- Cases of severe bronchospasm following CPB have been reported in both adults and children.
- Severe bronchospasm following CPB frequently occurs in the absence of cardiovascular collapse and other manifestations of an acute allergic reaction such as edema, urticaria and cutaneous vasodilatation.
- Severe bronchospasm following CPB has been reported in patients with a history of

asthma or atopy. In many cases however, there is no readily identifiable etiology.

- Full anticoagulation and CPB should be maintained.
- Further attempts to establish adequate ventilation should be resisted. Continued ventilation in the face of severe bronchospasm and air-trapping may result in severe pulmonary barotrauma and/or damage to local structures such as a left internal mammary artery graft.
- The immediate administration of several types of bronchodilator is associated with a favorable outcome.
- A diagnosis of bronchospasm should only be made after excluding other reasons for failure to re-establish mechanical ventilation prior to separation from cardiopulmonary bypass.

Acknowledgements

The author thanks Ajeet D Sharma, MD for his assistance in the preparation of this chapter, and R Duane Davis, MD and Stephen R Large FRCP FRCS for their permission to publish case history details.

References

1. Ecoff SA, Miyahara C, Steward DJ. Severe bronchospasm during cardiopulmonary bypass. *Can J Anaesth* 1996;**43**:1244–8.

2. Casella ES, Humphrey LS. Bronchospasm after cardiopulmonary bypass in a heart-lung transplant recipient. *Anesthesiology* 1988;**69**:135–8.

3. Buckingham RE Jr, Rogers TR, Sampson IH. Case 1989–1. A 55-year-old male undergoing CABG develops severe bronchospasm at the end of cardiopulmonary bypass. *J Cardiothorac Anesth* 1989;**3**: 9–18.

4. Neustein SM, Bronheim D. Severe bronchospasm following cardiopulmonary bypass in an asthmatic. *J Cardiothorac Vasc Anesth* 1992;**6**:609–11.

5. Hentz JG, De Armendi AJ, Schaeffer R. A new case of bronchospasm under extracorporeal circulation. *Ann Fr Anesth Reanim* 1986;**5**:157–9. [French]

6. Simpson JI, Eide TR, Clagnaz JF. Cold-induced bronchospasm during coronary artery bypass surgery. *Anesthesiology* 1993;**79**:180–3.

7. Hentz J, Levy M, Bauer MC et al. Bronchospasm during extracorporeal circulation. *Ann Fr Anesth Reanim* 1984;**3**:219–24. [French]

8. Shiroka A, Rah KH, Keenan RL. Bronchospasm during cardiopulmonary bypass. *Anesth Analg* 1982;**61**:538–40.

9. Tuman KJ, Ivankovich AD. Bronchospasm during cardiopulmonary bypass. Etiology and management. *Chest* 1986;**90**:635–7.

10. Vanetti A, Andrivet S, Razafinombana A et al. Severe bronchial spasm during heart surgery under extracorporeal circulation *Ann Chir Thorac Cardiovasc* 1973;**12**:163–4. [French]

11. Inoue Y, Fukutome T, Uehara J, Koujiro M. Severe bronchospasm induced by extracorporeal circulation for cardiac surgery. *Masui* 1994;**43**:395–9. [Japanese]

12. Durant PA, Joucken K. Bronchospasm and hypotension during cardiopulmonary bypass after preoperative cimetidine and labetalol therapy. *Br J Anaesth* 1984;**56**:917–20.

13. Johnston WE, Moss J, Philbin DM et al. Management of cold urticaria during hypothermic cardiopulmonary bypass. *New Engl J Med* 1982;**306**:219–21

14. Kyosola K, Takkunen O, Maamies T et al. Bronchospasm during cardiopulmonary bypass: a potentially fatal complication of open-heart surgery. *Thorac Cardiovasc Surg* 1987;**35**:375–7.

15. Hardy PA. Bronchospasm and hypotension following cardiopulmonary bypass. *Br J Anaesth* 1985;**57**:720–1.

16. Mills R, Leadbeater M, Ravalia A. Intravenous magnesium sulphate in the management of refractory bronchospasm in a ventilated asthmatic. *Anaesthesia* 1997;**52**:782–5.

20
Neurological complications of cardiopulmonary bypass

Michael J O'Leary and David J Bihari

Introduction

Although improvements in surgical, perfusion and anesthetic techniques have led to a reduction in the morbidity and mortality associated with cardiac surgery, neurological injury remains an important cause of postoperative morbidity and is responsible for an increasing proportion of perioperative deaths. Despite knowledge of many of the risk factors associated with the development of neurological complications after cardiac surgery there are, as yet, few effective preventative strategies, other than the prevention of hypoxia and hypotension, which can be employed. Management of patients with neurological injury following cardiac surgery is essentially supportive, however these patients present a specific management challenge to their physicians to deliver care that ensures the chance of recovery is optimized whilst not producing severely brain damaged survivors with poor quality of life. In a number of cases the ethical dilemmas of withholding and withdrawing treatment may need to be visited.

Case history

A 78-year-old male presented for coronary artery bypass graft surgery. He had a past history of an inferior myocardial infarct 10 years previously and a 6-month history of exertional angina with dyspnea on walking 100 meters. The electrocardiogram suggested an old inferior transmural infarction and left ventricular hypertrophy. Cardiac catheterization revealed severe triple vessel coronary artery disease and good left ventricular function.

A standard anesthetic technique was used. Premedication was with morphine 10 mg and midazolam 2.5 mg IM an hour before transfer to theater. A radial artery cannula, peripheral venous cannula and subclavian triple-lumen central venous catheter were inserted under local anesthesia. Following preoxygenation, anesthesia was induced with thiopental 100 mg, fentanyl 0.5 mg and pancuronium 12 mg, and the trachea intubated with a size 9.0 cuffed endotracheal tube. Anesthesia was maintained with isoflurane ≤1% (inspired) in oxygen and nitrous oxide (FiO_2 0.3), and incremental doses of fentanyl (total 2.5 mg including induction dose) until cardiopulmonary bypass (CPB) was instituted when isoflurane was replaced with propofol 4 mg kg^{-1} hour^{-1}.

Saphenous vein and the left internal mammary artery were harvested. Full anticoagulation (target Celite activated clotting time >450 seconds) with heparin was achieved. The proximal aorta was found to be grossly atheromatous with multiple areas of calcification and the surgeon reported considerable difficulty identifying a suitable position to place the aortic cross-clamp and aortic root cardioplegia cannula using digital examination. However, sites were eventually located that seemed to be free of disease and hypothermic (32°C), non-pulsatile CPB was established between the right atrium and ascending aorta. Antegrade cold crystalloid (St Thomas' I) cardioplegia was used for myocardial protection and a total of four coronary artery bypass grafts were performed. Spontaneous

Past medical history	Hypertension for 20 years. Left hemisphere cerebrovascular accident 2 years previously with good recovery. Hypercholesterolemia.
Regular medications	Atenolol 50 mg OD, lisinopril 10 mg OD, aspirin 150 mg OD, simvastatin 20 mg OD, isorbide dinitrate 30 mg TDS, glyceryl trinitrate 0.5 mg PRN
Examination	Weight 92 kg, Height 1.75 m. BMI 30 kg m^{-2}. Pulse 60 min^{-1} regular, BP 145/85 mmHg. No carotid bruits. No abnormality on neurological examination.
Investigations	Blood count within normal limits. [Na$^+$] 140 mmol l^{-1}, [K$^+$] 4.1 mmol l^{-1}, urea 24 mg dl^{-1} (8.5 mmol l^{-1}), creatinine 1.7 mg dl^{-1} (150 μmol l^{-1}) **CXR**: Heart size at upper limit of normal, lung fields clear. **ECG**: Sinus bradycardia. Voltage criteria for left ventricular hypertrophy, Q waves in leads II, III and aVF. **Carotid Doppler ultrasound**: Normal. **Cardiac catheterization**: Left anterior descending (LAD) artery — long 50% proximal stenosis and two 80% distal stenoses. Circumflex artery — 50% proximal stenosis and occlusion of the first obtuse marginal branch at its origin with slow retrograde filling. Right coronary artery — 90% proximal stenosis. Distal vessels were diffusely diseased. Left ventricular function was good. Mild mitral regurgitation.

return of cardiac activity occurred upon rewarming. Separation from CPB was aided with a low-dose epinephrine infusion ($\leq$1.5 μg min^{-1}). The total CPB and aortic cross-clamp times were 90 and 55 minutes, respectively. The remainder of the surgical procedure was uneventful. Following CPB the lungs were ventilated with oxygen in air (FiO$_2$ 0.3) and propofol by infusion was continued until delivery of the patient to the intensive care unit (ICU).

The patient arrived in the ICU still anesthetized. The propofol infusion was discontinued and a morphine infusion commenced at 2 mg h^{-1}. The epinephrine infusion was weaned off over 20 minutes. Nasopharyngeal temperature was 34.5°C and active rewarming was instituted using warmed intravenous fluids and a forced warm-air blanket (Bair Hugger, Actamed, Wakefield, UK). Three hours after admission to the ICU the blood pressure climbed to 160/70 mmHg, and an infusion of sodium nitroprusside (SNP) was commenced; however, this was weaned over the next 6 hours. Five hours following admission to the ICU the bedside nurse contacted the ICU resident as she was concerned that the patient 'was not waking up'.

On examination the patient was still endotracheally intubated but breathing spontaneously on 10 cmH$_2$O pressure support and 5 cmH$_2$O positive end expiratory pressure. The morphine infusion had been discontinued 1 hour previously. The patient opened his eyes to voice but would not obey commands. The best motor response was flexion of the upper limbs and withdrawal of the lower limbs to painful stimulus, but not localizing (Glasgow Coma Score (GCS) 6'T' — E3, V-intubated 'T', M3). Pupils were both small and reactive. He was generally hypertonic with uniformly brisk reflexes and bilateral extensor plantar responses. Cardiovascular examination was unremarkable with a blood pressure of 125/75 mmHg with SNP 83 μg min^{-1}. Respiratory and abdominal examinations were within normal limits for a patient in the early postoperative phase following cardiac surgery. Cranial computed tomography (CT), performed the following morning, showed evidence of an old left lacunar infarct and a small left parietal infarct with no acute changes.

The patient's condition was essentially unchanged 18 hours after surgery. He opened his eyes to voice and his best motor response was weak flexion to deep painful stimuli. There was persistent, generalized hypertonicity. No further opiates or sedatives were given. Breathing was spontaneous on pressure support ventilation.

Mediastinal and pleural blood loss was minimal and the drains were removed as per protocol. A nasogastric tube was inserted and nasogastric feeding commenced. Atenolol 50 mg daily and aspirin 150 mg daily were recommenced.

A conference was held with his wife, son and daughter. The patient's son explained that in recent months his father's quality of life had been significantly reduced by both angina and severe dyspnea. He had decided to proceed with surgery because he had become so dissatisfied with life as it was. He claimed that his father would not accept life severely limited by neurological disability and was keen to receive an estimate of the prognosis of his father's condition. The cardiac surgeon explained that in these cases, the prognosis is always uncertain, that significant improvement often occurs and that, in his opinion full support should continue.

A neurologist was asked to review the patient. His impression was that the patient's condition was consistent with either global cerebral hypoxia or multiple cerebral emboli and that the prognosis was guarded. He commented that the patient would be unlikely to survive if extubated, but that this might be a valid management option. A magnetic resonance imaging (MRI) scan of the brain demonstrated multiple bilateral cerebral and cerebellar infarcts in the posterior frontal and parietal lobes, the occipital lobes bilaterally, the deep periventricular white matter, the head of the caudate nucleus on the left, the temporal lobe on the right and the cerebellar hemispheres on both sides. Emboli were thought the most likely cause for these changes.

The family were initially keen that the patient be extubated and kept comfortable; however, on the morning of the third post-operative day he was found to be able to obey commands by hand-squeezing on both sides. The patient's wife was now not comfortable with limiting treatment. A percutaneous tracheostomy was performed and the nasogastric tube replaced with a fine-bore tube and he was successfully weaned from the ventilator over the next 12 hours and discharged to the ward.

Ten days later he was able to stand with assistance, had a strong cough and was mouthing words. He was cortically blind. To facilitate aspiration of secretions, the tracheostomy was removed and a minitracheostomy inserted. After 4 weeks the patient was discharged to a rehabili-tation unit. His blindness had improved to bitem-poral hemianopias, he had good upper limb power (4/5 on the right, 3/5 on the left) but poor co-ordination. He was able to walk with assistance and speak occasional words.

Discussion

Neurological injury remains a relatively common complication after CPB. Whilst damage may occur to the brain, spinal cord or peripheral nervous system this discussion will be limited to intracranial pathology only. The spectrum of intracranial neurological injury ranges from major neurological deficit (such as stroke), which is thankfully relatively rare, with a reported incidence of about 3%,[1] to subtle neuropsycho-logical changes, only detectable with specific testing, which may be present in up to 90% of patients one week following operation.[2] In the early weeks following cardiac surgery depres-sion has been reported to occur with a frequency of up to 20%.[3, 4] Some have suggested that this incidence mainly reflects the high prevalence of depression in patients awaiting cardiac surgery,[4] although this remains controversial. The presence of depressive illness may make evalua-tion of cognitive impairment difficult. There does not, however, appear to be a correlation between depression and cognitive decline per se, which suggests that depression alone cannot account for cognitive decline.[4] The incidence of cognitive decline at 3 months has been reported as being up to 50% by which time it is likely to be perma-nent.[5] For the purposes of this discussion the terms 'neurological injury' or 'neurological deficit' will be used to encompass all types of adverse neurological or neuropsychological outcomes.

Management of major neurological injury following cardiac surgery

As in the case presented, most cases of major neurological injury associated with cardiac surgery and CPB present acutely in the immedi-ate postoperative period as failure to awaken from anesthesia. Common clinical features are cerebral obtundation, hypertonicity and seizures. A minority of cases will present later during the postoperative period following initial lucid interval or uneventful recovery, usually as the development of transient ischemic attack, stroke or reduced level of consciousness. In the former group, the cause of the deficit will be either embolic phenomena or cerebral hypoperfusion and unfortunately there are presently no specific therapeutic interventions that can be offered to these patients. In the latter group, intracardiac thrombi and aortic plaque fissure and thrombus generation are the important sources of emboli. The presence of perioperative atrial fibrillation (AF) is closely associated with the subsequent development of stroke. New onset AF increases the risk of stroke two to three-fold, and the role of anticoagulants in this setting is unclear. Early cardioversion within 24 hours of the onset of the arrhythmia can probably be safely performed without anticoagulation, however anticoagulants should be commenced if AF persists beyond 48 hours.[6]

Imaging techniques offer diagnostic and, possibly, prognostic information, and rarely need to be performed urgently except where intracranial hemorrhage is suspected. Clinical features suggestive of intracranial hemorrhage include lateralizing neurological signs or signs of raised intracranial pressure. A high index of suspicion should prevail, of course, in those receiving therapeutic anticoagulation. Patients with confirmed intracranial hemorrhage should be considered for urgent surgical evacuation. Early CT scanning of the brain will almost universally be performed. Scans obtained within 24 hours of injury may frequently appear 'normal' in the presence of embolism or infarction, with lesions only becoming visible on repeat scanning after 48 hours. The distribution and extent of lesions may permit some prediction of the degree of neurological deficit, but give no information regarding likely functional recovery. MRI may allow earlier quantification of cerebral damage. In particular, diffusion-weighted and perfusion-weighted cerebral blood flow imaging may in the future allow more precise identification of early injury, better characterization of regional blood flow and identification of cerebral edema secondary to hypoxia or ischemia[7] Whilst this information may usefully guide local or general thrombolytic therapies in the general clinical

setting of stroke it is at present unclear how this information might affect treatment or prognosis in stroke following cardiac surgery. Of interest, in a study investigating changes on MRI in association with CPB 60% of patients had age-related or ischemic changes on the preoperative examination.[8] In this study there were no adverse neurological outcomes and no changes seen on serial perioperative MRI.

In the absence of a surgical lesion, management is essentially supportive with attention to the airway, oxygenation, ventilation and hemodynamic stability. The significant risk of hemorrhage from the surgical site precludes the use of thrombolytic agents such a streptokinase or tissue plasminogen activator.[7] Cardiac arrhythmias should be controlled, and echocardiography performed to exclude an intracardiac source of emboli, the presence of which should mandate systemic anticoagulation. Seizures, when they occur, should be controlled with anticonvulsant medication. Myoclonus suggests a profound cerebral hypoxic injury and is commonly difficult to control. Although commonly advocated as a treatment for myoclonus, clonazepam is in our experience rarely effective. Piracetam has been shown to be effective in the treatment of myoclonus of differing etiologies, including acute stroke[9, 10] and may, therefore, be considered. Baclofen may help reduce muscle spasm in chronic cases but is rarely indicated in the acute phase. In general, the natural history of myoclonic seizures in the setting of cerebral hypoxic injury is for spontaneous resolution within 24–36 hours. Electroencephalography may be warranted in individual cases. The presence of fever should prompt a search for infection, however, as fever itself may be harmful to the injured brain antipyretics such as paracetamol or aspirin should be given, and in selected cases the use of more aggressive cooling strategies such as a cooling blanket may be indicated.[11]

The outcome from major neurological injury following cardiac surgery is very variable. Significant recovery, even from apparently extensive lesions on initial presentation has been frequently described. A major neurological injury is none the less a devastating complication of cardiac surgery, which presents major challenges to the patient, their relatives and the cardiac surgical team. Elderly patients are often quite aware that their decision to undergo surgery has a risk attached, however this decision is frequently made because they believe their current quality of life to be unacceptable. Similarly, survival with severe neurological disability may therefore be wholly unacceptable to many of these patients. Unfortunately it is often not possible to directly ascertain the patient's wishes at this time. It is important to hold an early 'case conference' with the family, intensivists, the surgical team and, where appropriate, neurologists and rehabilitation specialists to make a plan for on-going care and set management limits. It should not be forgotten that the physician's primary responsibility is to the patient and that decisions should be made in the light of what is known about the patient's aspirations and their premorbid health and functional status, balanced with realistic prognostic estimates of likely temporary and permanent disabilities.

Approximately half of deaths following stroke will be due to medical complications. Ongoing airway management is perhaps the major supportive issue for many of these patients. Cerebral obtundation is frequent, and inability to cough, swallow and clear secretions adequately predisposes to nosocomial pneumonia which is the most common mechanism leading to death. Where the neurological injury is devastating and the patient's premorbid condition poor, it may be appropriate to wean from mechanical ventilatory support, extubate the trachea and provide comfort care only. Otherwise, a definitive airway and secretion management strategy is needed. The introduction of percutaneous tracheostomy procedures into intensive care practice has simplified management of these patients.[12] This procedure can be performed by the intensive care specialist at the bedside; it has advantages over minitracheostomy in that a cuffed tube of large internal diameter is used. This allows safe administration of nasogastric or oral feeding, easy access for mechanical ventilatory support when required and optimum secretion management. Moreover, percutaneous tracheostomy has been shown to be associated with a reduced incidence of postoperative complications such as hemorrhage and late infection when compared with a standard surgical approach,[13] and tracheostomy does not appear to increase the risk of sternotomy infection or mediastinitis.[14]

Early introduction of enteral nutrition via a nasoenteric tube has been shown to reduce infectious morbidity in a variety of populations of patients with critical illness[15] and should be employed.

Etiology of neurological injury following cardiopulmonary bypass

Perhaps the factor most strongly predictive of adverse neurological outcome following cardiac surgery employing CPB is patient age[1] (Table 20.1). In recent years the average age of patients undergoing cardiac surgical procedures has increased steadily. The influence of age on outcome is in all probability multifactorial. Elderly patients may have a reduction in baseline cerebral function, and in the presence of pre-existing limitations to normal cerebral function even minor new impairments of neurological or neuropsychological functioning are likely to have significant impact and thus to come to the attention of attending physicians. Furthermore, the incidence of previous cerebrovascular events is higher in an elderly population and patients who have suffered previous stroke or transient ischemic attack are more likely to sustain a perioperative stroke.[16] Elderly patients are much more likely to have significant aortic and cerebrovascular atherosclerotic disease than are young patients, factors also shown to be predictive of neurological injury.

Whilst there are many factors contributing to neurological dysfunction after cardiac surgery, cerebral hypoperfusion and cerebral embolization are the most important factors implicated. Cerebral hypoperfusion, as judged by jugular venous oxygen desaturation, has been demonstrated to occur during the rewarming phase of CPB, and to be associated with postoperative cognitive decline.[17] Hypoperfusion may not always be associated with reduced cerebral blood flow (CBF). Cerebral blood flow measured by xenon (^{133}Xe) clearance is reduced during CPB but increased in the postoperative period,[18] whereas jugular venous desaturation was shown to continue postoperatively. Although intuitively the presence of hypotension or hypoperfusion of the brain ought to correlate with poor neurological outcome, in practice there is little evidence to

Table 20.1 Risk factors for neurological injury following cardiopulmonary bypass

Patient factors	Operative factors

Age	Cerebral macroembolism
	  Aortic atheromatous disease
	  Carotid disease

Male sex	

(Although females have worse outcome overall after cardiac surgery this may primarily reflect higher risk profiles. Risk stratified, male sex is an independent predictor of worse neurological outcome)	Cerebral microembolism
	  Gas bubbles
	  Particulate matter:
	  coagulation component aggregates, fat, calcium, cellular aggregates, atheroma, valve debris, foreign matter from surgical material and bypass circuit

Poor LV function	Valve surgery

Prior cerebrovascular disease, occult or manifest.
  Symptomatic or significant carotid stenosis
	Cerebral hypoperfusion
	  Perfusion pressure
	  Cerebral blood flow

Diabetes mellitus	Hyperglycemia
Genetic factors (Apolipoprotein E e4 allele)	Temperature (?hypothermia protective)
Reduced baseline cognitive function	pH-stat blood gas management
	Nitric oxide generation
	Glutamate excitotoxicity
	Systemic inflammatory response

support targeting any specific perfusion pressure, flow level or flow characteristic over any other. A causal relationship between long CPB duration and the development of neurological deficit has been suggested by some workers; however, in most cases long CPB duration reflects greater complexity of the surgical procedure. Use of hypothermia as part of the myocardial protection strategy during CPB has potential cerebral protective advantages. Recent interest in warm perfusion techniques have led to the concern that they might be associated with increased risk of neurological deficit, and there is some evidence to suggest this may be the case.[19] Finally, the employment of 'α-stat' versus 'pH-stat' acid–base management may theoretically reduce the risk of neurological deficit (Table 20.2). Pressure-flow autoregulation in the cerebral circulation is better maintained during moderate hypothermia when α-stat acid–base management is employed compared with the use of pH-stat management. There are a number of clinical studies confirming fewer major neurological adverse outcomes when the α-stat approach is employed,[20] however

one study has reported more cognitive impairment in patients with bypass times greater than 90 minutes managed using the α-stat approach.[21]

Macroembolism is most likely the cause of major neurological injuries such as stroke. Macroemboli can arise from atheromatous aortic plaques, intracardiac air or thrombus and calcific debris dislodged during valve excision. There is a recognized relationship between aortic atheromatous disease and cerebral embolization during cardiac surgery, and atheroembolism from aortic plaque is thought to be responsible for approximately one-third of strokes after coronary bypass grafting.[6] Aortic cross-clamping, cannulation through an aortic plaque and 'scouring' of the aortic wall during perfusion may all cause embolization. Preoperative, non-invasive testing to identify high-risk patients has variable accuracy. The intraoperative use of transesophageal echocardiography (TEE) or epicardial ultrasound, however, may allow identification of significant plaques such that they may be safely avoided. In severe disease, a no 'cross-clamp' fibrillation strategy or a 'beating heart' non-CPB

Table 20.2 Principle of (α-stat versus pH-stat blood gas management strategies during cardiopulmonary bypass

pH-stat	α-stat
As temperature falls $\downarrow$ $PaCO_2$ & $\uparrow$ pH	Optimum pH during cooling $\equiv$ Elecrochemical neutrality of water
Blood gas electrodes measure at 37°C	(pH of water rises linearly maintaining constant $[OH^-]:[H^+]$ ratio)
	Maintenance of this ratio preserves charged state of α-imidazole buffers
	$\Rightarrow$ optimum enzyme function and maintenance of cell volume
Correct pH to 7.4 at patient temperature	Correct to pH 7.4 at 37°C
$\Rightarrow$ hypercapnia & acidosis at electrode temperature	$\Rightarrow$ CO_2 rapidly diffuses into cells $\Rightarrow$ pH reflected intracellularly
$\uparrow$ cerebral blood flow with cooling	Cerebral autoregulation maintained

strategy may need to be employed. The risk of stroke is significantly greater in patients undergoing valve surgery in comparison with coronary artery grafting alone.[22]

Gas or particulate emboli are a virtually universal feature of CPB and there is evidence that the incidence of postoperative neuropsychiatric dysfunction correlates with microembolic load.[23] It is common to observe air bubbles with TEE in association with aortic cannulation, and gas bubbles may be generated within the extracorporeal circuit throughout the bypass period from the blood–gas interface and related to perfusion events such as when the perfusionist is sampling or flushing from the CPB circuit. Particulate emboli are most frequently seen in association with aortic manipulations but may also occur due to blood component aggregates, debris from the operative site (e.g. thrombus, tissue) and occasionally particulate debris from the extracorporeal circuit (e.g. polyvinyl chloride or silicone particles) or surgical site (e.g. swab fibers). Lipid microembolization may be associated with the use of cardiotomy suction.[24] The amount of gaseous and particulate microemboli reaching the brain can be quantified by transcranial Doppler sonography of the middle cerebral artery.[23] The use of a 40 μm arterial line filter in the CPB circuit and use of membrane rather than bubble oxygenators may help reduce microembolization.

Several other factors have been implicated in post-CPB neurological dysfunction including genetic predisposition and hyperglycemia (Table 20.1).[25] Patients with diabetes mellitus appear to do worse following stroke in general, a finding which has been linked to an effect of hyperglycemia on the injured brain. Hyperglycemia appears to worsen neurological outcome in both global and focal cerebral ischemia. Most centres now avoid the use of glucose-containing priming solutions in the bypass circuit, and intraoperative hyperglycemia is treated aggressively with insulin. It is not known, however, if there is a threshold blood glucose level above which treatment is mandatory. Diabetic patients require careful monitoring in the perioperative period when undergoing cardiac surgery to ensure control of hyperglycemia and because of their high incidence of hypertension, vascular and renal disease.

The incidence of neurological deficit following cardiopulmonary bypass has been prospectively evaluated by Roach and colleagues.[1] In their study population non-fatal stroke, transient ischemic attack, stupor or coma at time of discharge, or death caused by stroke or hypoxic encephalopathy had an incidence of 3.1%. Independent risk factors identified for these outcomes were proximal aortic atherosclerosis, past history of neurological disease, use of intraaortic balloon counterpulsation, diabetes mellitus, history of hypertension, unstable angina and age (Table 20.3). Neuropsychiatric changes (defined as new deterioration in intellectual function, confusion, agitation, disorientation, memory deficit or seizure without evidence of focal injury) also occurred in 3% of patients, however these definitions appear to represent more severe injury than the cognitive changes studied by other workers and reported to occur with much greater frequency. Risk factors for adverse neuropsychiatric outcomes were different to those associated with major neurological deficit and included age, hypertension on admission (systolic blood pressure >180 mmHg or administration of antihypertensive medication), alcohol abuse, previous coronary artery surgery and history of cardiac arrhythmia. Of interest, these authors were unable to demonstrate a relationship between adverse neurological or neuropsychiatric outcomes and perioperative hypotension.

Detection and management of reversible conditions that may cause or worsen poor neurological outcome following CPB is clearly an important goal. The presence of a carotid bruit or demonstration of carotid artery stenosis by angiography or by Doppler sonography may be associated with increased risk of perioperative stroke (up to 20% with a greater than 80% stenosis). It appears that the risk of stroke is only moderately increased by the presence of asymptomatic carotid disease however, with factors such as embolism or hypoperfusion being more important. Which patients will benefit from preoperative carotid screening therefore remains controversial.[6] Patients who are elderly, female, have peripheral vascular disease, past history of TIA or stroke or have left main stem coronary disease are at increased risk of significant carotid stenosis. Most commonly carotid and cardiac operations will be performed in a staged manner, although recently a combined approach has gained favor. Increased rate of stroke is found if the carotid surgery is delayed to follow the cardiac operation.

Since it appears that most of the neurological injury seen after cardiac surgery has its etiology in the technique and management of CPB, there is increasing interest in undertaking CABG on a beating heart without CPB. This surgical technique avoids aortic cross-clamping and aortic cannulation; however, partial aortic clamping is still required for the proximal coronary anastomoses. Two non-randomized studies comparing traditional surgery using CPB with 'beating heart' operations have been published, with conflicting results. Murkin and colleagues found that patients undergoing 'beating heart' operations demonstrated a reduction in cognitive impairment (50 vs 5%) 3 months after surgery.[26] The CPB group had a greater number of coronary anastomoses performed than the 'beating heart' group, however, which suggests a greater overall degree of atherosclerotic disease and thus higher risk of neurological dysfunction per se. In contrast, Taggart and colleagues showed no advantage of 'beating heart' operations on cognitive outcome.[27] 'Beating heart' CABG surgery does seem to be associated with markedly reduced cerebral microembolic load[28] and possibly less cerebral injury, as assessed by reduced circulating levels of serum astroglial protein $S100\beta$.[29] It should be noted, however, that $S100\beta$ is released from sites other than the brain. Not all patients requiring CABG will be suitable for 'beating heart' surgery, however, as coronary lesions must be technically suitably positioned. Moreover, there are still few adequate trials confirming that comparable

Table 20.3 Adjusted odds ratios (95% confidence intervals) for major neurological injury and neuropsychiatric changes associated with selected risk factors. Adapted with permission from Roach et al[1]

Risk factor	Major neurological injury	Neuropsychiatric changes
Aortic atherosclerosis	4.53 (2.52–8.09)	
Past cerebrovascular event	3.19 (1.65–6.15)	
Intra-aortic balloon counterpulsation	2.60 (1.21–5.58)	
Diabetes mellitus	2.59 (1.46–4.60)	
Hypertension or systolic BP >180 mmHg	2.31 (1.20–4.47)	3.47 (1.41–8.55)
Unstable angina	1.83 (1.03–3.27)	
Age (per additional decade)	1.75 (1.27–2.43)	2.20 (1.60–3.02)
Previous coronary surgery		2.18 (1.14–4.17)
Alcohol abuse		2.64 (1.27–5.47)
Arrhythmia on day of surgery		1.97 (1.12–3.46)

quality revascularization can be achieved with 'beating heart' surgery. To answer the question whether this operative technique is truly associated with better neurological outcome will require large randomized controlled trials.

Pharmacologic strategies to prevent neurological injury

It might be anticipated that CPB would provide an ideal situation in which neuroprotective strategies could be employed as the potential agent can be administered before the neurological insult occurs. There is a wealth of literature describing potential neuroprotective pharmacological strategies for patients subjected to CPB; however none has as yet entered routine clinical practice. Thiopental reduces cerebral metabolic rate for oxygen (CMRO$_2$) and has for long been promoted as a neuroprotective agent. An early study suggested that the incidence of neuropsychiatric dysfunction was reduced by the use of thiopental by infusion during CPB, but this finding has not been confirmed by all.[21] Problems with the use of thiopental by infusion relate to its long half-life and consequent accumulation. This delays awakening and tracheal extubation and increases requirements for inotropic support in the postoperative period, making it inappropriate for use in routine cases. Thiopental is used as a neuroprotective in many centres during aortic root surgery or other deep hypothermic arrest procedures. Propofol has similar effects to thiopental on CMRO$_2$ without the problem of accumulation and delayed awakening but there are as yet no studies addressing its efficacy in this situation.

The calcium channel antagonist nimodipine has been shown to improve outcome following aneurysmal subarachnoid hemorrhage, but not in other situations involving intracranial hemorrhage. A controlled trial in cardiac valve surgery patients was terminated early due to lack of efficacy and increased adverse events in the treatment group.[30] The effect on neurological outcome of a variety of agents that affect blood coagulation and platelet function have been evaluated in cardiac surgical patients. No benefit was found from the use of prostacyclin, however a reduction in the incidence of perioperative

stroke was seen in a meta-analysis of studies evaluating aprotinin.[31] The competitive glutamate antagonist, remacemide hydrochloride, has been shown to improve neuropsychological outcome following CPB,[32] as has lignocaine by infusion.[33] A trend to improved neurological outcome was seen with the non-specific neuroprotectant GM$_1$-ganglioside.[20] These latter studies suggest that pharmacological treatments may have a role in the prevention of neurological injury in these patients in the future, however large multicenter randomized trials are needed before confident recommendations can be made.

Conclusions and learning points

- Neurological and neuropsychological complications remain relatively common following CPB despite improvements in anesthetic, surgical and perfusion techniques.
- Patient age, past cerebrovascular events, aortic atherosclerotic disease and diabetes mellitus are the main risk factors for a major neurological event.
- No pharmacological neuroprotective strategy has been convincingly demonstrated as efficacious in prevention.
- Intraoperative imaging techniques to help avoid aortic atheromatous plaques during cannulation may be effective in reducing cerebral embolization.
- Prevention of hyperglycemia and the use of α-stat acid–base management are recommended.
- CABG surgery avoiding CPB may be associated with reduced incidence of neurological dysfunction.
- Management of neurological injury is essentially supportive, with attention to the airway and to nutritional support of importance. Cerebral imaging is of diagnostic value and may permit some prognostic estimation but will rarely influence management. An early case-conference and management plan with setting of therapeutic limits where appropriate is required for patients with major neurological injuries.

References

1. Roach GW, Kanchuger M, Mora Mangano C et al. Adverse cerebral outcomes after coronary bypass surgery. Multicenter Study of Perioperative Ischemia Research Group and the Ischemia Research and Education Foundation Investigators. N Engl J Med 1996;335:1857–63.

2. Shaw PJ, Bates D, Cartlidge NE et al. Neurologic and neuropsychological morbidity following major surgery: comparison of coronary artery bypass and peripheral vascular surgery. Stroke 1987;18:700–7.

3. Timberlake N, Klinger L, Smith P et al. Incidence and patterns of depression following coronary artery bypass graft surgery. J Psychosom Res 1997;43:197–207.

4. McKhann GM, Borowicz LM, Goldsborough MA et al. Depression and cognitive decline after coronary artery bypass grafting. Lancet 1997;349:1282–4.

5. Roach GW, Newman MF, Murkin JM et al. Ineffectiveness of burst suppression therapy in mitigating perioperative cerebrovascular dysfunction. Multicenter Study of Perioperative Ischemia (McSPI) Research Group. Anesthesiology 1999;90:1255–64.

6. Eagle KA, Guyton RA, Davidoff R et al. ACC/AHA guidelines for coronary artery bypass graft surgery: executive summary and recommendations: a report of the American College of Cardiology/American Heart Association Task Force on Practice Guidelines (Committee to revise the 1991 guidelines for coronary artery bypass graft surgery). Circulation 1999;100:1464–80.

7. Brott T, Bogousslavsky J. Treatment of acute ischemic stroke. N Engl J Med 2000;343:710–22.

8. Simonson TM, Yuh WT, Hindman BJ et al. Contrast MR of the brain after high-perfusion cardiopulmonary bypass. Am J Neuroradiol 1994;15:3–7.

9. Koskiniemi M, Van Vleymen B, Hakamies L et al. Piracetam relieves symptoms in progressive myoclonus epilepsy: a multicentre, randomised, double blind, crossover study comparing the efficacy and safety of three dosages of oral piracetam with placebo. J Neurol Neurosurg Psychiatry 1998;64:344–8.

10. Genton P, Guerrini R, Remy C. Piracetam in the treatment of cortical myoclonus. Pharmacopsychiatry 1999;32 (Suppl 1):49-53.

11. Ginsberg MD, Busto R. Combating hyperthermia in acute stroke: a significant clinical concern. Stroke 1998;29:529–34.

12. Westphal K, Byhahn C, Rinne T et al. Tracheostomy in cardiosurgical patients: surgical tracheostomy versus ciaglia and fantoni methods. Ann Thorac Surg 1999;68:486–92.

13. MacCallum PL, Parnes LS, Sharpe MD, Harris C. Comparison of open, percutaneous, and translaryngeal tracheostomies. Otolaryngol Head Neck Surg 2000;122:686–90.

14. Stamenkovic SA, Morgan IS, Pontefract DR, Campanella C. Is early tracheostomy safe in cardiac patients with median sternotomy incisions? Ann Thorac Surg 2000;69:1152–4.

15. Jolliet P, Pichard C, Biolo G et al. Enteral nutrition in intensive care patients: a practical approach. Working Group on Nutrition and Metabolism, ESICM. European Society of Intensive Care Medicine. Intensive Care Med 1998;24:848–59.

16. Rorick MB, Furlan AJ. Risk of cardiac surgery in patients with prior stroke. Neurology 1990;40:835-7.

17. Croughwell ND, Newman MF, Blumenthal JA et al. Jugular bulb saturation and cognitive dysfunction after cardiopulmonary bypass. Ann Thorac Surg 1994;58:1702–8.

18. Venn GE, Sherry K, Klinger L et al. Cerebral blood flow during cardiopulmonary bypass. Eur J Cardiothorac Surg 1988;2:360–3.

19. Mora CT, Henson MB, Weintraub WS et al. The effect of temperature management during cardiopulmonary bypass on neurologic and neuropsychologic outcomes in patients undergoing coronary revascularization. J Thorac Cardiovasc Surg 1996;112:514–22.

20. Arrowsmith JE, Grocott HP, Reves JG, Newman MF. Central nervous system complications of cardiac surgery. Br J Anaesth 2000;84:378–93.

21. Murkin JM. Etiology and incidence of brain dysfunction after cardiac surgery. J Cardiothorac Vasc Anesth 1999;13:12–7.

22. Wolman RL, Nussmeier NA, Aggarwal A et al. Cerebral injury after cardiac surgery: identification of a group at extraordinary risk. Multicenter Study of Perioperative Ischemia Research Group (McSPI) and the Ischemia Research Education Foundation (IREF) Investigators. Stroke 1999;30:514–22.

23. Pugsley W, Klinger L, Paschalis C *et al.* The impact of microemboli during cardiopulmonary bypass on neuropsychological functioning. *Stroke* 1994;**25**:1393–9.

24. Brooker RF, Brown WR, Moody DM *et al.* Cardiotomy suction: a major source of brain lipid emboli during cardiopulmonary bypass. *Ann Thorac Surg* 1998;**65**:1651–5.

25. Newman S. The incidence and nature of neuropsychological morbidity following cardiac surgery. *Perfusion* 1989;**4**:93–100.

26. Murkin JM, Boyd WD, Ganapathy S *et al.* Beating heart surgery: why expect less central nervous system morbidity? *Ann Thorac Surg* 1999;**68**:1498–501.

27. Taggart DP, Browne SM, Halligan PW, Wade DT. Is cardiopulmonary bypass still the cause of cognitive dysfunction after cardiac operations? *J Thorac Cardiovasc Surg* 1999;**118**:414–20.

28. Watters MP, Cohen AM, Monk CR *et al.* Reduced cerebral embolic signals in beating heart coronary surgery detected by transcranial Doppler ultrasound. *Br J Anaesth* 2000;**84**:629–31.

29. Anderson RE, Hansson LO, Vaage J. Release of S100B during coronary artery bypass grafting is reduced by off-pump surgery. *Ann Thorac Surg* 1999;**67**:1721–5.

30. Legault C, Furberg CD, Wagenknecht LE *et al.* Nimodipine neuroprotection in cardiac valve replacement: report of an early terminated trial. *Stroke* 1996;**27**:593–8.

31. Smith PK, Muhlbaier LH. Aprotinin: safe and effective only with the full-dose regimen. *Ann Thorac Surg* 1996;**62**:1575–7.

32. Arrowsmith JE, Harrison MJ, Newman SP *et al.* Neuroprotection of the brain during cardiopulmonary bypass: a randomized trial of remacemide during coronary artery bypass in 171 patients. *Stroke* 1998;**29**:2357–62.

33. Mitchell SJ, Pellett O, Gorman DF. Cerebral protection by lidocaine during cardiac operations. *Ann Thorac Surg* 1999;**67**:1117–24.

21
Anterior spinal artery syndrome following coronary artery bypass graft surgery

Virinder S Sidhu

Introduction

Anterior spinal artery (ASA) syndrome has been reported following cardiac surgery only in association with intra-aortic balloon counterpulsation.[1] A case history is described in which ASA syndrome occurred in a patient following coronary artery bypass graft (CABG) surgery in which intra-aortic balloon counterpulsation was not used.

Case history

A 71-year-old woman with a 10-year history of hypertension and mild chronic renal impairment (hypertensive nephropathy) was transferred from a nearby hospital. She had been admitted to the referring hospital following an episode of acute left ventricular failure secondary to an acute subendocardial myocardial infarction. She had also developed a *Staphylococcus epidermidis* septicemia and had required intermittent hemodialysis. During the remainder of her stay she suffered from unstable angina. On admission, she was in sinus rhythm, her arterial pressure was 200/90 mmHg and neurological examination was normal. She was no longer in acute left ventricular failure or septicemic. She had been commenced on infusions of heparin and glyceryl trinitrate. Coronary angiography revealed left main stem stenosis and occlusion of the left anterior descending and circumflex arteries, and subtotal occlusion of the right coronary artery. Transthoracic echocardiography revealed a normal left ventricular ejection fraction and anterolateral hypokinesia. In view of her clinical condition and angiographic findings, CABG surgery was planned. General anesthesia was induced with diazepam 2 mg, alfentanil 7.5 mg, etomidate 8 mg, pancuronium 6 mg and maintained with oxygen, nitrous oxide and isoflurane. A glyceryl trinitrate infusion was used to maintain cardiovascular stability prior to cardiopulmonary bypass (CPB). Papaveretum 1 ml (7.7 mg) was given immediately preCPB and during rewarming with diazepam 3 mg and pancuronium 2 mg. Saphenous vein grafts to the obtuse marginal and posterior descending arteries, and grafting of the left internal mammary to the left anterior descending artery, were performed using moderate hypothermic (33°C) CPB with intermittent aortic cross-clamping and fibrillation. A non-pulsatile flow rate of 2.4 l min^{-1} and mean arterial pressure of 50–60 mmHg was maintained during CPB. The patient was successfully weaned from CPB without requiring inotropic support. The duration of CPB was 75 min. and the estimated total ischemic time 30 min.

The immediate postoperative period was complicated by hypotension, minimum systolic arterial pressure 75 mmHg. Hemodynamic stability was achieved initially with fluid and subsequently with an infusion of epinephrine 0.2 μg kg^{-1} min^{-1}. Pulmonary artery catheter-derived hemodynamics revealed: CO 3.5 l min^{-1};

systemic vascular resistance (SVR) 900 dyne s cm^{-5} and pulmonary capillary wedge pressure (PCWP) 20 mmHg. An infusion of dobutamine 10 µg kg^{-1} min^{-1} was added. An electrocardiogram (ECG) revealed sinus rhythm and anteroinferior ischemia. Echocardiography excluded cardiac tamponade. She was sedated, intubated and mechanically ventilated. Worsening oliguria prompted the instigation of continuous venovenous hemofiltration. On the third postoperative day sedation was discontinued and inotropic support weaned. On the fourth postoperative day she was alert and orientated, not requiring cardiovascular or respiratory support. Neurological examination revealed normal upper limb function, bilateral lower limb flaccidity with hyporeflexia with loss of pain and temperature sensation to the level of T_6 with preservation of joint position sense. An MRI scan confirmed ischemic damage to the thoracic spinal cord. On the 12th postoperative day she was discharged to the renal unit requiring intermittent hemodialysis. Three days later she developed an acute septicemic episode, rapidly deteriorated and died. There had been minimal neurological recovery. A post-mortem examination was not performed.

Anterior spinal artery syndrome

The ASA syndrome was first described in a patient with ASA thrombosis;[2] an infarct was noticed at autopsy in the anterior part of the spinal cord, extending from C_4 to T_3. Subsequently it was found that this syndrome could also be the result of a fall in perfusion pressure,[3] or local interference with spinal cord blood supply.[4]

The blood supply of the spinal cord was first described in 1882, by Adamkiewicz. Further studies have added to an understanding of the variable arterial supply to this area.[3, 5] The blood supply (Figure 21.1) is provided by one ASA and two smaller posterior spinal arteries (PSA). The ASA supplies at least 75% of the spinal cord, supplying the anterior and lateral columns. The PSAs supplying 25% or less, providing blood flow to the dorsal columns. The cervical part of the ASA is primarily formed by branches of the vertebral arteries, with collateral flow from the

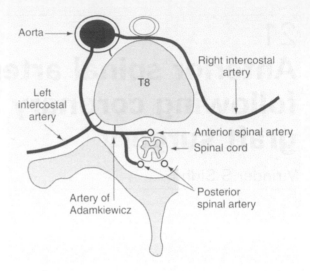

Figure 21.1

Transection of the spine showing the relationship between the artery of Adamkiewicz and the anterior spinal artery. Modified and reproduced from Djurberg and Haddad[6] with permission.

deep or ascending cervical artery and a few anterior radicular arteries. (Figure 21.2) The lumbosacral part of the ASA is supplied by radicular branches from the internal iliac arteries. The remainder of the ASA blood flow is supplied by six to eight radicular arteries, which are branches of the intercostal arteries — the largest being the artery of Adamkiewicz. The origin of the artery of Adamkiewicz is variable and may originate on the left side in 80% of subjects and from any level between T_5 and L_4. In 85% of patients the artery arises between T_9 and L_2. The two posterior spinal arteries also arise from the vertebral arteries and receive 10–20 radicular branches which anastomose freely with each other and with the posterior spinal artery. The collateral blood supply to the posterior spinal arteries makes segmental arterial injury in their distribution uncommon.

The anterior spinal artery territory of the spinal cord is particularly vulnerable to infarction if one of the main contributory vessels is damaged. This being especially common around T_4 where collateral blood flow is poor. Clinically the onset is abrupt often associated with pain and paresthesia followed by flaccid paralysis with loss of

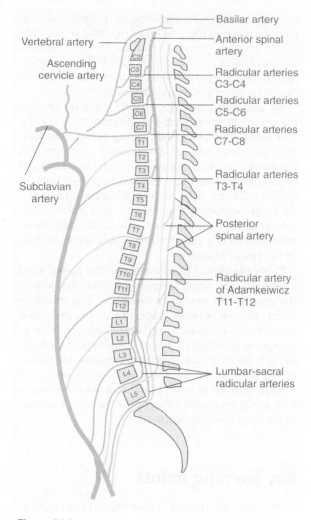

Figure 21.2

Blood supply of the spinal cord showing the anterior and posterior radicular branches shown in lateral view. Modified and reproduced from: Djindjian[7] with permission.

pain and temperature sensation below a variable level but with preservation of light touch, position and vibration sense — a 'dissociated' sensory loss. Initially there is flaccid paralysis of the lower limbs and later spastic paraparesis develops. There is usually retention of urine and feces in the early stages but automatic bladder and bowel control may eventually be achieved.

The diagnosis of ASA syndrome is clinical and supported by radiological imaging. Magnetic resonance imaging (MRI) scanning is the imaging modality of choice to demonstrate spinal cord infarction, associated vascular and bony abnormalities.[8] However, in the early phase no abnormality may be visible.

Following traumatic spinal injury, the early administration of steroids may reduce the extent of damage to the spinal cord however, there is no evidence that treatment other than nursing care is of value following spinal-cord infarction. Foo and Rossier reported improvement in motor function in 60 % of patients, but complete function was never regained.[9] Outlook for recovery was less favorable in patients with aortic occlusive disease (33%), or other aortic disease (20%).

Discussion

The clinical signs observed in our patient are consistent with ASA syndrome and were supported by MRI findings. There are currently 17 reports of paraplegia following myocardial revacularization.[1] All have been related to the use of intra-aortic balloon counterpulsation. Two pathophysiological mechanisms have been considered for this complication in association with the device. The first suggests that an aortic dissection or a hematoma of the advential layer can lead to occlusion of a major radicular branch leading to infarction of the spinal cord. The second suggests local occlusion of the artery of Adamkiewicz with atheromatous material could occur without a traumatic localized dissection of the aorta or hematoma. A common factor in the majority of the cases is the presence of atheromatous disease of the aorta.

The exact mechanism responsible for ASA syndrome in our patient is unclear. There was evidence of widespread atheromatous disease. The spinal arteries were likely to have been stenosed. It is conceivable that a relative fall in perfusion pressure to the spinal cord during non-pulsatile CPB was the cause. Hypotension in the immediate postoperative period may have aggravated the condition, but may not be solely responsible. Autoregulation of spinal cord blood flow has been demonstrated in animals to occur between a mean arterial pressure of 60 and 160 mmHg.[10] In the absence of any other clinical evidence of embolism, local occlusion to the artery of Adamkiewicz due to embolic atheromatous material following cannulation/decanulation/intermittent aortic cross-clamping remains an outside possibility.

Implications for neuraxial blockade

In recent years there has been growing interest in neuraxial blockade for CABG surgery.[11, 12] The perioperative use of thoracic epidural (TE) analgesia in patients undergoing cardiac surgery may beneficially affect outcome by producing stress-response attenuation,[13] thoracic cardiac sympathectomy,[14] intense postoperative analgesia[15] and facilitated fast-track recovery compared with systemic opioid administration.[16–18] However, hypotension[19] and myocardial depression,[20] may occur following TE local anaesthetics. Intrathecal (IT) opioids, although producing reliable postoperative analgesia after cardiac surgery, cannot however reliably attenuate the associated stress response.[21] Well-designed trials with adequate numbers of patients that investigate the ability of IT and TE analgesia to affect morbidity and mortality of patients following cardiac surgery are required.

Serious neurological problems that may be considered attributable to neuraxial blockade include: (1) inadvertent injection of the wrong drug; (2) direct trauma to the spinal cord or roots; (3) epidural hematoma or abscess formation; and (4) ASA syndrome due to prolonged hypotension. Giebler, Schere and Peter's study[22] on the incidence of neurological complications in more than 4000 patients receiving TE analgesia for abdominothoracic surgery, reported no evidence of permanent sensory or motor deficit attributable to epidural catheterization and no evidence of epidural hematoma. The maximum risk of permanent neurological deficit following TE was calculated to be 0.07 %. The estimated risk of epidural hematoma formation following epidural catheterization is of the order of 1:150 000 and 1:200 000 following IT injection.[23] The risk is increased in patients with coagulation disorders and those treated with anticoagulants.[24] The risk of epidural hematoma in a patient undergoing neuraxial blockade prior to systemic heparinization required for CPB may be as high as 0.35%.[25] Paradoxically, safe epidural catheterizations have been performed in patients with known coagulopathies,[26] on aspirin therapy[27] and thrombocytopenia.[28] Furthermore, spontaneous epidural hematoma may occur in the absence of neuraxial blockade.[29]

As yet there are no reports of any serious neurological complications related to IT or TE analgesia in patients undergoing cardiac surgery. The development of paraplegia in a patient following cardiac surgery in whom neuraxial blockade has been used warrants urgent investigation. CT or MRI will distinguish between epidural hematoma formation and spinal cord infarction. If spinal cord infarction has been demonstrated it could conceivably be attributed to neuraxial blockade.

This case report demonstrates that spinal cord infarction can occur following cardiac surgery in the absence of neuraxial blockade. The development of paraplegia secondary to the ASA syndrome is devastating with little chance of complete recovery. Careful consideration of the benefit of neuraxial blockade should be established against the potential risk, in patients with widespread atherosclerosis or in whom circulatory assistance with intra-aortic balloon counterpulsation could be required.

Key learning points

- The ASA syndrome in association with cardiac surgery is rare.
- It has previously been reported only in association with intra-aortic balloon counterpulsation.
- The ASA syndrome can occur following cardiac surgery in the absence of neuraxial blockade.
- The risk versus benefit of neuraxial blockade should be considered in patients with widespread atherosclerosis.

References

1. Benicio A, Moreira LF, Auler JO et al. Paraplegia following intraaortic balloon counterpulsation. Arq Bras Cardiol 1999;4:490–2.

2. Spiller WG. Thrombosis of the cervical anterior median spinal artery; syphilitic acute anterior poliomyelitis. *J Nerv Ment Dis* 1909;**36**:601–3.

3. Garland H, Greenberg J, Harriman DG. Infarction of the spinal cord. *Brain* 1966;**89**:645–62.

4. Weisman AD, Adams RD. The neurological complications of dissecting aortic aneurysm. *Brain* 1944;**67**:69–92.

5. Henson RA, Parsons M. Ischaemic lesions of the spinal cord: an illustrated review. *Q J Med* 1967;**36**:205–22.

6. Djurberg H, Haddad M. Anterior spinal artery syndrome. *Anaesthesia* 1995;**50**:347.

7. Djinjian R. Arteriography of the spinal cord. *Am J Roentgenol* 1969;**107**:461.

8. Yuh WT, Marsh EE, Wang AK *et al*. MR imaging of spinal cord and vertebral body infarction. *Am J Neuroradiol* 1992;**13**:145–54.

9. Foo D, Rossier AB. Anterior spinal artery syndrome and its natural history. *Paraplegia* 1983;**21**:1–10.

10. Griffiths IR. Spinal cord blood flow in dogs: the effect of blood pressure. *J Neurol Neurosurg Psychiatry* 1973;**36**:914–20.

11. Desborough JP. Thoracic epidural analgesia in cardiac surgery. *Anaesthesia* 1996;**51**:805–7.

12. Chaney M. Intrathecal and epidural anaesthesia and analgesia for cardiac surgery. *Anesth Analg* 1997;**84**:1211–21.

13. Moore CM, Cross MH, Desborough JP *et al*. Hormonal effects of thoracic extradural analgesia for cardiac surgery. *Br J Anaesth* 1995;**75**:387–93.

14. Blomberg S, Curelaru I, Emanuelsson H *et al*. Thoracic epidural anaesthesia in patients with unstable angina pectoris. *Eur Heart J* 1989;**10**:437–44.

15. Liem TH, Booij LH, Hasenbos MA, Gielen MJ. Coronary artery bypass grafting using two different anesthetic techniques: Part I: Hemodynamic results. *J Cardiothorac Vasc Anesth* 1992;**6**:148–55.

16. Joachimsson PO, Nystrom SO, Tyden H. Early extubation after coronary artery surgery in efficiently rewarmed patients: a postoperative comparison of opioid anesthesia versus inhala-tional anesthesia and thoracic epidural analgesia. *J Cardiothorac Anesth* 1989;**3**:444–54.

17. Liem TH, Hasenbos MA, Booij LH, Gielen MJ. Coronary artery bypass grafting using two different anesthetic techniques: Part 2: Postoperative outcome. *J Cardiothorac Vasc Anesth* 1992;**6**:156–61.

18. Turfrey DJ, Ray DA, Sutcliffe NP *et al*. Thoracic epidural anaesthesia for coronary artery bypass graft surgery. Effects on postoperative complications. *Anaesthesia* 1997;**52**:1090–5.

19. Stenseth R, Bjella L, Berg EM *et al*. Thoracic epidural analgesia in aortocoronary bypass surgery. I: Haemodynamic effects. *Acta Anaesthesiol Scand* 1994;**38**:826–33.

20. Stenseth R, Berg EM, Bjella L *et al*. Effects of thoracic epidural analgesia on coronary hemodynamics and myocardial metabolism in coronary artery bypass surgery. *J Cardiothorac Vasc Anesth* 1995;**9**:503–9.

21. Chaney MA, Smith KR, Barclay JC, Slogoff S. Large-dose intrathecal morphine for coronary artery bypass grafting. *Anesth Analg* 1996;**83**:215–22.

22. Giebler RM, Scherer RU, Peters J. Incidence of neurologic complications related to thoracic epidural catheterization. *Anesthesiology* 1997;**86**:55–63.

23. Vandermeulen EP, Van Aken H, Vermylen J. Anticoagulants and spinal-epidural anesthesia. *Anesth Analg* 1994;**79**:1165–77.

24. Dickman CA, Shedd SA, Spetzler RF *et al*. Spinal epidural hematoma associated with epidural anesthesia: complications of systemic heparinization in patients receiving peripheral vascular thrombolytic therapy. *Anesthesiology* 1990;**72**:947–50.

25. Owens EL, Kasten GW, Hessel EA. Spinal subarachnoid hematoma after lumbar puncture and heparinization: a case report, review of the literature, and discussion of anesthetic implications. *Anesth Analg* 1986;**65**:1201–7.

26. Odoom JA, Sih IL. Epidural analgesia and anticoagulant therapy. Experience with 1000 cases of continuous epidurals. *Anaesthesia* 1983;**38**:254–9.

27. Blomberg S, Emanuelsson H, Ricksten SE. Thoracic epidural anesthesia and central hemodynamics in patients with unstable angina pectoris. *Anesth Analg* 1989;**69**:558–62.

28. Waldman SD, Feldstein GS, Waldman HJ *et al.* Caudal administration of morphine sulfate in anticoagulated and thrombocytopenic patients. *Anesth Analg* 1987;**66**:267–8.

29. Markham JW, Lynge HN, Stahlman GE. The syndrome on spontaneous spinal epidural hematoma. Report of three cases. *J Neurosurg* 1967;**26**:334–42.

22
Anesthesia for left ventricular volume reduction surgery

Stephen J Pryn

Introduction

Surgery for patients in end-stage heart failure secondary to dilated cardiomyopathy is reserved for those refractory to medical therapy.[1] Left ventricular volume reduction (LVVR) aims to reduce the diameter of the dilated ventricle, altering the mechanics, resulting in a lower myocardial wall tension according to Laplace's law. Symptomatic improvement and improved ventricular contractility follow,[2,3] though the precise reasons for improvement are not established.[4–6] One of the options, partial left ventriculectomy (PLV), involves surgically removing a segment of ventricular wall, reducing its diameter, often in conjunction with mitral and tricuspid valvular repairs, and right ventricular plication.[7] This surgical approach has been used as an alternative to heart transplantation, or as a bridge to transplantation.[1] Two cases of partial left ventriculectomy are presented here.

Case history 1

A 57-year-old male with a 7 year history of progressively worsening exertional dyspnea — secondary to idiopathic dilated cardiomyopathy — presented with dyspnea at rest. He had no history of either ischemic heart disease or excessive alcohol intake. Coronary angiography 1 year previously had demonstrated normal coronary arteries. He had been receiving conventional medication for heart failure as an outpatient, however his condition had deteriorated despite

recent escalation of his diuretic therapy. On admission he was found to have chronic renal impairment. A transthoracic echocardiogram (TTE) revealed a grossly dilated poorly functioning left ventricle with an ejection fraction of 15%.

Cardiac transplantation was considered, but was rejected on account of the patient's renal failure. He was referred to the cardiac surgical team for LVVR surgery. Surgery was postponed for 7 days while renal function was optimized by cautious reduction in diuretic therapy as an inpatient. The serum concentrations of creatinine and urea fell to 1.6 mg dl^{-1} (138 µmol l^{-1}) and 24 mg dl^{-1} (8.6 mmol l^{-1}) respectively.

Two hours prior to surgery, the patient received oral sedative premedication (lorazepam 3 mg), together with 40% oxygen via a face mask. In addition to routine monitoring, both an arterial and pulmonary artery catheter were inserted under local anesthesia prior to the induction of anesthesia. Baseline thermodilution studies revealed pulmonary hypertension and a low cardiac output state: mean arterial pressure (MAP) 77 mmHg; central venous pressure (CVP) 13 mmHg; pulmonary capillary wedge pressure (PCWP) 35 mmHg; pulmonary artery pressure (PAP) 60/40 mmHg; cardiac index (CI) 1.7 l min^{-1} m^{-2}; stroke volume (SV) 36 ml; systemic vascular resistance (SVR) 1640 dyne s cm^{-5}, SvO$_2$ 52%. Anesthesia was induced in the operating theater with midazolam 2 mg, fentanyl 1 mg and pancuronium 12 mg. Following tracheal intubation the lungs were ventilated with oxygen in air (FiO$_2$ 0.5). Anesthesia was maintained with isoflurane (0.2–0.5%) and incremental doses of fentanyl (total dose 50 µg kg^{-1}). Moderate

Past medical history	Seven years progressively worsening LVF — now NYHA class IV. Atrial fibrillation with LBBB chemically cardioverted to sinus rhythm with first degree block and LBBB as outpatient. Previous surgery for varicose veins, inguinal hernias and benign prostatic hypertrophy. Non-smoker. No known drug allergies.
Regular medications	Lisinopril 5 mg OD, digoxin 125 µg OD, amiodarone 200 mg BD, bumetanide 8 mg BD, spironolactone 50 mg OD, isosorbide mononitrate M/R 30 mg OD.
Examination	Weight 67kg. Body mass index 25.6 kg m^{-2}. Pulse 85 regular, BP 95/60 mmHg, jugular venous distension, dependent edema, 5 cm palpable liver edge, fine bilateral basal inspiratory crackles, dyspneic on minimal exertion.
Investigations	Hb 11.5 g dl^{-1}, WBC 8.6 × 10^9 l^{-1}, platelets 214 × 10^9 l^{-1}, [Na$^+$] 135 mmol l^{-1}, [K$^+$] 5.1 mmol l^{-1}, urea 99 mg dl^{-1} (35.3 mmol l^{-1}), creatinine 3.7 mg dl^{-1} (331 µmol l^{-1}), INR 1.7, APPT ratio 1.0. **CXR**: Cardiomegaly with pulmonary edema. **ECG**: Sinus rhythm, left atrial hypertrophy, first degree block, LBBB. **Renal ultrasound**: Normal-sized kidneys with no hydronephrosis. **Cardiac catheterization**: Normal coronaries, dilated poorly functioning LV, moderate mitral regurgitation **TEE**: Dilated globally impaired LV, no regional wall motion abnormalities. No intracardiac thrombi. LVEDD 8.0 cm. LVEF 15%. Moderate central mitral regurgitation, mild tricuspid regurgitation.

hypotension (80/45 mmHg) prior to cardiopulmonary bypass (CPB) was treated with boluses of ephedrine 3 mg and intravenous crystalloid (500 ml lactated Ringer's solution). In anticipation of difficulties in weaning the patient from CPB an intra-aortic counter pulsation balloon pump (IABP) was inserted via the left femoral artery prior to sternotomy; in addition triiodothyronine 20 µg was administered intravenously. Conventional CPB was established using mild hypothermia (32°C), and anesthesia maintained with a propofol infusion (2mg kg^{-1} hour^{-1}).

Myocardial protection during the 34-minute period of aortic cross-clamping was provided using two doses of cold antegrade blood cardioplegia, followed by a single antegrade dose of warm blood cardioplegia prior to reperfusion. The surgical procedure consisted of an intrapapillary resection of an 'hour glass-shaped' segment of left ventricular wall, preserving the mitral apparatus, with a two-layered closure supported by an external Teflon patch held in

position by tissue glue. In addition the mitral valve was repaired using a single central stitch as described by Alfieri — thereby leaving two mitral orifices in a figure of eight pattern.[8] Ten minutes after reperfusion, and in preparation for weaning from CPB, a loading dose of enoximone 500 µg kg^{-1} was administered over 20 minutes, followed by a maintenance dose of 2 µg kg^{-1} min^{-1}. In addition an infusion of norepinephrine 0.05–0.1 µg kg^{-1} min^{-1} was given in order to avoid excessive systemic vasodilatation and maintain SVR at around 800 dyne s cm^{-5}. The heart reverted spontaneously to a sinus rate of 60 following aortic unclamping. In anticipation of a small stroke volume the heart rate was increased to 90 with atrial pacing using temporary epicardial wires. As prophylaxis for potentially 'irritable' ventricular arrhythmias, a loading dose of magnesium sulfate 12 mmol was administered. Weaning from CPB was achieved using pharmacological support in addition to the IABP. Extreme care was taken to avoid overdistension of the heart upon separation from CPB. The mean arterial blood pressure was restored to 65 mmHg, and thermodilution studies demonstrated improved hemodynamics: CVP 8 mmHg; PCWP 17 mmHg; PAP 45/25 mmHg; CI 2.6 l min^{-1} m^{-2}, SV 51 ml, SVR 990 dyne s cm^{-5}, SvO$_2$ 65%. Initial intraoperative TEE revealed trivial mitral regurgitation and a slightly reduced left ventricular diameter (now 7.2 cm). Two units of packed red blood cells were required to elevate the hemoglobin concentration to 10 g dl^{-1}.

Postoperative care involved continued sedation with propofol 0.5–1.5 mg kg^{-1} h^{-1} and alfentanil 0.25–0.5 μg kg^{-1} min^{-1} together with positive pressure ventilation for 48 hours. After successful weaning from mechanical ventilation and the tracheal extubation, the patient required intermittent mask CPAP for a further 2 days to treat hypoxemia. The IABP remained in situ for 4 days. Hemodynamic support was maintained with enoximone 2–3 μg kg^{-1} min^{-1} for a total of 5 days, together with norepinephrine ≤0.1 μg kg^{-1} min^{-1}, titrated to achieve SVR 800 dyne s cm^{-5}. Digoxin 125 μg OD, amiodarone 200 mg OD, frusemide 80 mg BD and spironolactone 50 mg OD were restarted on the first postoperative day, while losartan 25 mg OD was withheld until the enoximone was weaned. There were no major postoperative complications, in particular renal

function returned to normal in the early postoperative period. The patient was discharged after 20 days in hospital. At follow-up 1 year after surgery, the patient's symptom status had improved to NYHA class II, with echocardiographic evidence of greatly improved myocardial function (LVEDD 6.5 cm, LVEF 40%).

Case history 2

A 67-year-old male with a 6-year history of progressively worsening exertional dyspnea, secondary to idiopathic dilated cardiomyopathy, presented with dyspnea at rest. Similar to the previous case described, he had no history of either alcohol abuse or ischemic heart disease, coronary angiography performed a month before admission had demonstrated normal coronary arteries, and he had been receiving conventional medication for heart failure as an outpatient. Initial investigation revealed very poor left ventricular function and chronic renal impairment. He was considered not to be a suitable candidate for heart transplantation and was referred to the cardiac surgical team for LVVR surgery.

Past medical history	Six years progressively worsening LVF - now NYHA class IV. No previous surgery. Gout. Non-smoker. No known drug allergies.
Regular medications	Captopril 12.5 mg TDS, digoxin 125 μg OD, bumetanide 4 mg BD, amiloride 10 mg BD, isosorbide mononitrate 20 mg BD, probenecid 250 mg BD, warfarin 3 mg OD
Examination	Weight 91 kg. Body mass index 28.8 kg.m^{-2}. Pulse 110 regular, BP 100/65 mmHg, no jugular venous distension, mild dependent edema, chest clear to auscultation, dyspneic on minimal exertion.
Investigations	Hb 10.5 g dl^{-1}, WBC 6.4 × 10^9 l^{-1}, platelets 202 × 10^9 l^{-1}, [Na$^+$] 139 mmol l^{-1}, [K$^+$] 3.5 mmol l^{-1}, urea 24 mg dl^{-1} (8.7 mmol l^{-1}), creatinine 1.7 mg dl^{-1} (151 μmol l^{-1}), INR 2.3, APPT ratio 1.0. **CXR:** Cardiomegaly with pulmonary edema. **ECG:** Sinus tachycardia, left atrial hypertrophy, LBBB. **Cardiac catheterization:** Normal coronaries, dilated poorly functioning LV, moderate mitral regurgitation **TEE:** Dilated globally impaired LV, no regional wall motion abnormalities. LVEDD 7.7 cm. LVEF 25%. Moderate eccentric mitral regurgitation, mild tricuspid regurgitation. **MUGA scan:** LVEF 20%

Oral sedative premedication was given (lorazepam 3 mg), together with 40% oxygen via a face mask, 2 hours before surgery. On arrival in the anesthetic room, routine monitoring was established, together with the insertion of both an arterial and pulmonary artery catheter under local anesthesia prior to the induction of anesthesia. Baseline thermodilution studies revealed pulmonary hypertension and a low cardiac output state: MAP 75 mmHg, CVP 13 mmHg, PCWP 42 mmHg, PAP 60/35 mmHg, CI 1.5 l min^{-1} m^{-2}, SV 28 ml, SVR 1480 dyne s cm^{-5}, SvO$_2$ 38%. Anesthesia was induced in the operating theater with midazolam 4 mg, fentanyl 1.5 mg and pancuronium 12 mg. Maintenance anesthesia consisted of IPPV isoflurane (0.2–0.5%) in 60% oxygen in air, together with further fentanyl (total dose 50 µg kg^{-1}). Hemodynamics were well maintained (±20% baseline) following induction of anesthesia without need for further medication, and with only minimal crystalloid fluid replacement (500 ml lactated Ringer's solution). In anticipation of a potentially difficult wean from CPB, an IABP was inserted prior to initiation of CPB; in addition triiodothyronine 20 µg was administered intravenously. Conventional CPB was established using mild hypothermia (35°C), and anesthesia maintained with a propofol 2mg kg^{-1} hour^{-1}.

The aorta was cross-clamped for 41 minutes and myocardial protection provided by two doses of antegrade cold blood cardioplegia followed by a single dose of antegrade warm blood cardioplegia. Surgery consisted of an intrapapillary resection of a segment of left ventricular wall, preserving the mitral apparatus, and used a two-layered closure. The surgical procedure was complicated by the presence of an accessory middle papillary muscle, which made the resected segment rather small. Ten minutes after reperfusion a loading dose of enoximone 500 µg kg^{-1} was administered over 20 minutes, followed by a maintenance dose of 5 µg kg^{-1} min^{-1}. In addition norepinephrine 0.05 µg kg^{-1} min^{-1} was required to avoid excessive vasodilatation (target SVR 800 dyne s cm^{-5}). Magnesium sulfate 10 mmol was given to prevent ventricular arrhythmias. Initially the ECG showed complete heart block necessitating epicardial atrioventricular sequential pacing, however, after a few minutes a sinus tachycardia (110 bpm) supervened.

On attempting to wean from CPB it became apparent that there was globally poor biventricular function, and the heart could not maintain an output compatible with survival. TEE revealed that the left ventricle had not been reduced sufficiently in size (LVEDD 7.4cm), and the presence of moderate mitral and tricuspid regurgitation. It was decided to repair the tricuspid valve using an annuloplasty technique, and to revise the left ventricular resection. Inotropic support was stopped, full CPB re-established, and the aorta re-cross-clamped for a further 39 minutes using antegrade blood cardioplegia as before. Following tricuspid repair, the left ventricle was reopened along the same incision. The left ventricular resection segment was enlarged to include the papillary muscle and mitral valve. The mitral valve was replaced with a 27 mm Sorin bi-leaflet mechanical prosthesis, and the ventricular wall closed in two layers supported by a Teflon patch glued in place. Once again, following reperfusion, electrical activity returned in sinus tachycardia (105 bpm), and inotropic support was recommenced (enoximone 5 µg kg^{-1} min^{-1} and norepinephrine 0.1 µg kg^{-1} min^{-1}). Weaning from CPB was successful the second time with the aid of the IABP, and care was taken to avoid overdistension of the heart. Initially the cardiac output remained a little low with a mean arterial pressure of 55 mmHg, necessitating the addition of an epinephrine infusion (0.1 µg kg^{-1} min^{-1}) for the first 4 hours post-bypass. The TEE demonstrated that the left ventricle had been dramatically reduced in size (LVEDD 5.5 cm) and that there was no longer any mitral or tricuspid regurgitation. Thermodilution studies at this time demonstrated improved hemodynamics: MAP 60 mmHg, CVP 15 mmHg, PCWP 22 mmHg, PAP 45/25 mmHg, CI 2.1 l min^{-1} m^{-2}, SV 36 ml, SVR 780 dyne s cm^{-5}, SvO$_2$ 55%.

Postoperative care involved positive pressure ventilation for 48 hours and sedation with propofol 0.5–1.5 mg kg^{-1} hour^{-1} and alfentanil 0.25–0.5 µg kg^{-1}.min^{-1}. Following the discontinuation of mechanical ventilation and tracheal extubation, a minitracheostomy tube was inserted under local anesthesia to facilitate secretion clearance. The IABP remained in situ for 3 days. Hemodynamic support was maintained with enoximone 2–5 µg kg^{-1} min^{-1} for a total of 3 days, together with norepinephrine 0.025–0.05 µg kg^{-1} min^{-1}, titrated to achieve SVR 800 dyne s cm^{-5}. Supraventricular tachycardia was a problem for the first 3 days requiring oral amiodarone 200 mg TDS reducing to 200 mg OD, in addition to restarting digoxin 125 μg OD. Bumetanide 4 mg BD and spironolactone 50 mg BD, together with warfarin (target INR 3.0), were recommenced on the first postoperative day, while the addition of lisinopril 2.5 mg OD increasing to 10 mg OD was delayed until the enoximone infusion had been discontinued. The patient's renal function deteriorated in the early postoperative period, although renal replacement therapy was not required and renal function returned to baseline prior to hospital discharge. The serum creatinine concentration peaked at 2.9 mg dl[-1] (252 μmol l[-1]) on the third postoperative day and the serum urea concentration peaked at 59 mg dl[-1] (20.9 mmol l[-1]) on the fifth postoperative day. The patient was discharged after 19 days in hospital. At that stage a TTE revealed greatly improved myocardial function (LVEDD 5.5 cm, LVEF 40%). Seven months after surgery the patient's symptom status had improved to NYHA class II.

Discussion

Preoperative optimization of patients requiring LVVR surgery should always be considered. Although neither case presented here required preoperative inotropic or mechanical circulatory support, these modalities have been used in around 30% patients (0–57%) in the internationally reported series.[9–17] Over-aggressive diuretic therapy — causing hypovolemia and worsening renal function is not uncommon. The first case presented clearly demonstrates the benefit of a cautious reduction in the dose of loop diuretic. In addition, preoperative correction of diuretic induced hypokalemia and hypomagnesemia would be prudent with a view to reducing the incidence of perioperative dysrhythmia. Some patients presenting for LVVR surgery will be anticoagulated with warfarin to prevent the formation of mural thrombi (30% incidence of embolic episodes over a two year period) despite the fact that a significant number will be 'auto-anticoagulated' as a result of hepatic congestion (cf. case history 1). Although undoubtedly well intended, the use of warfarin in this context is not of proven benefit as no trial has defined the morbidity of warfarin therapy in this patient

group.[18] Our strategy is to discontinue warfarin 2 days prior to surgery to facilitate the control of postoperative coagulopathy. We also electively omit diuretics and angiotensin-converting enzyme inhibitor therapy on the morning of surgery to avoid hemodynamic decompensation secondary to hypovolemia following induction of anesthesia, and to avoid excessive postoperative hemodilatation.

Perioperative monitoring of patients undergoing LVVR should include placement of invasive intravascular (arterial, central venous and pulmonary arterial) lines under local anesthesia prior to induction of general anesthesia. Not only can baseline measurements be made with which to compare the postoperative result, but they also enable early detection and rational treatment of any hemodynamic decompensation occurring during anesthetic induction and maintenance. We have found the use of a pulmonary artery catheter with oximetric function and continuous thermodilution cardiac output (Baxter Vigilence; Baxter Healthcare Corporation; Santa Ana, CA, USA) to be extremely useful especially in the postoperative period.

TEE is essential for surgical planning,[16, 19] though the probe need only be placed after the induction of anesthesia. Valvular regurgitation must be carefully appraised and, in particular, mitral valve morphology accurately assessed to determine whether repair is feasible. In addition, TEE can be used to determine both the exact site and extent of surgical resection. LVVR surgery, though originally described as a resection on the lateral LV wall,[20] can also be achieved by anterior resection similar to left ventriculectomy,[13] or by a procedure to exclude the septum (Dor technique or endoventricular circular patch plasty[21]) or by mitral valve annuloplasty with an undersized ring.[22] These alternative techniques are especially attractive if the areas to be excluded are akinetic, thus preserving the better functioning areas of ventricular wall. Preoperative TEE must accurately delineate any areas of LV wall akinesia to determine the surgical approach to be used; for example the classical lateral 'Batista operation', or anteroseptal exclusion of akinetic area. Suma and colleagues[16] have reported increased success of the operation when ventricular incisions are guided by TEE. When determining the extent of ventricular resection the surgeon aims to reduce LVEDD to around 6 cm; the width of the resection specimen required equals the difference in LVEDD required multiplied by 3.14 (π). Echocardiographic measurement of the distance between the papillary muscles in the LV short axis will predict whether the necessary size of resection can be achieved between the papillary muscles (classical 'Batista operation' or intrapapillary resection), or whether this excision will have to be extended to include the papillary musculature and mitral valve (extrapapillary resection). Inadequate resection, in an attempt to preserve the mitral valve apparatus, invariably results in a poor hemodynamic response and should be avoided.[23] Following separation from CPB, TEE is again essential to check that surgically repaired valves are functionally competent (cf. case history 2).

Anesthetic management of patients with dilated cardiomyopathy is based upon modest afterload reduction, optimization of preload, and minimal myocardial depression.[24] Our experience has been that fentanyl (in doses up to 50 μg kg^{-1}) with a 'sleep' dose of midazolam followed by small doses of isoflurane or a propofol infusion is well tolerated. Care must be taken to avoid bradycardia, which would seriously compromise the cardiac output. We use pancuronium as our standard muscle relaxant if renal function is not greatly compromised, and augment the heart rate with glycopyrrolate if necessary. Many patients will have some degree of pulmonary edema with low pulmonary compliance, and ventilatory management in the operating room can be facilitated by a high FiO_2 together with judicious use of PEEP with pressure controlled ventilation.[25]

The management of CPB for LVVR surgery is largely conventional using a bicaval cannulation technique. Many patients will have large circulating blood volumes secondary to heart failure and renal impairment, and consideration should be given to hemofiltration during CPB. However, we have found this not to be necessary as a routine in our operative series. Myocardial protection can either be provided by the avoidance of aortic cross-clamping, as originally described by Batista,[4] or more commonly by aortic cross-clamping and blood cardioplegic arrest. The technique used must minimize intraoperative myocardial stunning. We have found a system of intermittent antegrade cold blood cardioplegia (blood:St Thomas' crystalloid base ratio 4:1), followed by a single antegrade dose of warm blood with potassium supplementation just prior to aortic declamping to be entirely satisfactory.[7]

The strategy necessary for successful weaning from CPB must respect the long ventricular suture line in the presence of persistently elevated myocardial wall tension. Dehiscence of the ventricle is a documented complication of this procedure[14, 15] albeit occurring early in the 'learning curve' of both these groups. It is important to avoid excessive inotropic stimulation, systolic hypertension and overdistension of the heart, as these factors will elevate the LV wall stress further. Batista described a strategy of aggressive afterload reduction using sodium nitroprusside without inotropic support,[9] however we have abandoned this method — as have many other groups. We prefer to use a longer-acting vasodilator with mild inotropic properties (i.e. enoximone), together with norepinephrine if necessary to fine-tune the degree of vasodilatation.[26] In contrast to the Batista series, the Cleveland Clinic group found that most of their patients were already vasodilated and indeed required pressor support with norepinephrine, with less that half requiring additional inotropes.[25] The aim is for vasodilatation (SVR 600–800 dyne s cm^{-5}), with the lowest mean arterial pressure necessary for satisfactory systemic perfusion (60–70 mmHg). Commonly the contractile strength recovers progressively over 20–30 minutes following weaning from CPB. It is important during this weaning phase not to overfill the heart with blood from the cardiotomy reservoir, as postoperative LV elastance is high. In addition to vasodilatation we also use an IABP placed pre-emptively prior to CPB. Our unit also uses tri-iodothyronine electively to correct the acute hypothyroidism associated with chronic heart failure.[27] Heart rate control is another important facet of weaning from CPB. We elevate the heart rate to 90–110 min^{-1} with either glycopyrollate or atrioventricular sequential pacing to optimize the cardiac output.

The principle postoperative problems encountered in the ICU are persistent intractable heart failure (15–30%),[9–11, 13–15, 17] supraventricular or ventricular dysrhythmia (up to 22%),[10] pulmonary complications (19%),[10] renal failure (13.5%),[10] and hemorrhage (5%).[10, 14, 15]

Postoperative hemodynamic management in the ICU continues on the same lines as that described for weaning from CPB: maintenance of a relative tachycardia (90–110 min^{-1}), adequate preload — yet avoidance of hypervolemia, maintenance of systemic vasodilatation (SVR 600–800 dyne s cm^{-5}), avoidance of excessive inotropy, and tolerance of the lowest MAP necessary for satisfactory systemic perfusion (60–70 mmHg). There is often a transient deterioration in myocardial function around 24 hours after surgery,[7] for this reason it is prudent to continue use of the IABP for at least 48 hours. Once cardiac function begins to improve again, the SVR is allowed to rise to 800–1200 dyne s cm^{-5}, and the MAP to 70–80 mmHg. Aggressive antifailure therapy with digoxin, diuretics and ACE inhibitors, is recommenced early in the postoperative period and maintained indefinitely.[26] Persistent intractable cardiac failure occurs in 15–30% patients[9–11, 13–15, 17] and is the cause of most in-hospital postoperative deaths. The Cleveland Clinic has the largest reported series of any western center and has used left ventricular assist device (LVAD) rescue in 17%, with the majority of these patients being relisted for heart transplantation.[17]

Respiratory function may well be compromised in the initial postoperative period due to long-standing preoperative pulmonary edema, though early extubation is desirable for improved hemodynamics.[25] The incidence of pulmonary complications has been reported as 19%,[10] though if heart failure can be controlled it is not a major cause of mortality.

Transient renal failure is also a relatively common postoperative complication, occurring in 13.5%,[10] and contributing an additional 5% to the overall mortality in a Brazilian center where no renal replacement therapy was available.[9]

Catastrophic hemorrhage from ventricular wall dehiscence has been reported early on in the experience with PLV,[14, 15] though changes in surgical technique[7] together with fastidious control of postoperative LV wall stress should minimize the incidence.

Perioperative dysrhythmia is common,[10] and the sudden onset of ventricular dysrhythmia contributes significantly to late postoperative mortality. The prophylactic postoperative use of amiodarone is commonly reported, although this does not seem to provide adequate protection. Empirical implantation of a cardiac defibrillator may ultimately become an essential adjunct of heart reduction surgery, similar to the conclusions drawn in the cardiomyoplasty experience.[1]

Overall, the perioperative mortality reported in this group of patients is high. In centers without access to LVAD, perioperative mortality is 20–30%,[9–11, 14] whereas western centers, with full LVAD rescue and transplant program support, report a mortality of 3–6%.[12, 15, 17] Sumo and colleagues[6] reported a dramatic fall in mortality from 33 to 6.9% as surgical experience increased and when TEE was used to guide the choice of surgical technique. Late survival is reported at 82–86% (12-month Kaplan–Meier) in the best western centers,[12, 15, 17] but only 30–70% in the other published series.[10, 11, 14, 16] However, of those long-term survivors, 85–90% have improved symptoms and are in NYHA class I or II,[10, 11, 14, 16] this figure is reduced to 67% when patients who have been salvaged by LVAD and relisted for transplantation are included.[1] The main causes of late deaths are progressive heart failure and sudden arrhythmias. The success of the procedure seems related to the extent of pre-existing myocyte damage,[9, 10] and preoperative myocardial biopsy may well become essential for rational patient selection.[10] The survival figures after PLV are comparable to those of heart transplantation,[12] and seem especially attractive when considering the diabolical mortality on the transplantation waiting list associated with shortage of donor supply (12-month Kaplan–Meier survival 75% whilst on waiting list).[12]

The precise applicability of LVVR surgery in the management of heart failure has yet to be fully elucidated; some see these procedures as promising potential alternatives to cardiac transplantation,[1] while others suspect that they may serve better as a bridge to transplantation rather than definitive therapy.[12] There is, however, a consensus that further randomized studies are required.[1, 28, 29] It follows that many more anesthetists and intensivists will be faced with the challenges of caring for these complex cases.

Conclusions and learning points

- LVVR surgery for patients in end-stage heart failure, secondary to dilated cardiomyopathy, is reserved for those refractory to medical therapy.
- Partial left ventriculectomy (PLV) involves surgically removing a segment of the wall of

the dilated ventricle, reducing its diameter, often in conjunction with valvular repairs.
- Preoperative optimization is often required.
- TEE is an essential perioperative monitor.
- Anesthetic management is based upon modest afterload reduction, optimization of preload, and minimal myocardial depression.
- The strategy necessary for successful weaning from CPB must avoid further elevation of myocardial wall tension.
- The principal postoperative problems are persistent intractable heart failure and ventricular dysrhythmia.
- Perioperative morbidity and mortality is high, and a significant proportion of survivors have worsening heart failure on long-term follow-up.
- Long-term survivors can have dramatically improved symptoms.
- LVVR surgery remains an experimental surgical technique.

References

1. Starling RC, Young JB. Surgical therapy for dilated cardiomyopathy. *Cardiol Clin* 1998;**16**:727–37.

2. Batista R. Partial left ventriculectomy – the Batista procedure. *Eur J Cardiothorac Surg* 1999;**15 (Suppl 1)**:S12-9.

3. Salerno TA, Bhayana J. Volume reduction surgery in the treatment of end-stage heart diseases. *Adv Card Surg* 1997;**9**:87–95.

4. Dickstein ML, Spotnitz HM, Rose EA, Burkhoff D. Heart reduction surgery: an analysis of the impact on cardiac function. *J Thorac Cardiovasc Surg* 1997;**113**:1032–40.

5. Ratcliffe MB, Hong J, Salahieh A *et al*. The effect of ventricular volume reduction surgery in the dilated, poorly contractile left ventricle: a simple finite element analysis. *J Thorac Cardiovasc Surg* 1998;**116**:566–77.

6. Green GR, Moon MR, DeAnda A Jr *et al*. Effects of partial left ventriculectomy on left ventricular geometry and wall stress in excised porcine hearts. *J Heart Valve Dis* 1998;**7**:474–83.

7. Birdi I, Bryan AJ, Mehta D *et al*. Left ventricular volume reduction surgery. *Int J Cardiol* 1997;**62 (Suppl 1)**:S29-35.

8. Fucci C, Sandrelli L, Pardini A *et al*. Improved results with mitral valve repair using new surgical techniques. *Eur J Cardiothorac Surg* 1995;**9**:621–6.

9. Kawaguchi AT, Bergsland J, Ishibashi-Ueda H *et al*. Partial left ventriculectomy in patients with dilated failing ventricle. *J Card Surg* 1998;**13**:335–42.

10. Stolf NA, Moreira LF, Bocchi EA *et al*. Determinants of midterm outcome of partial left ventriculectomy in dilated cardiomyopathy. *Ann Thorac Surg* 1998;**66**:1585–91.

11. Izzat MB, Kabbani SS, Suma H *et al*. Early experience with partial left ventriculectomy in the Asia-Pacific region. *Ann Thorac Surg* 1999;**67**:1703–7.

12. Etoch SW, Koenig SC, Laureano MA *et al*. Results after partial left ventriculectomy versus heart transplantation for idiopathic cardiomyopathy. *J Thorac Cardiovasc Surg* 1999;**117**:952–9.

13. Calafiore AM, Gallina S, Contini M *et al*. Surgical treatment of dilated cardiomyopathy with conventional techniques. *Eur J Cardiothorac Surg* 1999;**16 (Suppl 1)**:S73–8.

14. Angelini GD, Pryn S, Mehta D *et al*. Left-ventricular-volume reduction for end-stage heart failure. *Lancet* 1997;**350**:489.

15. Konertz W, Khoynezhad A, Sidiropoulos A *et al*. Early and intermediate results of left ventricular reduction surgery. *Eur J Cardiothorac Surg* 1999;**15 (Suppl 1)**:S26–30.

16. Suma H, Isomura T, Horii T *et al*. Nontransplant cardiac surgery for end-stage cardiomyopathy. *J Thorac Cardiovasc Surg* 2000;**119**:1233–44.

17. McCarthy JF, McCarthy PM, Starling RC *et al*. Partial left ventriculectomy and mitral valve repair for end-stage congestive heart failure. *Eur J Cardiothorac Surg* 1998;13:337-43.

18. O'Connell JB, Moore CK, Waterer HC. Treatment of end stage dilated cardiomyopathy. *Br Heart J* 1994;**72 (6 Suppl)**:S52–6.

19. Blanche C, Frota Filho JD, Trento A, Lucchese F. Technical considerations for partial left ventriculectomy (Batista operation). *J Cardiovasc Surg (Torino)* 1998;**39**:829–32.

20. Batista RJ, Santos JL, Takeshita N *et al*. Partial left ventriculectomy to improve left ventricular function in end-stage heart disease. *J Card Surg* 1996;**11**:96–7. [Erratum in *J Card Surg* 1997;**12**:ix]

21. Dor V, Saab M, Coste P *et al*. Left ventricular aneurysm: a new surgical approach. *Thorac Cardiovasc Surg* 1989;**37**:11–9.

22. Bolling SF, Pagani FD, Deeb GM, Bach DS. Intermediate-term outcome of mitral reconstruction in cardiomyopathy. *J Thorac Cardiovasc Surg* 1998;**115**:381-6; discussion 7-8.

23. Lim KH, Callaway M, Angelini GD. Left ventricular volume reduction for end-stage heart failure: intra-papillary or extrapapillary resection, mitral valve repair or replacement? *J Heart Valve Dis* 1998;**7**:484–7.

24. Oliver WC, De Castro MA, Strickland RA. Uncommon diseases and cardiac anesthesia. In: Kaplan JA (ed) *Cardiac anesthesia*. 4th edn. Philadelphia: Saunders, 1999.

25. Aronson SL, Hensley FA, Jr. Case 1 – 1998. Anesthetic considerations for the patient undergoing partial left ventriculectomy (Batista procedure). *J Cardiothorac Vasc Anesth* 1998;**12**:101–10.

26. Izzat MB, Buckley T, Khaw KS *et al*. Perioperative care in left ventricular volume reduction. *J Card Surg* 1999;**14**:136–40.

27. Broderick TJ, Wechsler AS. Triiodothyronine in cardiac surgery. *Thyroid* 1997;**7**:133–7.

28. McCarthy PM. Ventricular remodeling: hype or hope? *Nat Med* 1996;**2**:859–60.

29. Carpentier A. Does surgical reduction of heart size reduce heart failure? *Lancet* 1997;**350**:456.

23
Neuraxial analgesia for thoracic surgery: high-risk thoracic surgical patients with bleeding disorders

Mark Stafford-Smith

Introduction

Neuraxial anesthesia and analgesia strategies have been embraced as a routine part of patient management for major thoracic surgery at many institutions due to the improved pain control and reduced morbidity attributed to these techniques.[1] However, a consensus has not been reached on the use of epidural and intrathecal procedures in operative patients with bleeding disorders. A careful analysis of patient risk and potential benefit is always warranted when introducing a therapy, but this is particularly pertinent when considering neuraxial intervention in a patient with abnormal coagulation.

Case history

A 63-year-old man, previously healthy except for a history of mild type I von Willebrand's disease

(VWD), was admitted to hospital for resection of a newly diagnosed adenocarcinoma of the distal esophagus. Planned surgery involved a combined right thoracotomy and laparotomy approach (Ivor Lewis esophagogastrectomy).

A son with a similar history had been diagnosed with type I VWD, prompting the patient's recent investigation and diagnosis.

Baseline laboratory investigations included factor VIII (F_{VIII}) level 26% (normal 54–195%), von Willebrand factor (VWF) activity 79% (normal 71–160%), and VWF antigen 95% (normal 71–210%). Following a trial administration of desmopressin (DDAVP 25 mg SC) the patient's F_{VIII} level was 123%. VWF multimer analysis was normal, confirming the type I variant of the disease.

A preadmission hematology consult was obtained because of the potential for life threatening bleeding associated with VWD in the setting of major surgery. Primary recommendations included:

Past medical history	Type I von Willebrand's disease. Childhood epistaxis. Prolonged bleeding following tonsillectomy and dental extractions. No transfusions required.
Regular medications	None
Examination	Weight 83 kg. Otherwise unremarkable.
Investigations	Hb 11.8 g dl^{-1}, platelets 253 × 10^9 l^{-1}. PT 12.3 s, APTT 22 s. Blood group: O rhesus positive.

1. Hospital admission on the day prior to surgery.
2. Complete avoidance of non-steroidal anti-inflammatory drugs (NSAIDs), heparin and low molecular weight heparin in the perioperative period.
3. Frequent perioperative monitoring of F_{VIII} levels, and other relevant coagulation tests.
4. Perioperative antihemophilic factor (AHF) administration to maintain specific target F_{VIII} levels (>70% during surgery; 80–100% on postoperative days 1–4; 50–80% on postoperative days 5–8 50; ≥50% on postoperative days 9–12).
5. Use of DDAVP on postoperative days 8–12 if necessary.
6. Intermittent pneumatic leg compression for deep venous thrombosis prophylaxis.

In addition to the usual issues discussed during the preoperative anesthetic visit, regional anesthesia and transfusion strategies were specifically addressed. The patient was counseled that insertion of a thoracic epidural catheter and other neuraxial procedures were not recommended; however, preoperative thoracic paravertebral blocks (PVBs) were offered as an adjunct to parenteral narcotics for postoperative pain control.

Three hours before surgery, the patient received 2000 units of high purity AHF (Humate P, Aventis, Strasbourg, France). Laboratory assessment of F_{VIII} level, VWF activity, ristocetin cofactor activity, complete blood count, PT and APTT were performed prior to, and 1 hour after AHF administration, and then 6 hourly after surgery. Pre- and 1 hour postAHF administration F_{VIII} levels were 56 and 81%, respectively.

No premedication was given. Prior to anesthesia induction, two large-bore intravenous cannulae, a right radial arterial line and a right internal jugular triple lumen catheter were placed. Light sedation was achieved using midazolam 0.5 mg, with subsequent increments of propofol 10–20 mg as needed. In addition, six right PVBs (from T_4 to T_{10}) were performed, with 4 ml bupivicaine 0.5% injected at each site.

After routine monitoring was established, anesthesia induction was achieved using standard dosing regimens for intravenous fentanyl, thiopental, and succinylcholine. A right-sided double lumen endotracheal tube was placed with the aid of fiberoptic bronchoscopy and lung isolation confirmed. Anesthesia was then maintained with isoflurane 1% in oxygen and fentanyl 50–100 µg as necessary. After return of muscle tone, continued relaxation was achieved with pancuronium bromide. Normothermia was maintained using intravenous fluid warming and a forced-air lower body warmer (Bair Hugger, Augustine Medical Inc., Eden Prairie, MN, USA). The 4-hour surgery proceeded without difficulty, the anesthetic course was stable, being notable only for a 105-minute period of one-lung anesthesia. A total of 450 µg fentanyl was administered during surgery. Residual neuromuscular blockade was reversed with neostigmine 2.5 mg and glycopyrollium 0.5 mg. Although subsequent emergence and tracheal extubation were uncomplicated, the patient complained of significant discomfort upon regaining consciousness. Despite the intravenous administration of a further 150 µg fentanyl in 25 µg increments, the patient continued to have moderate pain, and was stable but somnolent. The decision was made to transfer the patient from the operating room to the ICU for further pain management.

Upon arrival in the intensive care unit, the patient remained uncomfortable and dyspneic with apparent chest wall splinting. Arterial blood gas (ABG) analysis while breathing 100% oxygen revealed: pH 7.28; pCO_2 60 mmHg (7.9 kPa), pO_2 280 mmHg (36.8 kPa). The patient received numerous further increments of intravenous fentanyl over the following 3 hours with improved pain relief; however, he was noted to be markedly somnolent and bradypneic. ABG analysis revealed: pH 7.18; pCO_2 78 mmHg (10.3 kPa), pO_2 116 mmHg (15.3 kPa). Effluent from wound drains was moderate, but considered acceptable.

There was a consensus among the attending surgical, anesthesiology, hematology and acute pain service physicians that the respiratory insufficiency that threatened the patient's recovery was related to inadequate analgesia and opioid-induced somnolence. Insertion of a thoracic epidural catheter was reconsidered. The opinion of the hematologist was that the risk of a significant spinal hemorrhage with a neuraxial procedure in the setting of 'all measurable clotting activity being normal' should be considered to be 'roughly equivalent to that of a patient without a bleeding history or bleeding disorder', further that 'clotting activity would be maintained as normal as possible for as long as medically necessary'. Following a discussion of these issues with the patient and his family, an epidural catheter was placed at the $T_{7/8}$ interspace without difficulty using a left paramedian approach. It was agreed that clotting activity would be maintained as close to normal as possible until after the epidural catheter was removed.

An epidural infusion for analgesia containing hydromorphone 0.005% (i.e. 0.05 mg ml⁻¹) and bupivicaine 0.125% was commenced at 3 ml h⁻¹, and 40 µg increments of intravenous naloxone were administered to reduce somnolence and bradypnea. The patient's level of consciousness, comfort, and respiratory effort significantly improved soon after the institution of the epidural infusion. One hour following insertion of the epidural catheter, ABG measurements were considerably improved, having already warranted reduction of the inspired oxygen concentration: pH 7.32; pCO_2 48 mmHg (6.3 kPa), pO_2 96 mmHg (12.6 kPa). Effluent from wound drains continued to be significant but acceptable.

The patient subsequently made an uneventful recovery, being transferred from the intensive care unit to a ward bed 24 hours after surgery. The thoracic epidural analgesia infusion provided good pain relief until the seventh postoperative day, at which time the epidural catheter was removed, normal coagulation parameters having been confirmed. Levels of F_{VIII} ranged between 108 and 173% during the first 8 postoperative days. Intravenous AHF 500–1000 u day⁻¹ was required during the first 6 postoperative days only. Perioperative blood product transfusion was limited to 6280 units Humate P and 2 units of packed red blood cells. The patient was discharged home without further difficulties on the tenth postoperative day.

Discussion

The case presented reviews some of the dilemmas faced in the management of a patient presenting for major thoracic surgery with a history of abnormal coagulation. Postoperative mortality for some thoracotomy procedures exceeds 5%; in many

cases respiratory complications contribute significantly to postoperative mortality and morbidity.[2] The potential advantages of employing neuraxial analgesia for these procedures to improve postoperative respiratory function, in addition to other benefits, are obvious. Although evidence suggests improved overall respiratory and general outcome with epidural versus parenteral pain relief[3, 4] serious complications of neuraxial procedures can be catastrophic (e.g. spinal hematoma), making the decision to use neuraxial analgesia in the setting of abnormal coagulation all the more controversial.

A preoperative risk/benefit assessment for the patient discussed resulted in a clinical plan combining regional block and intravenous opioid analgesics for postoperative pain control; however, this decision was re-evaluated by attending physicians in the context of significant respiratory complications in the early postoperative period felt to be related to failure of this analgesic strategy. In the setting of monitored improvement in coagulation status, the decision was made to place a thoracic epidural catheter. While there is little literature to guide pain management in patients with this set of problems, the consensus of the attending physicians was that the inclusion of epidural analgesia in the clinical management was warranted.

VWD involves deficient or defective VWF, and is the commonest hereditary procoagulant disorder (0.5–1.0% incidence).[5] The type I variant of this disease is most frequent and has an autosomal dominant inheritance, usually presenting in the heterozygous form. Patients with the type I variant generally give a history of mild bleeding problems such as those described in this case (e.g. epistaxis and bleeding after tonsillectomy or dental extractions). However the potential for life-threatening bleeding with major surgery is real, therefore a hematologist should be involved in management when surgery is contemplated.

Principles include strict avoidance of agents that further impair hemostasis, and the administration of high purity AHF for major, or DDAVP for minor surgical procedures to maintain adequate F_{VIII} and VWF levels.[5] It should be noted that laboratory testing in VWD is notoriously variable, and that those with blood group O (such as the patient) have lower VWF levels than other blood groups. In type I variants, measured levels of VWF are in the low normal to low range, however multimer patterns and haemostatic properties of the protein are normal.[6] Due to the function of VWF as a carrier for F_{VIII}:C, reduced levels of this procoagulant factor are also present. Humate P is a product derived from purification of human cryoprecipitate which contains F_{VIII}:C and VWF. In April 1999, the FDA approved Humate P for the treatment of bleeding episodes in severe VWD and in mild to moderate VWD where the use of DDAVP is known or suspected to be inadequate. DDAVP (0.3 µg kg^{-1} IV, administered over 15–30 minutes) improves hemostasis by inducing release into the circulation of endothelial stores of F_{VIII}:C and VWF; however, this method has significant interpatient variability and tachyphylaxis, and therefore is often not sufficient for the hemostatic requirements of major surgery.

Spinal hematoma is a rare but catastrophic complication of neuraxial procedures that may cause major neurological injury or death. In the setting of abnormal hemostasis, anesthesia-related neuraxial procedures, including epidural catheter removal, have been frequently associated with spinal hematomas.[7–10] Although surgical treatment of spinal hematoma may reverse some neurological sequelae, results are generally poor unless intervention occurs within 6 hours of the onset of symptoms.[11] This has led to a consensus that neuraxial procedures are unwarranted in patients with existing (or imminent, i.e. less than 1 hour from the procedure) coagulation impairment. The patient described has an inherited coagulation disorder that was considered 'corrected' (by exogenous Humate P) during the period for which epidural analgesia was contemplated. However, this assumption can only be based on laboratory investigation in the absence of outcome or safety data.

Postoperative pulmonary dysfunction is ubiquitous following abdominal and thoracic surgical procedures.[12] Although postoperative respiratory dysfunction is a multifactorial problem, a significant component is due to reflex diaphragmatic paralysis.[13, 14] Intravenous narcotic analgesia does not predictably improve diaphragmatic and pulmonary function, and may aggravate respiratory insufficiency as occurred in this case. However, pain relief achieved using epidural local anesthetic or narcotic reliably coordinates diaphragmatic excursions, and improves lung volumes and respiratory function.[15, 16] In the case presented, withdrawal of the systemic effects of parenteral narcotics using intravenous increments of naloxone, accompanied by the introduction of epidural analgesia improved level of consciousness, optimized pain relief and corrected respiratory acidosis.

Consideration of alternate regional analgesic approaches that avoid the spinal canal altogether are warranted in the setting of abnormal coagulation, and include selective paravertebral or intercostal nerve blocks. In the patient discussed, PVBs were employed to achieve postoperative unilateral chest wall analgesia. Peripheral nerves exit from the spinal cord into the paravertebral space, an area bounded anteriorly by the parietal pleura, inferiorly and superior by the heads of associated ribs, and posteriorly by the superior costotransverse ligament. Technical considerations for PVBs have been well described elsewhere.[17] Sequential thoracic PVB injections (e.g. T_4–T_{10}, injecting 0.5% bupivicaine 4 ml per space) can produce unilateral chest wall anesthesia lasting 18–24 hours. Advantages of this technique include avoidance of neuraxial opioid side-effects and hypotension related to sympathetic block, with no risk of neuraxis hematoma. Reduced requirements for intraoperative opioids may be anticipated with successful PVB placement.

Generally following a thoracotomy, PVBs must be supplemented with other analgesic modalities to achieve full comfort. However, despite the fact that postoperative right chest wall anesthesia was documented in this case, the contribution of PVBs to overall analgesia was not sufficient to avoid the requirement for significant doses of intravenous opioid.

Sequential intercostal blocks (e.g. T_4–T_{10}) can contribute to unilateral postoperative chest wall analgesia. Intercostal nerve block (ICB) involves depositing local anesthetic (e.g. 0.5% bupivicaine, 4 ml per nerve) at the inferior border of the associated rib near the proximal intercostal nerve. ICBs may be placed by the surgeon under direct vision within the chest, or percutaneously by the anesthesiologist before or after surgery. Similar proposed advantages exist for ICBs and PVBs compared to neuraxial analgesia. However, when compared to PVBs, ICBs recede more rapidly (6–12 hours) than PVBs and do not block the posterior ramus of the intercostal nerve. PVBs are preferred over ICBs at our institution because of the more extensive block and prolonged duration offered by the former.

Recent polymorphism research and the clinical availability of selective inhibitors of cyclo-oxygenase-2 (COX-2) may lead to improvements and modifications of existing analgesia strategies. Rofecoxib and celecoxib are COX-2 inhibitors that are already clinically available for postoperative analgesia.[18, 19] These agents are taken orally, and have similar analgesic efficacy compared to standard NSAIDs. Most of the COX-1-associated side-effects caused by NSAIDs can be avoided (i.e. platelet, gastrointestinal and renal effects).[18–20] However, the effects of COX-2 on hemostasis in the setting of VWD has yet to be evaluated. A new generation of parenteral COX-2 inhibitor agents are likely to be available in the near future that may be useful for clinical situations cases as the one discussed.[21]

Genetic polymorphisms lead to unpredictable effects of some opioid medications. Codeine-containing preparations are discouraged at our institution, since analgesic efficacy with this drug is genotype-dependent and not reliable.[22] This is due to genetic polymorphism of the cytochrome P_{450}-2D6 enzyme that converts codeine to morphine — the active moiety.[23] For example, approximately 8% of caucasians are 'poor metabolizers' and therefore gain little or no pain relief from codeine.[22] Recently recognized effects of serotonin-1_B receptor polymorphism on morphine antinociception in a murine model may represent another genotype-related explanation for the highly variable opioid requirements for effective analgesia seen in humans.[24]

Conclusions and learning points

- The role of neuraxial procedures for anesthesia and analgesia always requires careful evaluation of potential for risk and anticipated benefits, particularly in the patient with abnormal hemostasis where they are relatively contraindicated.
- Postoperative respiratory complications are very common following major thoracic surgery, and measures of pulmonary function after these procedures are generally improved with neuraxial analgesia.
- Constant re-evaluation of analgesic strategies

are an important part of patient care and recovery in the period immediately following major thoracic surgery.
- In care of the postoperative patient with coagulation abnormalities where neuraxial analgesic strategies have not been used, these may be reconsidered in the setting of a delayed recovery thought to be associated with poor pain control, particularly when hemostasis can be further optimized.
- Vigilance for symptoms of spinal hematoma must be part of monitoring for all patients following neuraxial procedures.
- Future developments in pain management for thoracic surgical patients with bleeding disorders may include the introduction of COX-2 inhibitors as analgesic agents without platelet effects, and clinical ability to identify polymorphisms that influence the analgesic effect of currently available analgesic agents.

References

1. Lui S, Carpenter RL, Neal JM. Epidural anesthesia and analgesia. Their role in postoperative outcome. *Anesthesiology* 1995;**82**:1474–506.

2. Watson A, Allen PR. Influence of thoracic epidural analgesia on outcome after resection for esophageal cancer. *Surgery* 1994;**115**:429–32.

3. Peeters-Asdourian C, Gupta S. Choices in pain management following thoracotomy. *Chest* 1999;**115 (5 Suppl)**:122S–124S.

4. Ballantyne JC, Carr DB, deFerranti S *et al*. The comparative effects of postoperative analgesic therapies on pulmonary outcome: cumulative meta-analyses of randomized, controlled trials. *Anesth Analg* 1998;**86**:598–612.

5. Slaughter TF, Greenberg CS. Practice guidelines and treatment of patients with von Willebrand's disease. *Anesthesiology* 1996;**85**:441–2.

6. Slaughter TF, Parker JK, Greenberg CS. A rapid method for the diagnosis of vonWillebrand's disease subtypes by the clinical laboratory. *Arch Path Lab Med* 1995;**119**:148–52.

7. Vandermeulen EP, Van Aken H, Vermylen J. Anticoagulants and spinal-epidural anesthesia. *Anesth Analg* 1994;**79**:1165–77.

8. Ruff RL, Dougherty JH, Jr. Complications of lumbar puncture followed by anticoagulation. *Stroke* 1981;**12**:879–81.

9. Ruff RL, Dougherty JH Jr. Evaluation of acute cerebral ischemia for anticoagulant therapy: Computed tomography or lumbar puncture. *Neurology* 1981;**31**:736–40.

10. Brem SS, Hafler DA, Van Uitert RL *et al.* Spinal subarachnoid hematoma: A hazard of lumbar puncture resulting in reversible paraplegia. *N Engl J Med* 1981;**303**:1020–1.

11. Lawton MT, Porter RW, Heiserman JE *et al.* Surgical management of spinal epidural hematoma: relationship between surgical timing and neurological outcome. *J Neurosurg* 1995;**83**:1–7.

12. Ford GT, Whitelaw WA, Rosenal TW *et al.* Diaphragm function after upper abdominal surgery in humans. *Am Rev Respir Dis* 1983;**127**:431–6.

13. Ford GT, Rosenal TW, Clergue F, Whitelaw WA. Respiratory physiology in upper abdominal surgery. *Clin Chest Med* 1993;**14**:237–52.

14. Simonneau G, Vivien A, Sartene R *et al.* Diaphragm dysfunction induced by upper abdominal surgery. Role of postoperative pain. *Am Rev Respir Dis* 1983;**128**:899–903.

15. Bromage PR, Camporesi E, Chestnut D. Epidural narcotics for postoperative analgesia. *Anesth Analg* 1980;**59**:473–80.

16. Pansard JL, Mankikian B, Bertrand M *et al.* Effects of thoracic extradural block on diaphragmatic electrical activity and contractility after upper abdominal surgery. *Anesthesiology* 1993;**78**:63–71.

17. Greengrass R, Steele S. Paravertebral blocks for breast surgery. *Techniques in Regional Anesthesia & Pain Management* 1998;**2**:8–12.

18. Ehrich EW, Dallob A, De Lepeleire I *et al.* Characterization of rofecoxib as a cyclooxygenase-2 isoform inhibitor and demonstration of analgesia in the dental pain model. *Clin Pharmacol Ther* 1999;**65**:336–47.

19. Geis GS. Update on clinical developments with celecoxib, a new specific COX-2 inhibitor: what can we expect? *Scand J Rheumatol Suppl* 1999;**109**:31–7.

20. Catella-Lawson F, McAdam B, Morrison BW *et al.* Effects of specific inhibition of cyclooxygenase-2 on sodium balance, hemodynamics, and vasoactive eicosanoids. *J Pharmacol Exp Ther* 1999;**289**:735–41.

21. Cheng Z, Nolan AM, McKellar QA. Measurement of cyclooxygenase inhibition in vivo: a study of two non- steroidal anti-inflammatory drugs in sheep. *Inflammation* 1998;**22**:353–66.

22. Persson K, Sjostrom S, Sigurdardottir I *et al.* Patient-controlled analgesia (PCA) with codeine for postoperative pain relief in ten extensive metabolisers and one poor metaboliser of dextromethorphan. *Br J Clin Pharmacol* 1995;**39**:182–6.

23. Mikus G, Somogyi AA, Bochner F, Eichelbaum M. Codeine O-demethylation: rat strain differences and the effects of inhibitors. *Bioch Pharmacol* 1991;**41**:757–62.

24. Hain HS, Belknap JK, Mogil JS. Pharmacogenetic evidence for the involvement of 5-hydroxytryptamine (serotonin)-1B receptors in the mediation of morphine antinociceptive sensitivity. *J Pharmacol Exp Ther* 1999;**291**:444–9.

24
Lung volume reduction surgery

Stuart J Gold and David JR Duthie

Introduction

Otto Brantigan first introduced lung volume reduction surgery (LVRS) as a treatment for end-stage chronic obstructive pulmonary disease (COPD) in the 1950s at the University of Maryland. The procedure was abandoned because of the unacceptably high postoperative mortality (16%).[1-3] Interest in LVRS has been reawakened by Joel Cooper as a palliative procedure for severe emphysema, using modern surgical techniques to decrease post-operative complications: in particular, air leak at the suture lines.[4,5]

The main challenge for the cardiothoracic anesthetist lies with patient selection for surgery and an anesthetic technique, which will expedite painless return to spontaneous ventilation at the end of surgery with minimal respiratory depression.

Case history

A 69-year-old Caucasian male presented with a 6-year history of increasing exertional dyspnea (MRC grade 4), persistent dry cough and occasional wheeze. He gave a history of an exercise tolerance of only 20 yards before he had to rest due to dyspnea. The patient had stopped smoking 2 years earlier having smoked 20–30 cigarettes a day for 50 years.

Pulmonary function tests revealed a severe obstructive ventilatory defect with air trapping. There was no significant change in either FEV_1 or FVC following bronchodilator therapy. Despite 2 weeks of intensive rehabilitation, there was no improvement in either the shuttle walk test (SWT) or the endurance shuttle walk test (ESWT).

The decision to proceed with surgery was made by the patient following extensive discussion with the respiratory medicine and thoracic

Past medical history	Long smoking history.
Regular medications	Combined salbutamol/ipratropium bromide metered-dose inhaler (MDI) 2 puffs QDS, eformoterol MDI 2 puffs QDS, terbutaline MDI PRN, aminophylline SR 225 mg BD. No home oxygen therapy.
Examination	Weight 73.8 kg. BMI 24.1 kg m^{-2}.
Investigations	**Lung function tests:** FEV_1 0.47 l (15% predicted), FVC 1.41 l (35% predicted), FEV_1/FVC 34% (45% predicted). **Body plethysmography:** Total lung capacity 10.26 l. Expiratory reserve volume 1.08 l. Residual volume 7.89 l. **High resolution CT:** Diffuse pulmonary emphysema. **Shuttle walking test (SWT):** 150 m. SpO_2 fell from 93% (at rest) to 86%. **Endurance SWT:** 118 s at 3 km h^{-1}.

surgical staff regarding the potential risks and benefits of surgery. On the morning of surgery the patient was premedicated with oral temazepam 20 mg 1 hour before to transfer to the operating theater. Cannulae were placed in the right radial artery and a vein on the dorsum of the right hand under local anesthesia. Anesthesia was induced with fentanyl 100 µg, propofol 200 mg, and atracurium 50 mg. A 39-French left double-lumen tube was inserted easily and the position of the tube confirmed clinically. Anesthesia was maintained with isoflurane (0.5–1.5% inspired) in oxygen-enriched air. The right internal jugular vein was then cannulated with a triple-lumen catheter. A thoracic epidural was inserted with the patient in the right lateral position. Initial attempts made at T_{5-6} but were unsuccessful because of bony obstruction. The epidural was eventually successfully sited at T_{8-9} using a paramedian approach.

Right-sided video-assisted thorascopic lung volume reduction surgery was uneventful with the patient tolerating one lung ventilation on 100% oxygen. Manipulation of tidal volume and ventilator frequency allowed inflation with pressures no greater than 20 cmH$_2$O. Arterial oxygen saturation remained above 95% and maximum $F_{ET}CO_2$ was 55 mmHg (7.3 kPa). Two intercostal incisions (2 × 2 and 1 × 4 cm) were made and 148.9 g of the right upper lobe was excised, staples were buttressed with Peristrips, Goretex and 10 ml of Quixil glue (Omrix Biopharmeceuticals, Belgium). Apical (28 Fr) and basal (32 Fr) intercostal tube drains were connected to –37 mmHg (–5 kPa) suction. The entire procedure lasted 2 hours with an estimated blood loss of 500 ml. Two litres of crystalloid (compound sodium lactate solution) and 1 l colloid were given during this time. Bupivacaine 0.25%, 20 ml was administered epidurally during surgery.

Postoperatively the patient was extubated and treated in the thoracic high-dependency unit, using a patient-controlled epidural analgesia system (bupivacaine 0.1% and fentanyl 0.0005% at a background rate of 4 ml h^{-1}, a bolus dose of 2 ml and a 'lock-out' time of 30 minutes).

His initial recovery was reasonable but complicated by a persistent air leak that required intermittent negative pressure chest drainage to maintain lung expansion and 4 l min^{-1} oxygen via nasal cannulae to maintain SpO$_2$ ≥ 94%. He had an episode of pyrexia (38.4°C) that was treated — following venepuncture for blood cultures — as catheter-related sepsis, with vancomycin 1 g BD and ciprofloxacin 400 mg BD. Central venous, arterial and peripheral venous cannulae were removed and cultured.

The patient deteriorated on the eleventh day after surgery; developing a supraventricular tachycardia (SVT) of 180 beats min^{-1} associated with confusion and dyspnea. The SVT rate slowed to 110 beats min^{-1} following an infusion of amiodarone 300 mg, but a dramatic increase in air leak occurred with collapse of the right lung. Arterial blood gas analysis, on high-flow oxygen via a tight-fitting facemask revealed: pH 7.31; PaCO$_2$ 59 mmHg (7.9 kPa); PaO$_2$ 70 mmHg (9.3 kPa); HCO$_3$ 29.8 mmol l^{-1}; base excess 2.5 mmol l^{-1}. Due to increasing air leak and decreasing level of consciousness, it was decided to reintubate the trachea and ventilate the lungs using high-frequency jet ventilation.

Following preoxygenation and administration of etomidate 20 mg and suxamethonium 100 mg, the trachea was intubated with a single-lumen tube and lung ventilation achieved using synchronized intermittent mandatory ventilation (SIMV) and inspiratory pressure support (PS). High-frequency jet ventilation (HFJV) was then superimposed using a Monsoon Universal Jet Ventilator (Acutronic Medical Systems AG; Hirzel, Switzerland) at a rate of 150 min^{-1}, with an inspiratory time of 500 ms and 100% oxygen. The patient was sedated with infusions of propofol and alfentanil, and paralysed with an infusion of atracurium. During the course of this intervention there was a gradual decrease in arterial blood pressure that was thought to be secondary to vasodilation. A norepinephrine infusion was commenced to maintain a mean arterial pressure (MAP) >60 mmHg. Subsequent increases in requirements for inotropic support, however, necessitated the insertion of a pulmonary artery flotation catheter to guide therapy.

The surgical team did not feel that surgical intervention was appropriate at this time, therefore treatment was entirely supportive. Unfortunately microbiology cultures grew methicillin-resistant *Staphylococcus aureus* (MRSA) from the patient's pleural fluid, sputum, and central venous cannula tip. This was treated with vancomycin 1 g BD and imipenem 1 g TDS. Nasogastric feeding was commenced on the second ICU day. Until his sudden deterioration the patient had been eating well and had been seen by a dietician who remained involved throughout his stay in ICU.

After 3 days the air leak stopped and HFJV was decreased. The patient continued to be ventilated using pressure-controlled ventilation with a FiO_2 of 0.5. Cardiovascularly he became more stable, no longer requiring inotropes and a deliberate attempt was made to run the patient 'dry', to facilitate weaning for mechanical ventilation. It was not possible to wean the patient in the next 2 days and a tracheostomy was performed to facilitate this on the fifth ICU day.

Progress remained slow and during the following 12 days attempts to reduce respiratory support were all unsuccessful. He remained ventilator dependent, needing repeated suction and bronchoscopy to clear secretions. Seventeen days after ICU admission a right subclavian vein thrombosis occurred, due to long-term central venous cannulation. This was treated with an intravenous infusion of heparin. Weaning progressed to periods on a 'T-piece' with PEEP 7.5 cmH_2O lasting no longer than a few hours. Progress was further compromised by the development of a right-sided pneumonia with evidence of empyema.

Following a further fiberoptic bronchoscopy on the day 22, a decision was made to reparalyze and ventilate, with the patient in the left lateral position. This maneuver was discontinued after 2 days with no great clinical improvement. Over the next 22 days repeated attempts to wean ventilatory support were unsuccessful despite adequate nutritional support, oxygen delivery, fluid balance and cardiovascular parameters. Further attempts were made to wean on 'clinical grounds' with permissive hypercapnia but the right lung continued to contribute very little to gas exchange.

Forty one days after admission to the ICU a double-lumen tracheostomy tube was placed under fiberoptic guidance to allow differential ventilatory support with PS and continuous positive airway pressure (CPAP) for each lung. Right lung; PS 20 cm H_2O + CPAP 5 cm H_2O, left lung; PS 14 cm H_2O + CPAP 3 cm H_2O. After 24 hours of differential ventilation his condition again deteriorated and full, pressure limited (25 cm H_2O) ventilation via both bronchial lumens, and re-introduction of inotropic support (dobuta-mine 7 μg kg^{-1} min^{-1}) was necessary. Despite further attempts to improve ventilation over the next 24 hours, differential support was abandoned as it appeared to be making the situation worse.

Over the next 7 days the patient's renal function began to deteriorate. Over the following 15 days his acute renal failure was managed conservatively and a short course of high-dose methylprednisolone was administered. Although the use of endobronchial surfactant was considered, it was not given because of the lack of good evidence demonstrating clinical efficacy and cost. On day 66 continuous venovenous hemofiltration was instituted to remove excess fluid ahead of a determined attempt to wean from mechanical ventilation.

Spontaneous ventilation was not sustained and the patient died after 73 days of intensive care, 85 days after his lung volume reduction surgery. A post mortem examination confirmed that the patient had died from respiratory failure secondary to bilateral organizing pneumonia, adult respiratory distress syndrome (ARDS), and severe emphysema.

Discussion

Although the mechanisms of functional and physiological improvement seen after LVRS in patients with severe COPD are not known, a number of factors are likely to contribute. These include: a decrease in hyper-inflation,[6] an increase in elastic recoil,[7] improved thoracic wall movement[8] and improved diaphragmatic function.[9] These changes following LVRS combine to make the lung, diaphragm and chest wall a more effective 'pump'.[10]

Whatever its mechanism of action, LVRS has been shown to improve both subjective measures of quality of life and physiological variables. Due to the small number of patients receiving this novel surgery in any particular unit, case series are the only current source of data. A recent review article[11] identified 19 series with adequate preoperative assessment and postoperative follow-up data for a total of 567 patients. Improvements following LVRS included: an increase in FEV_1 from interquartile range (IQR) 0.64–0.73 l to IQR 0.91–1.07 l; an increase in

6-minute walking distance (6MWD) from IQR 241–290 m to IQR 306–434 m; and subjective improvement in dyspnea and quality of life scores. The review reported mortality rates to be IQR 0–6 % for early deaths (≤30 days after surgery) and IQR 0–8 % for late mortality (>30 days after surgery) at 3–6 months. As a case series, conclusions must be drawn from this review with caution. Sources of bias that affect these results include: publication bias; absence of control groups; and lack of blinding.

Intensive pulmonary rehabilitation can improve exercise tolerance, dyspnea and quality of life.[12, 13] This can even be undertaken successfully at home,[14] and most centers include this treatment for patients undergoing LVRS. All patients currently being enrolled into the National Emphysema Treatment Trial (NETT)[15] will undergo pulmonary rehabilitation. This government-funded, multicenter prospective randomized trial has been designed to compare maximal medical therapy with medical therapy plus LVRS. The primary outcome measures will be survival and maximum exercise capacity in a study population of 2500 patients.

There are several surgical techniques available to perform LVRS. The technique can be open, requiring median sternotomy or endoscopic, video-assisted thoracoscopic surgery (VATS). The lung excision can be either unilateral or bilateral. Although there is no surgical technique of choice, a study of 260 patients revealed that bilateral VATS using staples was associated with improved 2-year survival and lung function when compared to unilateral VATS.[16]

One of the biggest challenges in anesthesia for LVRS is patient selection and considerable effort has gone into identifying the characteristics of patients likely to have a successful outcome. The decision to proceed with LVRS should follow informed discussions between the patient, surgeon, anesthetist and respiratory physician. In the case described above, postoperative complications were poorly tolerated in a patient with little respiratory reserve.

A number of preoperative factors are known to be of value in predicting postoperative outcomes. Reduced mortality is associated with patient age <70 years, FEV_1 >0.5 l and PaO_2 >54 mmHg (7.2 kPa).[17] Pre-operative dynamic intrinsic positive end-expiratory pressure (PEEPi, dyn), ≥5 cmH_2O, correlates well with increased FEV_1 and improve-

ment in dyspnea score following LVRS.[18] Reduced preoperative expiratory strength and markedly elevated dead space ventilation is associated with increased short term mortality.[19] Patients with emphysema localized to an upper or lower lobe on computed tomography or perfusion scintigraphy have a better outcome after LVRS than patients with diffuse or homogenous emphysema.[20] Patients with chronic hypercapnia alone have no significant increase in mortality or morbidity and should not be denied LVRS on the basis of this alone.[21]

Patients with below normal body mass index (BMI) have increased morbidity compared to those who have normal BMI. In one study, 26% patients with low BMI required ventilatory support for more than 24 hours, compared to 4% patients with normal BMI.[22] The authors speculated that preoperative improvement of nutritional status may reduce morbidity; however, if the low BMI is caused by the 'pulmonary cachexia syndrome', improving nutritional status may not necessarily help. Low BMI has been identified as an independent indicator of advanced lung disease.[23] Patients with advanced lung disease are more likely to require mechanical ventilation of the lungs following LVRS.

Most patients who present for LVRS have pulmonary function tests and exercise tolerances that many anesthetists would feel preclude them from many types of elective surgery. An FEV_1 less than 1 l, would suggest a high risk of postoperative respiratory failure after lung resection. There are now many case reports of patients with severe emphysema and early stage lung cancer who would not previously have been offered surgery due to their poor respiratory reserve who have undergone surgery with improvement in pulmonary function postoperatively.[24] An interesting report describes a patient who underwent LVRS at the same time as repair of a thoracic aortic aneurysm, with postoperative improvement in pulmonary function.[25] This is analogous to patients having coronary revascularization at the same time as carotid endarterectomy.

Postoperative analgesia in patients who have had LVRS is extremely important to allow patients to cough, thus preventing atelectasis secondary to shallow breathing. Thoracic epidural analgesia offers good quality pain relief with limited systemic adverse effects. There is, however, no consensus on which drug combination 'maximizes' ventilation and 'minimizes' respiratory depression. Some argue that no opioids should be administered either epidurally or systemically, to prevent any respiratory depression.[26] We use a continuous infusion of bupivacaine 0.1% and fentanyl 0.0005% (5 µg ml^{-1}) at 4 ml h^{-1} with additional 2 ml 'on demand' boluses at up to 30 minutes intervals administered using a patient-controlled epidural analgesia (PCEA) pump. This produces less intercostal motor block than higher concentrations of bupivacaine. Low-dose fentanyl gives a good quality of analgesia without significant respiratory depression, permitting the use of a lower concentration of bupivacaine.

Conclusions and learning points

- LVRS is likely to become used increasingly as a treatment option for well-defined groups of patients with severe emphysema.
- Evidence for preoperative predictors of outcome is currently based on relatively small case series rather than prospective randomized controlled clinical trials.
- Patients who have advanced lung disease that is favorable for LVRS, may be able to undergo surgery for other thoracic conditions at the same time as LVRS.
- Postoperative complications are tolerated poorly in a population of patients with end-stage respiratory disease.
- Communication with surgical, respiratory medicine and anesthetic consultants is essential to ensure that only suitable patients are offered this potentially beneficial treatment.
- There is currently no one discriminatory test to identify patients who will benefit most from LVRS. With increasing experience of this type of surgery, a range of results of preoperative investigations are being used to predict likely surgical outcomes and advise patients on the risks and benefits of surgery. Over the range of results, limits are being identified, below which a patient will be considered to have disease too advanced to benefit from surgery, and above which disability is not severe enough to justify surgery. This case report suggests that improvement in physiological

parameters following rehabilitation may be as important as the absolute values of preoperative investigations. A lack of improvement during rehabilitation may indicate insufficient physiological reserve to survive the immediate effects of surgery.

References

1. Brantigan O, Mueller E. Surgical treatment of pulmonary emphysema. *Am Surg* 1957;**23**:789–804.

2. Brantigan O, Kress M, Mueller E. The surgical approach to pulmonary emphysema. *Dis Chest* 1961;**39**:485–501.

3. Brantigan O, Mueller E, Kress M. A surgical approach to pulmonary emphysema. *Am Rev Respir Dis* 1959;**80**:194–202.

4. Cooper J, Trulock E, Triantafillou A. Bilateral pneumectomy (lung reduction) for chronic obstructive pulmonary disease. *J Thorac Cardiovasc Surg* 1995;**109**:106–19.

5. Cooper J. Technique to reduce air leaks after resection of emphysematous lung. *Ann Thorac Surg* 1994;**57**:1038.

6. Klepetko W. Surgical aspects and techniques of lung volume reduction surgery for severe emphysema. *Eur Respir J* 1999;**13**:919–25.

7. Gelb AF, McKenna RJ, Brenner M *et al*. Lung function after bilateral lower lobe lung volume reduction surgery for alpha 1-antitrypsin emphysema. *Eur Respir J* 1999;**14**:928–33.

8. Fujimoto K, Kubo K, Haniuda M *et al*. Improvements in thoracic movement following lung volume reduction surgery in patients with severe emphysema. *Intern Med* 1999;**38**:119–25.

9. Lando Y, Bosselle PM, Shade D *et al*. Effect of lung volume reduction on diaphragm length in severe chronic obstructive pulmonary disease. *Am J Respir Crit Care Med* 1999;**159**:796–805.

10. Shade D Jr, Cordova F, Lando Y *et al*. Relationship between resting hypercapnia and physiologic parameters before and after lung volume reduction surgery in severe chronic obstructive pulmonary disease. *Am J Respir Crit Care Med* 1999;**159**:1405–11.

11. Young J, Fry-Smith A, Hyde C. Lung volume reduction surgery (LVRS) for chronic obstructive pulmonary disease (COPD) with underlying severe emphysema. *Thorax* 1999;**54**:779–89.

12. Crockoft AE, Saunders MJ, Berry G. Randomised controlled trial of rehabilitation in chronic respiratory disability. *Thorax* 1981;**36**:2003.

13. Goldstein RS, Gork EH, Stubbing D. Randomised controlled trial of respiratory rehabilitation. *Lancet* 1994;**334**:1394.

14. Debigare R, Maltais F, Whittom F *et al*. Feasibility and efficacy of home training before lung volume reduction. *J Cardiopulm Rehab* 1999;**19**:235–41.

15. Rational and design of the national emphysema treatment trial (NETT): a prospective randomised trial of lung volume reduction surgery. *J Thorac Cardiovasc Surg* 1999;**118**:518–28.

16. Serna DL, Brenner M, Osann KE *et al*. Survival after unilateral versus bilateral lung volume reduction surgery for emphysema. *J Thorac Cardiovasc Surg* 1999;**118**:1101–9.

17. Brenner M, McKenna RJ Jr, Chen JC *et al*. Survival following bilateral staple lung volume reduction surgery for emphysema. *Chest* 1999;**115**:390–6.

18. Tschernko EM, Kritzinger M, Gruber EM *et al*. Lung volume reduction surgery: preoperative functional predictors for post-operative outcome. *Anesth Analg* 1999;**88**:28–33.

19. Ferguson GT, Fernandez E, Zamora MR *et al*. Improved exercise performance following lung volume reduction surgery for emphysema. *Am J Respir Crit Care Med* 1998;**157**:1195–203.

20. Kazerooni EA. Radiologic evaluation of emphysema for lung volume reduction surgery. *Clin Chest Med* 1999;**20**:845–61.

21. Wisser W, Kleptko W, Senbalklavaci O *et al*. Chronic hypercapnia should not exclude patients from lung volume reduction surgery. *Eur J Cardiothorac Surg* 1998;**14**:107–12.

22. Mazolewski P, Turner JF, Baker M *et al*. The impact of nutritional status on the outcome of lung volume reduction surgery: a prospective study. *Chest* 1999;**116**:693–6.

23. Donahoe M. Nutritional support in advanced lung disease. *Clin Chest Med* 1997;**18**:547–61.

24. Mentzer SJ, Swanson SJ. Treatment of patients with lung cancer and severe emphysema. *Chest* 1999;**116**:477–9.

25. Zannini P, Carretta A, Chiesa R *et al*. Combined lung volume reduction surgery and thoracic aortic aneurysm resection. *J Cardiovasc Surg* 1998;**39**:509–10.

26. Klafta JM. http://dacc.uchicago.edu/default.html.

25

Bronchopleural fistula in the presence of empyema

Justiaan LC Swanevelder and Cindy Horst

Introduction

A direct communication between the tracheo-bronchial tree and the pleural cavity is called a bronchopleural fistula (BPF). If this communication extends through the chest wall to the outside it is called a bronchopleurocutaneous fistula. Empyema or pus in the pleural cavity often accompanies this condition. Most cases of BPF in the presence of empyema follow pulmonary resection. Other causes include: blunt and penetrating trauma; tumor invasion; chronic inflammatory disease; spontaneous rupture of an empyema or lung-cyst; and rupture of bronchus, bulla or parenchymal tissue as a result of barotrauma. The induction of anesthesia and perioperative management of such a patient needs thorough planning and several very important principles have to be considered.

Case history

A 59-year-old Caucasian male presented with increasing cough, foul blood-stained sputum and fever. Fourteen months earlier he had presented with mixed epithelioid-sarcomatous malignant mesothelioma (T2N0M0) and had undergone right radical pleuropneumonectomy with resection of the right hemidiaphragm and the pericardium.

On examination he was febrile, tachypneic and tachycardic. His peripheral oxygen saturation was 92% while breathing room air and arterial

Past medical history	Occupational asbestos exposure. Right radical pleuropneumonectomy.
Regular medications	Paracetamol 1 g QDS.
Examination	Weight 58 kg. BMI 18 kgm^{-2}. Cachectic. Temperature 38.6°C. HR 120 bpm. BP 135/80 mmHg. Cough productive of purulent sputum. Widespread coarse crackles and wheeze on left side. Transmitted breath sounds on the right.
Investigations	Hb 11.3 gd l^{-1}, WBC 13.0 × 10^9 l^{-1}, platelets 619 × 10^9 l^{-1}. [Na$^+$] 137 mmol l^{-1}, [K$^+$] 4.2 mmol l^{-1}, urea 9.5 mg dl^{-1} (3.4 mmol l^{-1}), creatinine 0.6 mg dl^{-1} (54 µmol l^{-1}) **ECG:** Sinus tachycardia. Right axis deviation. **CXR:** Air/fluid level on the right. Left lung field clear. **ABG:** pH 7.43, PO$_2$ 67 mmHg (8.9 kPa), PCO$_2$ 37 mmHg (4.9 kPa), [HCO$_3^-$] 27 mmol l^{-1}, base excess -3.0 mmol l^{-1}

blood gas analysis confirmed mild hypoxia. A plain chest radiograph revealed an air/fluid level that was lower than that seen on a radiograph performed in the outpatient clinic a week earlier. The patient's airway was assessed by an anesthetist, who considered it would be easy to place an endotracheal tube as necessary.

On the basis of the above, a diagnosis of BPF and empyema was made and a right intercostal chest drain was inserted under local anesthesia and connected to an underwater seal. From his chest 750 ml blood-stained fluid was drained and samples sent for microscopy and culture. These revealed no growth after several days. Intravenous cefuroxime 1.5 g TDS and flucloxacillin 1 g QDS were commenced. Supplemental oxygen was administered via a Hudson mask and the patient was nursed in the semi-recumbent position — with the left lung uppermost — and preparations were made for rigid bronchoscopy.

On the following day, the patient was transferred to the operating theater maintaining a semi-sitting position with his right side down. A suction catheter was at hand in case of overspill during tracheal instrumentation. After preoxygenation, induction of anesthesia was achieved using remifentanil 0.1 μg kg^{-1} min^{-1}, propofol by target-controlled infusion (TCI) pump aiming for a target concentration of 4 μg ml^{-1} and suxamethonium 1 mg kg^{-1}. Atropine was available in case of a bradycardia. The consultant thoracic surgeon was present with the bronchoscope ready, in case ventilation was problematic. When the patient was anesthetized the rigid bronchoscope was easily introduced into the trachea and oxygenation maintained with intermittent Venturi ventilation using a Sanders injector. Bronchoscopy revealed a fistula in the right bronchial stump to which tissue glue was applied. This established a reduction in the air leak but he still required the chest drain, which was subsequently connected to a drainage bag via a flutter valve. Postoperative recovery was complicated by diarrhoea. No pathogens were isolated from stool samples and *Clostridium difficile* toxin was not detected. A small air leak continued and after 6 days the patient was discharged home on metronidazole 500 mg TDS, with the chest drain in situ.

One month later the patient was readmitted for limited rib resection plus drainage and debridement of his right hemithorax as the infected postpneumonectomy space was not adequately drained through the intercostal drain. There was still a small air leak. The patient was assessed on the ward and premedication was not deemed necessary.

The patient was again maintained in the sitting position with the infected right side in the dependent position. A suction catheter was available. After establishing intravenous access, glycopyrrolate 400 μg was administered to decrease secretions. Local anesthesia of the upper airways was obtained with topical application of 10% lignocaine to the oropharynx and supraglottic area. Transtracheal injection of 4 ml lignocaine 2% was performed with a 21–gauge needle through the cricothyroid membrane. The patient was preoxygenated, and anesthesia was induced using a propofol TCI with a target concentration of 2 μg ml^{-1}. Spontaneous ventilation was maintained throughout. A left-sided 39–French double-lumen endotracheal tube (Bronchocath, Mallinckrodt Medical Inc; St Louis, MO, USA) was inserted and the right bronchial stump isolated. Correct positioning of the tube was confirmed using a fiberoptic bronchoscope. The left lung was ventilated with a tidal volume of 500 ml at 16 breaths per minute, while anesthesia was maintained using propofol TCI, fentanyl 200 μg and atracurium 40 mg. The use of topical anesthesia and the maintenance of spontaneous respiration allowed direct laryngoscopy, tracheal intubation and isolation of the left lung without the need for neuromuscular blockade and intermittent positive pressure ventilation. The patient was placed in the left lateral position and the position of the endotracheal tube rechecked with the fiberoptic bronchoscope.

A minithoracotomy and rib-resection were performed, and evacuation of the postpneumonectomy space and surgical closure of the BPF proceeded without incident. Before closure of the chest the right bronchial stump was checked for residual leaks by filling the chest cavity with warm saline, applying 30 cmH_2O pressure to the airway and looking for bubbling of air. At the end of the procedure the surgeon performed an intercostal block using 3 ml bupivacaine 0.5% infiltrating the thoracotomy and chest drain wounds with a total of 15 ml bupivacaine 0.5%. Residual neuromuscular blockade was antagonized with neostigmine 2.5 mg and glycopyrrolate 600 μg and, after satisfactory spontaneous ventilation was re-established, the trachea was extubated. The patient was recovered in the right lateral semi-sitting position. Supplemental humidified oxygen was administered by face-mask.

An intravenous morphine patient-controlled analgesia (PCA) device and oral diclofenac sodium 50 mg TDS were used for postoperative pain relief. Fluid drained from the chest cavity grew methicillin resistant *Staphylococcus aureus* (MRSA) and a course of intravenous vancomycin 1 g BD and ciprofloxacin 400 mg BD was commenced. The patient made an otherwise uneventful recovery and was discharged home in good condition, 3 weeks after surgery.

Discussion

Any infective process of the lung, such as pneumonia, tuberculosis or a lung abscess, can be complicated by the development of an infected pleural effusion or empyema.[1-3] This can also occur after thoracic surgery, thoracic trauma, or needle puncture of the pleural space. Pulmonary inflammation leads to irritation of the visceral pleura, an increased production of pleural fluid and a subsequent pleural effusion. This protein-rich exudate is an excellent culture medium for bacteria. The pus and fibrin deposits may form loculations and pleural thickening, which will cause partial collapse of the lung and interfere with normal ventilation. If this is not drained, a thick membrane forms, leading to entrapment of the lung and pus may erode into the airways creating a BPF, and eventually penetrate the chest wall.

Following lobectomy or pneumonectomy, an excessively long bronchial stump can collect secretions, which may become infected and ultimately cause dehiscence. Although in most cases this occurs within a few weeks after surgery, dehiscence and empyema may occur several years after pneumonectomy. The blood supply to the right bronchial tree is less than that of the left side, thus breakdown of the bronchial stump is more likely to occur after right rather than left pneumonectomy.[4] Although the incidence of BPF has decreased markedly over the past 20–30 years, the mortality associated with this condition remains high.

The patient with empyema typically presents with shortness of breath, fever and a cough productive of purulent sputum. In addition, patients may also complain of chest pain, subcutaneous emphysema and hemoptysis. On examination they will often be tachypneic, have dullness to chest percussion, decreased breath sounds and rhonchi. Following pneumonectomy the mediastinum is usually shifted *towards* the affected side. Bronchopleural fistula of acute onset, however, may present with tension pneumothorax and shift of the trachea and mediastinum *away* from the side of the pathology. Rarely in the presence of BPF and empyema the potentially rapidly fatal complication of pulmonary artery hemorrhage can occur. Management of this predicament is outside the scope of this discussion. The diagnosis of BPF and empyema is confirmed by a chest radiograph, which may reveal a falling air-fluid level,[5] and a diagnostic pleural aspiration. At bronchoscopy the diagnosis will be clear if fluid or pus is detected coming from the bronchial stump.

The treatment of empyema is surgical drainage of the infected fluid and re-expansion of the residual lung tissue.[6-9] In the initial stages this may be achieved with insertion of an intercostal chest drain. Most fistulae will close spontaneously; healing with conservative treatment, tube drainage of the pleural cavity, and time. Small fistulae can be sealed with bronchoscopic application of tissue glue.[10, 11] If the fistula is large or the empyema presents at a later stage – when organisation of the fibropurulent fluid has taken place – it is unlikely that resolution will occur with conservative management and formal surgical repair, by video-assisted thoracoscopy or lateral thoracotomy (with or without rib resection and decortication), is required.

In general these patients have two major problems:[12] Firstly, the remaining 'healthy' lung can be soiled by the overflow of pus or infected fluid from the dehisced bronchial stump, resulting in a lung with reduced gas exchange capacity. The remaining lung may have compromised function as a consequence of underlying pulmonary disease. Secondly, the patient's pulmonary function may be compromised because of a loss of tidal volume via the bronchopleural connection. If large enough this leads to a decrease in effective alveolar ventilation. During mechanical ventilation, increasing the delivered tidal volume or peak airway pressure merely increases the leak. Together these problems may lead to hypoxia and hypercarbia.

The size of a BPF and the magnitude of tidal volume loss can be quantified using several methods.[12] The commonest of these is to monitor the amount of air that bubbles from the chest drain. A small, intermittent leak during expiration indicates that the fistula is small, whereas larger amounts of air bubbling continuously indicates that the fistula is large. Measurement of the difference between inspired and expired tidal volumes can be used to quantify the size of a bronchopleural fistula. This can be done using a spirometer or pneumotachygraph attached to the endotracheal tube or, in the non-intubated patient, attached to a face-mask. Respiratory rate will tend to increase if the loss of tidal volume is sufficient to compromise alveolar ventilation. Worsening tachypnea, particularly when accompanied by hypoxia and hypercarbia, indicates that the fistula is substantial.

The perioperative management of the patient with BPF and empyema who requires thoracotomy can be divided in to three distinct stages: preoperative resuscitation and optimization, anesthesia and postoperative care. Basic resuscitation of the patient with the administration of intravenous fluids, antibiotics and supplemental oxygen, should commence as soon as possible.[2, 13] If necessary, surgery should be delayed until the patient's cardiorespiratory state can be optimized. A functional chest drain should be inserted under local anesthesia to drain any pus or infected fluid from the chest cavity and prevent it from spilling into the bronchial tree. By preventing the development of a positive pressure in the chest cavity, the chest drain will prevent mediastinal shift, compression of the remaining lung and hemodynamic instability. It is important to be cautious when applying suction to the chest drain because the alveolar ventilation may be severely impaired. Positioning of the patient in the semi-sitting position with the diseased side dependent is of the utmost importance, to prevent soiling the unaffected lung. If bronchoscopy and surgical correction is planned, the patient should be transported to the operating theater and anesthetized in this position.

The principle goals of anesthetic management are maintenance of oxygenation and isolation of the diseased lung.[12, 14, 15] To avoid tidal volume loss through the BPF, soiling of the remaining lung and expansion of pleural air spaces, the timing of lung isolation is very important.

Although selective isolation of the affected lobe or lung with a bronchial blocker placed with a bronchoscope is sometimes achieved, the most common practice is the placement of a double-lumen tube. The choice between a bronchial blocker and a double-lumen tube is usually a matter of personal preference of the anesthetist. A suction apparatus should be at hand at all times during anesthesia and tracheal manipulation. The airway should be cleared regularly during the procedure and before extubation.

Three approaches to airway management and lung isolation have been advocated: local anesthesia, general anesthesia with spontaneous ventilation, and general anesthesia with a short-acting neuromuscular blocking agent. Regardless of the approach used, an intravenous infusion and full physiological monitoring should be established in advance. In addition, many anesthetists use direct arterial pressure monitoring. Tracheal intubation and lung isolation under local anesthesia is achieved using a fiberoptic bronchoscope. Topical anesthesia of the mouth, tongue, pharynx and upper airways is supplemented by bilateral internal laryngeal nerve blocks and a transcricoid injection of 3–5 ml of lignocaine 2%. Mild sedation with a small dose of midazolam or diazepam and the use of glycopyrrolate to decrease secretions, will contribute to the success of this procedure. Lung isolation under general anesthesia with spontaneous ventilation requires that the patient be induced in the sitting position with the affected lung tilted in the dependent position. When combined with the local anesthetic technique described above, this technique provides excellent intubating conditions. The selection of induction agent is a matter for personal preference.[14, 16, 17] Intravenous induction with thiopental or propofol, or inhalational induction with halothane or sevoflurane are acceptable. It is important, however, to ensure that the rate of administration is such that spontaneous respiration is maintained until the lung is isolated. Drugs that impede spontaneous ventilation, such as opioids and neuromuscular blocking agents, should be withheld until after lung isolation. Lung isolation under general anesthesia with a short-acting muscle relaxant is controversial. In some centers this technique is routinely employed as the standard approach[4] while in others, the technique is reserved for patients with a small BPF and patients in whom tracheal intubation and lung isolation under local anesthesia or general anesthesia with spontaneous ventilation is unsuccessful.[15] Before embarking on this technique, however, the anesthetist must be convinced that lung isolation will be easily achieved. Following preoxygenation, anesthesia is induced with an intravenous induction agent and a short-acting muscle relaxant such as suxamethonium or mivacurium. A rigid bronchoscope and Sander's injector should be immediately available, in case rapid lung isolation is unsuccessful and it is not possible to establish adequate ventilation.

All of the above techniques have one aim in common, avoidance of intermittent positive pressure ventilation (IPPV) prior to lung isolation.[12] Bronchopleural fistula is an indication for high-frequency jet ventilation (HFJV) both during the procedure and in the postoperative period, should ventilatory support be necessary. HFJV will potentially reduce the magnitude of the air leak by ensuring lower peak airway pressures and a reduced tidal volume. At present there is still no evidence however, that any mode of ventilation is superior in the management of a bronchopleural fistula.[18]

During the procedure regular suctioning of both sides is essential to prevent soiling of the unaffected lung. The anesthetist should always be aware that the double-lumen tube can easily be displaced by surgical manipulation and that the original lung isolation may be lost. After completion of the BPF closure, ventilation of any residual lung tissue on the affected side should be initiated slowly under direct vision. This will decrease the risk of re-expansion pulmonary edema. Prior to chest closure, the surgeon may fill the affected hemithorax with warm sterile saline and test the integrity of the closure by looking for any residual air leak while continuous positive pressure is applied to the airway.

The quality of postoperative care has a significant influence on outcome following surgery for BPF and empyema.[4] It is important to achieve spontaneous ventilation at the end of the procedure and extubate the trachea if at all possible. To improve respiratory function positioning of the patient in the semi-sitting position is vital. Adequate pain relief is of the utmost importance to achieve good spontaneous tidal volumes and ventilation efforts. Techniques commonly used include: continuous epidural infusion; patient-controlled epidural anesthesia; and regional techniques such as paravertebral blockade. Postoperative IPPV and the application of positive end expiratory pressure (PEEP) may lead to further persistent air leaks and should be avoided if possible. If ventilation is required postoperatively or when surgical closure of the BPF is not an immediate option, a number of ventilation strategies can be used.[12, 19] If the compliance of the unaffected lung is good, pressure-controlled ventilation (PCV) with low peak airway pressures, without PEEP may be used. However, in cases where the 'unaffected' lung is poorly compliant as a consequence of pneumonia or the adult respiratory distress syndrome, PCV is of little use. Morbidity and mortality in this setting is significant. HFJV[18] has minimal effects on the cardiac output and may decrease the loss of tidal volume through the BPF. Gas exchange is not, however, always predictable and HFJV is poorly tolerated by the non-paralyzed conscious patient. Unless a bronchial blocker is used the unaffected lung is not protected against soiling. Selective intubation of the unaffected lung with a double-lumen tube and one-lung ventilation is a possibility, but not a very good long-term option. In particular, patients with associated lung pathology may develop a large trans-pulmonary shunt, which is not well tolerated. Differential lung ventilation (through a double-lumen tube) with two ventilators and independent ventilator settings for each lung has been used and may be of value, but has limitations.[20]

Conclusions and learning points

- Bronchopleural fistulae are most commonly an early postoperative complication of lobectomy and pneumonectomy.
- A bronchopleural or bronchopleurocutaneous fistula is often accompanied by empyema and the approach to such a patient should be carefully considered preoperatively.
- The management of such a patient is to control the air leak and protect the unaffected lung from soiling.
- If the unaffected lung is soiled with empyema pus from the diseased lung, it will lead to ventilation:perfusion mismatch and, ultimately, hypoxemia.

- In the presence of a large fistula there can be significant loss of tidal volume especially during positive pressure ventilation. This results in decreased alveolar ventilation and hypercarbia.
- Isolation of the unaffected lung with a double-lumen tube or a bronchial blocker, before airway manipulation or anesthesia, is of the utmost importance.
- After repair of the bronchopleural fistula it is vital to re-establish spontaneous ventilation, extubate the trachea and recover the patient in the sitting position.
- Postoperative care, particularly pain control, has a significant impact on clinical outcome.

References

1. Wright CD, Wain JC, Mathisen DJ, Grillo HC. Postpneumonectomy bronchopleural fistula after sutured bronchial closure: incidence, risk factors, and management. *J Thorac Cardiovasc Surg* 1996;**112**:1367–71.

2. Ferguson MK. Surgical management of intrapleural infections. *Semin Respir Infect* 1999;**14**:73–81.

3. Ferguson MK. Thoracoscopy for empyema, bronchopleural fistula, and chylothorax. *Ann Thorac Surg* 1993;**56**:644–5.

4. Gothard J, Kelleher A. *Essentials of cardiac and thoracic anaesthesia*. Oxford: Butterworth-Heinemann. 1999; 137–82.

5. Lauckner ME, Beggs I, Armstrong RF. The radiological characteristics of bronchopleural fistula following pneumonectomy. *Anaesthesia* 1983,**38**:452–6.

6. Wain JC. Management of late postpneumonectomy empyema and bronchopleural fistula. *Chest Surg Clin N Am* 1996;**6**:529–41.

7. Hollaus PH, Lax F, Wurnig PN *et al*. Videothoracoscopic debridement of the postpneumonectomy space in empyema. *Eur J Cardiothorac Surg* 1999;**16**:283–6.

8. Hollaus PH, Huber M, Lax F *et al*. Closure of bronchopleural fistula after pneumonectomy with a pedicled intercostal muscle flap. *Eur J Cardiothorac Surg* 1999;**16**:181–6.

9. Hollaus PH, Lax F, Wurnig PN, Pridun NS. Videothoracoscopic treatment of postpneumonectomy empyema. *J Thorac Cardiovasc Surg* 1999;**117**:397–8.

10. Eng J, Sabanathan S. Tissue adhesive in bronchial closure. *Ann Thorac Surg* 1989;**48**:683–5.

11. Bayfield MS, Spotnitz WD. Fibrin sealant in thoracic surgery. Pulmonary applications, including management of bronchopleural fistula. *Chest Surg Clin N Am* 1996;**6**:567–83.

12. Benumof JL. Anesthesia for Emergency Thoracic Surgery. In: Benumof JL (ed.) *Anesthesia for thoracic surgery*. 2nd edn. London: WB Saunders. 1994; 612–56.

13. Deschamps C, Pairolero PC, Allen MS, Trastek VF. Management of postpneumonectomy empyema and bronchopleural fistula. *Chest Surg Clin N Am* 1996;**6**:519–27.

14. Riley RH, Wood BM. Induction of anaesthesia in a patient with a bronchopleural fistula. *Anaesth Intensive Care* 1994;**22**:625–6.

15. Doolan L, Clarke P. Common peri-operative problems and complications: pulmonary haemorrhage/empyema/bronchopleural fistula/persistent air leaks. In: Ghosh S, Latimer R (eds) *Thoracic anaesthesia: principles and practice*. Oxford: Butterworth-Heinemann. 1999; 241–54.

16. Donnelly JA, Webster RE. Computer-controlled anaesthesia in the management of bronchopleural fistula. *Anaesthesia* 1991;**46**:383–4.

17. Crofts SL, Hutchison GL. General anaesthesia and undrained pneumothorax. The use of a computer-controlled propofol infusion. *Anaesthesia* 1991;**46**:192–4.

18. Spinale FG, Linker RW, Crawford FA, Reines HD. Conventional versus high frequency jet ventilation with a bronchopleural fistula. *J Surg Res* 1989;**46**:147–51.

19. Bateman CJ, Keogh BF. Specialized modes of respiratory support in thoracic surgical patients. In: Ghosh S, Latimer RD (eds) *Thoracic anaesthesia: principles and practice*. Oxford: Butterworth-Heinemann. 1999; 277–306.

20. Feeley TW, Keating D, Nishimura T. Independent lung ventilation using high-frequency ventilation in the management of a bronchopleural fistula. *Anesthesiology* 1988;**69**:420–2.

26
Living-related lobar lung transplantation

Katherine Grichnik

Introduction

Pulmonary transplantation is a viable option for adults and children with end-stage lung disease due to multiple etiologies. Survival, functional status and quality of life after cadaveric lung transplantation (CLT) are ever changing as the medical community gains experience in the care of this difficult group of patients and as the pressure to perform CLT has led to the use of more marginal donor organs. Despite these pressures, short-term survival following CLT has steadily improved. Long-term survival, however, has remained relatively unchanged. Most centers are reporting 70–80% survival at 1 year, 56–70% survival at 3 years and 41–49% survival at 5 years.[1-4] The most recent United Network for Organ Sharing (UNOS) is that from 1998.[5] Survival for CLT recipients was 70.6% at 1 year, 49.1% at 5 years, and 20% at 9 years. The factors having the greatest impact on mortality were diagnosis and poor preoperative condition, that is requiring intensive care or mechanical ventilatory support at the time of transplantation. The major cause of hospitalization and mortality in the first year is infection.[5, 6] Episodes of rejection and obliterative bronchiolitis (OB) continue to be a problem.[5] Efforts to address these issues are ongoing. One group reports the use of donor bone marrow infusion to decrease episodes of OB.[7] Another reports the use of 'panel-reactive antibodies' (PRA) to assess the degree of humoral sensitization in the recipient before CLT as means of predicting the probability of acute and chronic rejection.[8]

Functional results are important to the transplant process. Meyers and Patterson reported significant improvements in spirometry (FEV$_1$ increasing from 16–22% to 68–85% of predicted) in the immediate postoperative period.[9] At 5, 6 and 7 years after single lung transplantation, average FEV$_1$ was 75, 73 and 68% of predicted values.[10] The question of quality of life is poorly reported in the literature.[2] In 1997, UNOS reported hospital admissions, episodes of rejection, diagnosis of OB, and other morbidity following CLT.[11] Interestingly, 63% patients had no hospitalizations during a 3-year follow-up period after CLT. Due to the success of CLT, the number of people awaiting transplantation far exceeds the donor pool available. It is estimated that 30–50% of patients may die while on a waiting lists with current waiting list times ranging from 6 to 24 months at various institutions.[12, 13]

An alternative to CLT is living-related lobar lung transplantation (LRLLT). This concept was first developed in children.[14] Since then, the concept of lobar transplantation for children and small adults has been developed.[14] This mode of lung transplantation is being offered to patients with declining physical status with a limited life expectancy or those who are at significant risk of developing an absolute contraindication to transplantation such as irreversible non-pulmonary end-organ failure.

Case history

A 28-year-old female with end-stage pulmonary disease secondary to cystic fibrosis, presented for

LRLLT. A year earlier she had undergone transplant assessment and had been placed on the waiting list for CLT. Extensive investigation at the time revealed significantly impaired respiratory function consistent with bronchiectasis and bullous lung disease. Cardiac, renal and hepatic function was within normal limits. Standard transplant serological testing was negative except for the presence of *Varicella zoster* IgG antibody.

Unfortunately, over the next 5 months, the patient's condition progressively deteriorated with escalating oxygen requirements, more frequent pulmonary infections and decreasing exercise capacity. At this time, arterial blood gas analysis revealed: pH 7.45, PaO_2 41 mmHg (5.4 kPa) and $PaCO_2$ 52 mmHg (6.8 kPa). Repeat spirometry revealed a fall in FEV_1 from 27 to 19%

of predicted. She had lost 8 kg in weight. With this deterioration and in view of her blood group (O), it was felt that she would not survive the average wait of 12–24 months for this blood type for CLT. Thus, the option of LRLLT was discussed.

Five family members were willing to be potential living-related donors. These included her husband, parents, and two siblings. All were evaluated separately at Duke University Medical Center. Since they lived in another area of the country, the family temporarily moved to North Carolina for the preoperative assessments and surgical procedures.

During preoperative assessment of the donors, the patient's mother and husband were excluded due to medical conditions and their blood group typing. The father, sister and brother underwent

RECIPIENT	
Past medical history	Cystic fibrosis.
Regular medications	Theophylline 200 mg BD, co-amoxiclav 875 mg BD, metoclopramide 20 mg QDS, paroxetine 40 mg OD, tobramycin inhaler OD, Dornase Alfa (Pulmozyme®) nebulizer OD, pancrelipase (Pancrease®) 2 caps AC.
Examination	Weight 55 kg, height 1.63 m, BMI 21 kg m^{-2}.
Investigations	Hb 11.4 g dl^{-1}, WBC 15.1 × 10^9 l^{-1}, Platelets 561 × 10^9 l^{-1}. PT 12.3 s, aPTT 23.8 s. [Na$^+$] 142 mmol l^{-1}, [K$^+$] 3.9 mmol l^{-1}, urea 12 mg dl^{-1} (4.3 mmol l^{-1}), creatinine 0.7 mg dl^{-1} (62 µmol l^{-1}), glucose 125 mg dl^{-1} (6.9 mmol l^{-1}). Liver function tests — within normal limits. Varicella zoster IgG antibody — positive. Hepatitis C antibody, carcinoembryonic antigen assay, herpes simplex antibody, toxoplasma IgG antibody, and HIV antibody — all negative. **ABG:** pH 7.45, PaO_2 41 mmHg (15.4 kPa), $PaCO_2$ 52 mmHg (6.8 kPa), SpO_2 97% (FiO_2 0.21) **Spirometry:** FEV_1 0.83 l (19% predicted), FVC 2.07 l (54% predicted) **CXR:** Severe bilateral bronchiectasis with scattered heterogeneous pulmonary opacities. Pulmonary artery enlargement consistent with pulmonary hypertension. **Ventilation: perfusion scan:** Perfusion = right lung 69%, left lung 40%. **ECG:** Normal sinus rhythm. **Chest CT:** Expanded lung volumes with diffuse bronchiectasis and bullous changes in both apices. Multiple areas of bronchial wall thickening and mucous plugging. **Abdominal ultrasound:** Several small gallstones. No thickening of gallbladder wall. **Transthoracic echo:** Normal left ventricular and valvular function. **MUGA scan:** LVEF 54%. **Cardiac catheterization:** PA 37/15 mmHg, PCWP 9 mmHg. CO 5.6 l min^{-1}, PVR 2.38 Wood units (190 dyne s cm^{-5})

further pulmonary function testing, psychological testing, interviews with the anesthesiologist, the surgeon, the pulmonologist, and the social worker. They all had a general medical physical examination, determination of blood chemistries, serologies, plain chest radiography and computed tomography and blood type compatibility testing. The sister and brother were found to be acceptable as donors for LRLLT, with the father acceptable as a back-up donor. Both siblings were identical histocompatibility locus antigens (HLA) matches to the patient.

The sister was 29 years old and in good health. There was no significant medical history, physical examination was unremarkable and the results of all investigations within normal limits.

The brother was 23 years old and also in good health. There was no significant medical history and physical examination was unremarkable.

Serology was negative except for a positive hepatitis C antibody. However, his hepatitis C RNA was negative, as was a liver biopsy. Social work and psychology consults found both siblings to be an appropriate candidates for living-related lobe donation.

It was noted that in the previous month, *Burkholderia cepacia* (sensitive to meropenem and ciprofloxacin) and *Staphylococcus maltophilis* (sensitive to ciprofloxacin and trimethephan-sulfa) had been isolated in the patient's sputum. Since these bacteria were sensitive to available antibiotics, it was elected to proceed with operation. The patient was known to be allergic to sulfa medications and ceftazidime. Thus, she had to undergo a desensitization protocol to allow the use of these antibiotics for this operation.

A date for the LRLLT was chosen in which three operating rooms could be devoted to

SISTER	
Examination	Weight 100 kg, Height 1.70 m BMI 34.6 kg m^{-2}.
Investigations	Hct 39%, WBC 7.3 × 10^9 l^{-1}, Platelets 242 × 10^9 l^{-1}. INR 1.0, aPTT 23.5 s. [Na$^+$] 140 mmol l^{-1}, [K$^+$] 4.5 mmol l^{-1}, urea 9 mg.dl^{-1} (3.2 mmol l^{-1}), creatinine 0.8 mg dl^{-1} (78 μmol l^{-1}), glucose 88 mg dl^{-1} (4.9 mmol l^{-1}). Liver function tests — within normal limits **Serology:** Negative. **ABG:** pH 7.44, PaO$_2$ 80 mmHg (10.7 kPa), PaCO$_2$ 36 (4.8 kPa) SpO$_2$ 97% (FiO$_2$ 0.21). **CXR:** Normal heart size and pulmonary vasculature. Lung fields clear. **Spirometry:** FEV$_1$ 3.87 l (108% predicted), FVC 4.48 l (105% predicted) **Dobutamine echocardiogram:** Normal.

BROTHER	
Examination	Weight 82 kg, Height 1.825 m, BMI 24.6 kg.m^{-2}.
Investigations	Hct 39%, WBC 7.3 × 10^9 l^{-1}, Platelets 242 × 10^9 l^{-1}. INR 1.0, aPTT 23.5 s. [Na$^+$] 138 mmol l^{-1}, [K$^+$] 4.0 mmol l^{-1}, urea 13 mg dl^{-1} (4.6 mmol l^{-1}), creatinine 1.0 mg dl^{-1} (88 μmol l^{-1}), glucose 82 mg dl^{-1} (4.6 mmol l^{-1}). Liver function tests — within normal limits. **Serology:** Hepatitis C antibody positive. Hepatitis C RNA negative. **Liver biopsy:** Normal. **ABG:** pH 7.39, PaO$_2$ 90 mmHg (12 kPa), PaCO$_2$ 44 (5.8 kPa) SpO$_2$ 97% (FiO$_2$ 0.21). **CXR:** Normal heart size and pulmonary vasculature. Lung fields clear. **Spirometry:** FEV$_1$ 5.12 l (104% predicted), FVC 6.45 l (108% predicted) **Dobutamine echocardiogram:** Normal.

simultaneous thoracic surgical procedures. The patient and her siblings were admitted to the hospital on the day before the procedure. Although both donors were given the option of perioperative epidural analgesia, only the sister gave consent. A thoracic epidural catheter was sited on the evening before surgery on the grounds that heparin would be administered intraoperatively and that a bloody tap or a spinal hematoma would necessitate abandonment of the procedure.

It was anticipated that pleural adhesions due to cystic fibrosis might make dissection and removal of the recipient's lungs difficult. For this reason it was decided to start all three procedures at the same time. The brother was selected for donation of his right lower lobe and the sister for donation of her left lower lobe.

The conduct of anesthesia for the donors was similar. Both received oral methadone 10 mg premedication 1 hour before surgery. Intravenous and radial artery cannulae were placed under local anesthesia and midazolam 2–5 mg sedation. Anesthesia was induced with thiopental, fentanyl and pancuronium. Following tracheal intubation with a double-lumen endotracheal tube the lungs were ventilated with air and oxygen (FiO_2 0.4–0.8). Anesthesia was maintained with isoflurane (0.5–1.5%) and incremental doses of fentanyl and pancuronium. Heparin 5000 iu was administered prior to the application of vascular clamps in preparation for lobectomy. Once removed, the donor lobes were preserved and transported to the recipient's operating room. Removal of the sister's left lower lobe was complicated by the need for autologous pericardial patching of the main pulmonary artery as the superior segmental pulmonary artery and lingular arteries emerged at the same level. Upon completion of surgery, residual neuromuscular blockade was antagonized with neostigmine and glycopyrrolate. Following the return of spontaneous ventilation and tracheal extubation, the donors were transferred to the ICU for observation and discharged to the ward a few hours later. Neither donor had any significant postoperative complications — specifically hemorrhage, infection or persistent air leak. Both were discharged from hospital on the third postoperative day.

The anesthetic management of the recipient was similar to that of the donors. In addition to the procedures described above, a femoral arterial cannula and an oximetric continuous cardiac output pulmonary artery catheter were placed. She was placed in the supine position and access to the thoracic cavity gained via a subxiphoid 'clamshell' incision. As anticipated, dissection of the native lungs was difficult resulting in considerable hemorrhage. Packed red blood cells were administered in an attempt to maintain a hematocrit of 30%. The lowest hematocrit during dissection was 19%. At this point the recipient was heparinized and placed on cardiopulmonary bypass (CPB) via cannulation of the ascending aorta and the right atrial appendage. The native lungs were then resected. The right lower donor lobe anastomoses were performed first, followed by the left lower donor lobe. The recipient separated from CPB with the aid of dopamine and epinephrine infusions. The heparin was reversed with protamine and adequate surgical hemostasis was obtained, with the infusion of fresh frozen plasma, cryoprecipitate and platelets. The double-lumen endotracheal tube was replaced with a single-lumen tube and the patient transported to the ICU sedated and ventilated.

On the first postoperative day, the recipient was neurologically intact, hemodynamically stable and had good pulmonary function. In view of minimal surgical bleeding and a normal coagulation profile, a thoracic epidural catheter was placed. After establishment of adequate epidural analgesia with bupivacaine 0.125%, the patient was weaned from mechanical ventilation and the trachea extubated. She initially did well, but subsequently developed an ileus, a left sided pleural effusion, surgical emphysema and sputum retention. On the fifth day after surgery, respiratory distress and worsening hypercarbia ($PaCO_2$ 66 mmHg (8.8 kPa)) necessitated reintubation and ventilation. The initial ventilatory management consisted of pressure support (16–20 cmH_2O) and PEEP (5 cmH_2O) during daylight hours and pressure assist/control (rate, 6 min[-1]) overnight. Exhaled tidal volumes averaged 350 ml and mean airway pressures never exceeded 15 cmH_2O. A loculated left pleural effusion was drained under CT guidance. The ileus quickly resolved and nasogastric feeding was commenced. After 6 days she was eventually weaned to FiO_2 0.21, pressure support (10 cmH_2O) and PEEP (5 cmH_2O) and was extubated on postoperative day 14. She continued to improve and was discharged to home 3 weeks after surgery. A year after LRLLT the patient remains well and has resumed employment.

Discussion

Recipient criteria

The indications for lobar lung transplantation are the same as those for lung transplantation. These include cystic fibrosis, pulmonary fibrosis, primary pulmonary hypertension, viral bronchiolitis, bronchopulmonary dysplasia, posttransplantation obliterative bronchiolitis and primary ciliary dyskinesia.[15] In general, LRLLT is reserved for a younger population and thus those patients requiring lung transplantation due to emphysema do not usually qualify due to age.

Consideration of LRLLT may be prompted in the following circumstances: (1) when progression of the disease state is such that death could be expected before a reasonable probability of CLT. (2) When the patient has low priority on the list for lung transplantation in a given geographical area, has a difficult blood type compatibility match relative to available resources, or has had a deterioration in health status. (3) When retransplantation is proposed — as the decreased donor organ ischemic time might improve outcome.[16] Clearly, LRLLT must be proposed and planned *prior* to pulmonary deterioration to the point of making the recipient an unacceptable risk for transplantation at all. Contraindications to LRLLT include panresistent flora and significant irreversible end-organ damage.[14] Some centers consider severe cachexia, significant pleural adhesions, diabetes with end-stage organ dysfunction, cardiac dysfunction and long-term ventilatory support as relative contraindications to LRLLT.[13, 17] Because of the size of an adult lung lobe, the recipient must be a child or small adult — the lobe must reasonably fit the thoracic cage of the recipient and be capable of supporting the cardiopulmonary needs of the recipient. All recipients must have a support system and their psychological, emotional and educational status be of an adequate level to allow them to cope with this major surgery and its long-term sequelae. Further, the recipient must have compatible and willing family members to donate lung tissue.

Donor criteria

Initially, when LRLLT was first performed, parents were the only donors considered.[17] However, the criteria have been expanded to all extended relatives who wish to be considered for the preoperative evaluation process. Further, unrelated donors have been used.[18] All potential donors must be educated about the procedure, its risks for the donor and recipient, its benefits and the likely long-term outcomes. Appendix 26.1 is an example of an information letter given to potential donors and recipients for LRLLT. The preoperative work-up for donor includes complete physical examination, extensive pulmonary function testing, blood type testing, routine serological testing, sputum cultures, CT scans, CXR, ECG, echocardiogram, and exclusion of any significant comorbid disease states (see Table 26.1). The donor candidate must meet the anesthesiologist, the surgeon, the psychiatrist, the social worker, and the lung transplant coordinator. Importantly, the feasibility and relative ease of performing a thoracotomy for removal of a lobe must be assessed to minimize risk to the donor for this medically unnecessary (to the donor) procedure. The donor must not be coerced into donation by other family members. Thus, psychological evaluation must be done both as a group (to assess family dynamics) and individually. Consent must be given by the well-informed individual, after this extensive evaluation. Often, families will choose to move to the

Table 26.1 Donor testing for eligibility for living related lung transplant

1. Blood type and screen
2. Pulmonary function tests with arterial blood gas
3. Chest radiograph and chest computed tomography
4. Serum chemistries and liver function studies
5. Hematocrit, white blood cell count, platelet count, coagulation parameters
6. Serologies to rule out HIV, hepatitis B, and hepatitis C
7. Establish CMV, Herpes, and toxoplasmosis status
8. Dobutamine echocardiography
9. Interview with a transplant pulmonologist, surgeon and anesthesiologist
10. Interview with a non-transplant pulmonologist and surgeon — to assure non-coersion and allow a donor to decline if desired
11. Interview with a psychologist
12. Interview with a social worker

city in which the transplant is to take place to be together for the preoperative work-up process and to provide support to the recipient, both preoperatively and postoperatively. All other things being equal, the 'larger' donor is chosen for donation of the right lower lobe.[18]

Scheduling of surgery

The timing of surgery must be carefully considered. It is appropriate to take into account the donors wishes (such as finishing a semester at college or university prior to donation) if the recipient is stable enough to allow a waiting period. Ultimately, however, the health status of the recipient must dictate the timing of the transplant. Transplantation should occur prior to the recipient becoming critically ill and thus decreasing the probability for a good outcome from transplantation.

The day of transplantation must be considered so as to allow the simultaneous use of three operating rooms. All three patients should be taken in to the operating rooms at the same time. Because of the need to remove the lobe 'uninjured', donor thoracotomy and lobectomy inevitably takes more time than lobectomy for other indications. Similarly, the presence of significant adhesions may impede preparation of the recipient. Ideally the recipient's dissection and cannulation for CPB should take the same amount of time as the donors' lobectomies.

Surgery on the donors

The donors should be evaluated preoperatively by their primary anesthesia team. Monitoring should be dictated by the condition of the donor and may consist of the standard ASA monitors with arterial pressure monitoring and measurement of urine output. Central venous cannulation may be considered on an individual basis. The airway anatomy of the donors must be such that one lung ventilation can be achieved with a double-lumen endotracheal tube, an endobronchial blocker or endobronchial intubation. Postoperative analgesia should be planned in advance and may consist of thoracic epidural analgesia (preferred at our

institution for thoracotomy), paravertebral nerve blockade, intercostal nerve blockade, or intravenous (patient- or nurse-controlled) analgesia.

The technical aspects of donor lobectomy are described in detail elsewhere.[19] A vasodilator such as prostaglandin E_1 may be considered to dilate the pulmonary vascular bed. The right lower and left lower lobes are the lobes of choice for transplantation. Manipulation of the lobe is kept to a minimum during dissection of the bronchus, pulmonary artery and pulmonary vein. Heparin and methylprednisolone may be given at the time of lobectomy. The order of division of the vein, artery and bronchus are important to avoid vascular congestion of the lobe. The artery is divided first, followed by the vein and then the bronchus. The pulmonary artery and pulmonary vein of the donor lobe are then alternately perfused with a 'pneumoplegia' solution until uniform blanching and cooling of the lobe is achieved. At the same time the lobe is ventilated with room air to prevent atelectasis.

Surgery on the recipient

The recipient should be carefully evaluated prior to surgery by the primary anesthesiologist. Airway, intravenous access and other monitoring difficulties are common and should be anticipated with adequate preparation time. The appropriate antibiotics and immunosuppressive agents must be given prior to incision. Placement of a double-lumen endotracheal tube may facilitate the dissection portion of the operation. Dissection to free adhesions may be difficult and result in considerable blood loss. Further, in chronically infected patients (i.e. those with cystic fibrosis), a vasodilated state may occur with manipulation of this infected tissue.

After complete dissection and stabilization of the patient, the patient is placed on CPB. CPB is used to control the blood flow to the lobe implanted first. In a bilateral sequential lung transplant without CPB, the entire cardiac output in directed to a newly implanted lung while the second lung is being implanted. It is thought that a lobe (in contrast to an entire lung) would not be able to handle this perfusion and that reperfusion pulmonary edema will result. CPB also provides a measure of safety in critically ill patients who may not otherwise tolerate one lung anesthesia during a bilateral sequential lung transplant technique. The heart may beat through this procedure and aortic cross-clamping should not be required. The sequence of anastomosis is usually (1) the bronchus, (2) the vein and (3) the artery.

Separation from CPB may require inotropic support and bleeding should be anticipated. It has been suggested that separation from CPB in a slightly hypovolemic state may facilitate lung function postoperatively.[17] The patient may require the use of a ventilator capable of pressure support modes after transplantation. After chest closure, the double-lumen endotracheal tube is replaced with a large diameter single-lumen endotracheal tube. The recipient may be expected to have an unstable ICU course for the first 24–48 hours with bleeding and minor organ dysfunction being common.

Donor outcomes

Donor outcomes are very important to the success of a LRLLT program. One study[17] reported complications in 7 of 76 donors. These included postpericardiotomy syndrome in three patients, atrial fibrillation in one patient, and surgical re-exploration (for empyema, bleeding and persistent air leak) in three patients. Spirometry revealed 17% and 18% reduction in FVC and FEV$_1$, respectively, without functional impairment. Another study[18] reported only two complications in 16 donors; these were a prolonged air leak and surgical re-exploration for a hematoma. Woo et al[20] reported no major complications and a 16–18% reduction in FVC in donors for 17 pediatric LRLLT recipients. Other complications, which may occur, include bronchopleural fistula, wound infection, injury to the vagus or recurrent laryngeal nerves, and gastrointestinal tract bleeding.

The ethics of donor lobectomy have been debated. Essentially, the lives of three individuals are placed at risk for the benefit of one. There should be zero donor mortality and minimal morbidity to justify this procedure. However, there are no data available on the mortality and morbidity rates for lobectomies in otherwise healthy patients without lung cancer or other conditions leading to thoracic surgery. If a 5% mortality rate is accepted as the risk for thoracic surgery in patients aged 60 or less with lung cancer, then a reasonable estimate of mortality in a healthy younger donor with normal lung function being operated on by an experienced surgeon should be 1–3%.[21]

The reluctance to subject healthy individuals to thoracotomy and lobectomy has resulted in LRLLT being reserved for those recipients who are desperately ill and who are unlikely to survive until a cadaveric lung is available. Thus the outcomes from LRLLT may not be as good as those from CLT, adding further to the ethical debate. The potential advantages and disadvantages of LRLLT are listed in Table 26.2.

Table 26.2 Potential advantages and disadvantages of LRLLT[21]

Advantages	Disadvantages
• Potentially better short-term results due to less ischemic time and more careful lung preparation • Potential better long-term survival as tissue match among family members may be superior to cadaveric matching • Immunosuppression may need to be less aggressive due to better tissue matching • Avoidance of a long wait at a medical center far from the patient's home • Shorten the waiting time for others on the lung transplant list (private and public benefit). • Donor and recipient satisfaction with recipient survival and improvement in quality of life	• Risk of evaluation process to donors • Operative morbidity and mortality to donor • Long-term morbidity to donor such as exercise limitation, less pulmonary reserve with infection or trauma, possible pulmonary hypertension in later years • Psychological issues before and after transplant for donor and the recipient, especially if the procedure is not successful

Recipient outcomes

There is limited and variable literature on the results of LRLLT as it has only recently become more widely used in surgical practice. The surgical group led by Starnes[17] initially offered LRLLT only to severely ill patients awaiting CLT. They reported 14 deaths in 37 patients at 14 months postoperatively. The recipients had 30 episodes of rejection, all of which responded to steroid augmentation. Recipient postoperative pulmonary function improved to 72% predicted FVC, 73% predicted FEV_1, 92% of predicted mean mid-forced expiratory flow and 87% of predicted mean lung diffusion capacity. Of those patients (N=14) studied at 1 year, all had normal right heart pressures. Lymphoproliferative disease and OB were also diagnosed in two and three patients respectively.

Mendeloff et al[22] reported on bilateral lung transplantation with LRLLT considered only for patients with end-stage disease, who were not likely to survive until a cadaveric donor became available. Seven of the eight patients transplanted from living-related donors were reported to be early to mid-term survivors.

The Starnes group then reviewed their outcomes in pediatric LRLLT versus pediatric CLT.[23] They found no differences in overall rejection and 12-month pulmonary function testing. However, at 24 months, the LRLLT patients had a greater FEV_1 than the CLT recipients. There was no occurrence of OB in eight LRLLT patients compared to six of seven CLT recipients at 24 months. Survival at 24 months was 77% for the LRLLT recipients and 67% for CLT recipients.

In patients transplanted for indications other than cystic fibrosis, the Starnes group[16] reported 75% 1-year survival with a mean FVC 81% of predicted, and a mean FEV_1 76% of predicted. Even in patients with pre-existing pulmonary hypertension, postoperative pulmonary pressures normalized. In comparison, survival rates at 1-year for CLT recipients with cystic fibrosis are 70–85%.[20, 24–27] Clearly, the early LRLLT patients did not have the survival nor the reduction in rejection episodes that were predicted. This may have been due to the degree of deterioration of the patients who underwent initial LRLLT or the relative small size of the lobes transplanted.[17] It appears that, with experience and improvements in technique, survival in some series is reported to be similar to or better than CLT. However, these excellent outcomes need to be verified as they are primarily reported by one group. Others have noted lower corrected survival rates for LRLLT recipients as compared to CLT recipients and have thus called for performance of LRLLT only when cadaveric lungs are unlikely to become available.[17]

Alternatives to LRLLT

Currently, for those patients with a failing pulmonary system who are not expected to survive the wait for CLT, there are few options. Chronic prostaglandin infusion has been used for patients with disease characterized primarily by pulmonary hypertension. Xenotransplantation is yet in the initial laboratory investigative stages for heart and renal transplant.[28] There are significant barriers to solid organ xenotransplantation, such as hyperacute rejection, acute vascular rejection, cellular rejection, the physiological limits of the procured organ and the risks of transmission of an animal infectious agent (zoonosis).

Conclusions and key learning points

- LRLLT is a viable option for lung transplantation for recipients and donors willing to consider the procedure.
- LRLLT is usually considered for patients with end-stage lung disease, who are not expected to survive until a cadaveric organ becomes available. These patients have few other options.
- Extensive donor and recipient work-ups must be done.
- Donors must not be coerced into donation of a pulmonary lobe.
- The ethical considerations of placing two healthy patients at risk are significant.
- The initial outcomes for LRLLT recipients are comparable and possibly better than CLT. The short-term outcomes need to be verified and the long-term outcomes remain to be determined.

References

1. Trulock EP. Lung transplantation. *Am J Respir Crit Care Med* 1997;**155**:789–818.

2. Bhorade SM, Vigneswaran WT, Lanuza D, Garrity ER. Lung transplantation at Loyola University Medical Center. *Clin Transpl* 1999;281–8.

3. Meyers BF, Lynch J, Trulock EP *et al*. Lung transplantation: a decade of experience. *Ann Surg* 1999;**230**:362–70.

4. Milano CA, Buchan K, Perreas K, Wallwork J. Thoracic organ transplantation at Papworth Hospital. *Clin Transpl* 1999;273–80.

5. Keck BM, Bennett LE, Rosendale J *et al*. Worldwide thoracic organ transplantation: a report from the UNOS/ISHLT International Registry for Thoracic Organ Transplantation. *Clin Transpl* 1999;35–49.

6. Palmer SM, Alexander BD, Sanders LL *et al*. Significance of blood stream infection after lung transplantation: analysis in 176 consecutive patients. *Transplantation* 2000;**69**:2360–6.

7. Pham SM, Rao AS, Zeevi A *et al*. Effects of donor bone marrow infusion in clinical lung transplantation. *Ann Thorac Surg* 2000;**69**:345–50.

8. Lau CL, Palmer SM, Posther KE *et al*. Influence of panel-reactive antibodies on posttransplant outcomes in lung transplant recipients. *Ann Thorac Surg* 2000;**69**:1520–4.

9. Meyers BF, Patterson GA. Lung transplantation: current status and future prospects. *World J Surg* 1999;**23**:1156–62.

10. Chaparro C, Scavuzzo M, Winton T *et al*. Status of lung transplant recipients surviving beyond five years. *J Heart Lung Transplant* 1997;**16**:511–6.

11. Keck BM, Bennett LE, Fiol BS *et al*. Worldwide thoracic organ transplantation: a report from the UNOS/ISHLT International Registry for Thoracic Organ Transplantation. *Clin Transpl* 1998;39–52.

12. DeChesser AD. Organ donation: the supply/demand discrepancy. *Heart Lung* 1986;**15**:547–51.

13. Dark JH. Lung: living related transplantation. *Br Med Bull* 1997;**53**:892–903.

14. Starnes VA, Oyer PE, Bernstein D *et al*. Heart, heart-lung, and lung transplantation in the first year of life. *Ann Thorac Surg* 1992;**53**:306–10.

15. Yamamoto H, Kubo K, Nishizawa N *et al*. [Primary ciliary dyskinesia treated with living-donor lobar lung transplantation]. *Nihon Kokyuki Gakkai Zasshi* 1999;**37**:739–42.

16. Huddleston CB, Mendeloff EN, Cohen AH *et al*. Lung retransplantation in children. *Ann Thorac Surg* 1998;**66**:199–203; discussion 204.

17. Starnes VA, Barr ML, Cohen RG *et al*. Living-donor lobar lung transplantation experience: intermediate results. *J Thorac Cardiovasc Surg* 1996;**112**:1284–90.

18. Starnes VA, Barr ML, Schenkel FA *et al*. Experience with living-donor lobar transplantation for indications other than cystic fibrosis. *J Thorac Cardiovasc Surg* 1997;**114**:917–21.

19. Cohen RG, Barr ML, Schenkel FA *et al*. Living-related donor lobectomy for bilateral lobar transplantation in patients with cystic fibrosis. *Ann Thorac Surg* 1994;**57**:1423–7.

20. Woo MS, MacLaughlin EF, Horn MV *et al*. Living donor lobar lung transplantation: the pediatric experience. *Pediatr Transplant* 1998;**2**:185–90.

21. Kramer MR, Sprung CL. Living related donation in lung transplantation. Ethical considerations. *Arch Intern Med* 1995;**155**:1734–8.

22. Mendeloff EN, Huddleston CB, Mallory GB *et al*. Pediatric and adult lung transplantation for cystic fibrosis. *J Thorac Cardiovasc Surg* 1998;**115**:404–13.

23. Starnes VA, Woo MS, MacLaughlin EF *et al*. Comparison of outcomes between living donor and cadaveric lung transplantation in children. *Ann Thorac Surg* 1999;**68**:2279–83.

24. Egan TM, Detterbeck FC, Mill MR *et al*. Improved results of lung transplantation for patients with cystic fibrosis. *J Thorac Cardiovasc Surg* 1995;**109**:224–34.

25. Hasan A, Corris PA, Healy M *et al*. Bilateral sequential lung transplantation for end stage septic lung disease. *Thorax* 1995;**50**:565–6.

26. Starnes VA, Lewiston N, Theodore J *et al*. Cystic fibrosis. Target population for lung transplantation in North America in the 1990s. *J Thorac Cardiovasc Surg* 1992;**103**:1008–14.

27. Shapiro BJ, Veeraraghavan S, Barbers RG. Lung transplantation for cystic fibrosis: an update and practical considerations for referring candidates. *Curr Opin Pulm Med* 1999;**5**:365–70. [Erratum in *Curr Opin Pulm Med* 2000;**6**:170]

28. Platt JL. Prospects for xenotransplantation. *Pediatr Transplant* 1999;**3**:193–200.

Appendix 26.1: Living lobar lung transplant: donor information*

Letter of information about living-related lung transplantation for potential donors and recipients, Duke University Health System

Living lobar lung transplantation has been an acceptable option for selected patients who require lung transplant since the advent of this procedure in 1993. Patients receiving living lobar lung transplants have outcomes comparable to patients receiving traditional, cadaveric transplants. Duke University Health System performed its first living-related lobar lung transplant in 1997, with the recipient and donors continuing to do well to date.

Two donors are required for one living-related lobar lung transplant recipient. Each donor will give a lobe, or one section of one lung, either the right lower lobe or the left lower lobe. While no serious or life-threatening complications have been reported, potential donors should know that there are significant risks to donating:

• Overall decrease in lung function of about 18%.
• 1 in 20 chance of having minor complications such as:
    pain;
    bleeding;
    prolonged fluid leak;
    prolonged air leak;
    infection;
    irritation of the heart;
• 1 in 200 chance of dying during or immediately after the surgery.

Most donors are hospitalized for about 9 days. The total recovery time is likely to be 4–6 weeks, during which the donor will be unable to work or care for other family members. Donors will need to stay in Durham for about 1 week after leaving the hospital for follow-up with the doctors.

Potential donors must be closely related to the recipient, with biologic family members providing the best matches. Potential donors must:

• Be between 18 and 55 years of age.
• Have a compatible blood type with the recipient.
• Be 3–6 inches taller than the recipient.
• Have normal pulmonary function studies.
• Be in overall good health.
• Quit smoking and refrain from all tobacco products for the rest of their lives.
• Have had no previous chest surgery.

Evaluation as a potential donor requires a 1–2 week stay near Duke University Hospital. After a telephone interview with the Transplant Nurse Coordinator, confirmation of blood type and pulmonary function studies (to include spirometry, lung volumes, and diffusion capacity) should be faxed to the Transplant Office at 919-681-9571. Studies and appointments to be completed at Duke University Hospital include:

• Blood work.
• Pulmonary function studies and arterial blood gas.
• Chest X-ray and CT scan.
• Stress test.
• Assessment by the social worker.
• Assessment by the psychologist.
• Assessment by the transplant pulmonologist and surgeon.
• Assessment by the non-transplant pulmonologist and surgeon.

For further information about becoming a living lobar lung transplant donor please contact the Lung Transplant Office at 800-249-5864 or 919-684-2240.

*Printed with permission from the Lung Transplant Group, Duke University Medical Center.

27

Broad-complex tachycardias after coronary artery bypass surgery

Rana A Sayeed, Andrew J Ritchie and Andrew A Grace

Introduction

Tachycardia with *broad* QRS complexes (>120 ms duration) is a relatively uncommon but potentially fatal complication after coronary artery bypass graft (CABG) surgery. Prompt diagnosis and aggressive treatment are essential to reduce early mortality. Subsequent assessment and risk stratification allow the appropriate management of selected cases at high risk of late postoperative sudden cardiac death.

Case history

A 72-year-old man presented with a 14-year history of symptoms due to coronary artery disease. He had suffered three myocardial infarctions over a 10-year period, the most recent 4 years earlier, followed by postinfarct angina. His angina had deteriorated over the last 2 months to Canadian Cardiac Society (CCS) class IV with

more frequent episodes of chest pain following minimal exertion and at rest. A 99m-technetium methoxyisobutylisonitrile (99mTc-MIBI) myocardial perfusion scan 2 years earlier had shown reversible inferolateral ischemia and a fixed anteroseptal defect. He also complained of transient episodes of palpitations associated with mild angina and breathlessness but no loss of consciousness.

Ventriculography and coronary angiography revealed moderate impairment of LV function with anterior hypokinesia and severe coronary artery disease. The left anterior descending (LAD) artery was occluded after the origin of a diseased first diagonal branch and there were several severe stenoses of the left circumflex. The right coronary artery was ectatic but free from flow-limiting disease. An ambulatory 24-hour ECG recorded occasional ventricular premature beats and couplets but neither non-sustained or sustained ventricular tachycardia (VT) nor any supraventricular tachycardia (SVT).

Past medical history	Myocardial infarction (×3). Post infarction angina. Palpitations. Hypercholesterolemia. Cigarette smoker
Regular medications	Aspirin 75 mg OD, atenolol 50 mg OD, isosorbide mononitrate MR 120 mg OD, amlodipine 10 mg OD, nicorandil 20 mg BD, pravastatin 10 mg OD, glyceryl trinitrate 400 µg PRN.
Examination	Height 1.69 m. Weight 89.4 kg. BP 145/89 mmHg. Otherwise unremarkable.
Investigations	Hb 12.4 g dl^{-1}, WBC 6.19 × 10^9 l^{-1}, platelets 263 × 10^9 l^{-1}, [Na$^+$] 142 mmol.l^{-1}, [K$^+$] 4.4 mmol l^{-1}, urea 3.2 mmol l^{-1}, creatinine 0.84 mg dl^{-1} (74 µmol l^{-1}).

The patient was admitted for CABG. Examination on admission was unremarkable. The ECG (Figure 27.1) showed prominent M-shaped rSR' complexes in leads V_5 and V_6 interpreted as indicating left bundle branch block (LBBB) and deep Q-waves in leads II and III. The chest X-ray was unremarkable.

CABG surgery was uneventful. Following premedication with intramuscular morphine 15 mg and hyoscine 0.3 mg 1 hour before surgery, anesthesia was induced using fentanyl citrate 1 mg, midazolam 10 mg and pancuronium 8 mg and maintained with propofol 4 mg kg^{-1} h^{-1}. Perioperative antibiotic prophylaxis consisted of intravenous gentamicin 160 mg and flucloxacillin 1 g at induction and four further doses of flucloxacillin 1 g at 6-hour intervals after surgery. CPB was established between the right atrium and ascending aorta after full anticoagulation with heparin sodium (activated clotting time >450 s). A flow rate of 2.4 l min^{-1} m^{-2} was maintained with mean arterial pressure ≥50 mmHg and systemic hypothermia at 30°C. Cold

(4°C) blood cardioplegia infused into the aortic root provided myocardial protection. Three coronary artery bypasses were completed using reversed saphenous vein grafts applied to the first obtuse marginal branch of the left circumflex and the first diagonal branch of the LAD and the left internal mammary artery to the LAD. The proximal anastomoses were fashioned after removal of the aortic cross-clamp with the heart beating in sinus rhythm. Myocardial ischemic time was 31 minutes and CPB duration 53 minutes. The heart was weaned from CPB easily without inotropic support and the operation completed with the insertion of mediastinal drains and the placement of atrial and ventricular epicardial pacing wires.

After surgery the patient was transferred to the ICU. The initial recovery period was complicated by excessive mediastinal bleeding, requiring administration of additional protamine and transfusion of blood, platelets, and fresh-frozen plasma, and a relative bradycardia for which demand sequential atrioventricular (DDD) pacing

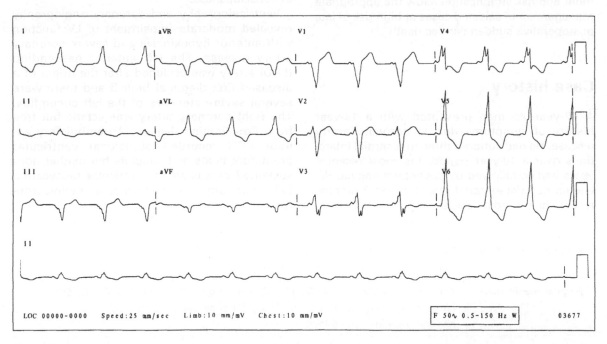

Figure 27.1

The obvious features on the admission 12-lead ECG are (1) the broad ventricular QRS complexes (QRS duration > 120 ms) with an M-shaped rSR pattern in V_5 and V_6 suggestive of left bundle branch block and (2) the deep Q waves in lead III (see Discussion for further details).

was started. On the first postoperative morning, the patient became febrile, producing thick yellow secretions on endotracheal suction, and had the radiographic signs of left lower lobe consolidation. An attempt at weaning from ventilation was unsuccessful because of poor arterial blood gases. He was started on ciprofloxacin 400 mg BD for presumed pneumonia and ventilation continued. Physiotherapy and antibiotic therapy improved his respiratory function enough to allow successful extubation onto continuous positive airway pressure (CPAP) on the second postoperative day.

Early on the third postoperative day, 60 hours after surgery, the patient unexpectedly developed a polymorphic broad-complex tachycardia (Figure 27.2a) at 180–200 bpm; despite the fast rate there was little hemodynamic compromise. Arterial blood gas analysis showed: [H+] 34.6 nmol l-1 (pH 7.46); PaCO$_2$ 30 mmHg (4.0 kPa); PaO$_2$ 59 mmHg (7.8 kPa; with FiO$_2$ 0.8); SaO$_2$ 92%; [HCO$_3$-] 22.8 mmol l-1; base deficit 1.9 mmol l-1; [K+] 4.1 mmol l-1; and hemoglobin 11.7 g dl-1. The working diagnosis was of a ventricular tachycardia. The arrhythmia persisted despite slow infusion of potassium (20 mmol KCl) and

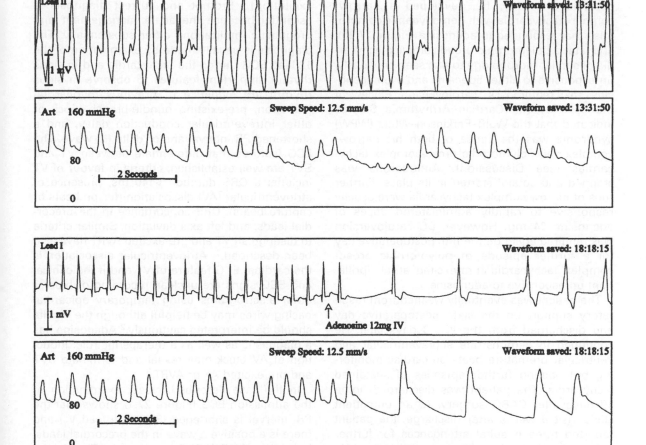

Figure 27.2

(a) Single-lead ECG recorded on the fourth postoperative day showing a polymorphic broad-complex tachycardia at 165–175 bpm (see Discussion for further details). (b) Single-lead ECG showing termination of a narrow-complex tachycardia by adenosine (12 mg rapid IV bolus).

magnesium (20 mmol $MgSO_4$) and intravenous amiodarone loading was started (300 mg over 1 hour, followed by 900 mg over the next 23 hours). The patient became increasingly distressed and tachypneic with a deteriorating PaO_2 and was electively reintubated and ventilated; sinus rhythm resumed spontaneously following intubation.

Continuous ECG monitoring showed frequent supraventricular and ventricular premature beats despite maintaining a serum $[K^+] \geq 4.5$ mmol l^{-1}, $PaO_2 \geq 68$ mmHg (9.0 kPa) and continuing amiodarone maintenance therapy. The serum ionized magnesium concentration was 2.6 mg dl^{-1} (1.07 mmol l^{-1}) — just above the normal range (1.7–2.4 mg dl^{-1}; 0.7–1.0 mmol l^{-1}). On the fourth postoperative day, he developed a narrow-complex tachycardia with hemodynamic compromise that responded to adenosine (Figure 27.2b), and later a polymorphic broad-complex tachycardia of similar morphology to that seen previously, unresponsive to either lidocaine and even adenosine, that required DC cardioversion. Review of the case by the Cardiac Arrhythmia Service indicated that the Wolff–Parkinson–White (WPW) syndrome was the cause of both his narrow-complex and polymorphic broad-complex tachycardias (see Discussion). Amiodarone was stopped and sotalol started in its place. Further runs of narrow complex tachycardia were usually responsive to rapidly administered doses of adenosine 24 mg. However, DC cardioversion was required again on the fifth postoperative day for a further episode of polymorphic broad-complex tachycardia (pre-excited atrial fibrillation) unresponsive to adenosine.

The patient was eventually weaned from respiratory support on the sixth postoperative day and discharged from the ICU 3 days later. He continued to demonstrate supraventricular and ventricular premature beats on cardiac monitoring but had no further episodes of sustained tachycardia. The patient was discharged home 19 days after CABG surgery. At an outpatient clinic visit 6 weeks after discharge, the patient reported three hospital attendances for further palpitations but otherwise a good recovery. He underwent electrophysiological study and radiofrequency ablation of his right posteroseptal accessory pathway; the postablation ECG showed a slightly prolonged PR interval and a normal QRS complex morphology.

Discussion

Broad-complex tachycardias complicating the WPW syndrome

The diagnosis of broad-complex tachycardia after CABG may present difficulties as highlighted in this case. The differential diagnosis for a tachycardia with broad ventricular complexes includes VT, SVT with aberrant conduction (pre-existing or rate-related), and antidromic atrioventricular re-entrant tachycardia (AVRT) or pre-excited atrial fibrillation (AF) in the WPW syndrome (with antegrade conduction down the accessory pathway and ventricular pre-excitation).[1] Prompt and correct diagnosis is essential because the acute management and prognostic implications differ substantially. The diagnosis is usually made by examination of the 12-lead ECG during the tachycardia and in sinus rhythm. Important features to observe in sinus rhythm are evidence of previous myocardial infarction, pre-existing bundle-branch block or other intraventricular conduction delay, and a shortened PR interval and/or delta (Δ) wave. The ECG features that differentiate between VT and SVT are well established; criteria in favour of VT include: a QRS duration >140 ms, presence of atrioventricular (AV) dissociation (fusion beats or capture beats), QRS concordance in the precordial leads; and left axis deviation. Similar criteria to distinguish VT and pre-excited AVRT have also been described.[1] Atrioventricular dissociation is the cardinal ECG feature of VT and if the clinical and ECG signs are unclear, recording of bipolar atrial electrograms using temporary epicardial pacing wires may be helpful although the results should be interpreted cautiously.[2] Adenosine has a diagnostic as well as a therapeutic role: induction of AV block may reveal and terminate SVT and pre-excited AF or AVRT.[3]

In the case described, closer examination of the admission ECG (Figure 27.1) shows that the PR interval is shortened (80 ms in lead V_1) and there is a positive Δ wave in the precordial leads, indicative of WPW ECG morphology. The slurred Δ wave gives rise to the LBBB-type morphology with QRS prolongation and a pattern of pre-excitation suggestive of a right posteroseptal location for the accessory pathway. The broad-complex tachycardia in Figure 27.2a is AF with ventricular pre-excitation by antegrade conduction via the accessory pathway; the irregular QRS morphology arises from the irregular pattern of atrial depolarization and the variable conduction down the accessory pathway.

The WPW syndrome is the commonest cause of ventricular pre-excitation. The prevalence of the WPW ECG morphology is not absolutely clear as pre-excitation may be intermittent. Between 0.1 and 3.1 per 1000 population have Δ waves seen at some point on ECG but most never experience palpitations and therefore do not strictly have the WPW syndrome, a description that also implies the symptoms of tachycardia.[4] The first presentation can occur at any age but symptoms usually emerge in the second and third decades. The usual arrhythmia associated with WPW is orthodromic AVRT with retrograde conduction via the accessory pathway; less commonly there is antegrade accessory pathway conduction leading to maximally pre-excited QRS complexes in antidromic AVRT[5] or pre-excited AF, as in this case. Adenosine aids the diagnosis by blocking conduction at the AV node and breaking the re-entry circuit (Figure 27.2b). Sotalol slows conduction in both the AV node and accessory pathway and is an effective treatment for tachycardias associated with WPW.[6] Radiofrequency ablation of the accessory pathway at the time of electrophysiological study provides definitive treatment.[4]

Broad-complex tachycardia after coronary surgery is usually due to VT

New-onset sustained ventricular tachycardia (defined as VT episodes longer than 30 seconds or causing hemodynamic compromise with a rate greater than 120 bpm) is a serious complication after CABG. The morphology may be monomorphic, with regular QRS morphology, or polymorphic, characterized by progressive beat-to-beat variation in the QRS axis such that the waveform 'twists' around the baseline and is easily mistaken for ventricular fibrillation.

Most studies of new-onset VT after CABG have been retrospective or based on reports from specialized arrhythmia services with often small cohorts in each series limiting the conclusions.

Early series reported an incidence of new-onset sustained VT after CABG from 0.41 to 1.4%,[7–10] but a more recent prospective study found an incidence of monomorphic VT as high as 3.1%.[11] A possible factor in this increase in incidence is the greater proportion of patients with previous myocardial infarction undergoing CABG.

The unexpected emergence of VT is often indicative of significant myocardial ischemia or perioperative myocardial infarction that may result from incomplete revascularization or graft occlusion. One series reported ECG signs of ischemia in 48% of patients for a week after CABG[12] and another found at least one occluded vein graft in 3/7 (43%) cases undergoing angiography for postCABG VT in the absence of symptoms of ongoing ischemia.[8] Myocardial ischemia induces alterations in both resting and action potentials of cardiac myocytes that lead to changes in the conduction and refractoriness of the myocardium; these changes are distributed heterogeneously across the ischemic zone, providing the *substrate* for ventricular arrhythmias by means of both re-entrant and non-re-entrant mechanisms.[13] Remote myocardial infarction also contributes to postoperative VT. Myocardial scar tissue represents a potential arrhythmogenic substrate, especially in patients with impaired LV function: successful revascularization may allow reperfusion of regions of 'electrical hibernation', bands of myocytes within myocardial scar tissue, that become the active substrate for re-entrant VT.[11, 14] The finding that placement of a bypass graft across a non-collateralized occlusion to an infarct zone independently predicts a higher risk of postCABG monomorphic VT supports this concept.[11]

Sustained monomorphic VT

Monomorphic VT is associated with the presence of an established anatomical arrhythmogenic substrate and/or revascularization of an area of old infarction. It is more likely in patients with a history of previous myocardial infarction, severe congestive heart failure (NYHA class III/IV), and reduced LV ejection fraction.[11, 14, 15] Monomorphic VT is often refractory to treatment and commonly inducible by programmed electrical stimulation. Polymorphic VT (and VF) is associated with acute myocardial ischemia or perioperative infarction and subsequent transient electrical instability; VT is less often inducible during electrophysiological studies.[14, 15]

Polymorphic VT

Polymorphic VT may be due either to ischemia or to 'torsades de pointes'. Torsades de pointes has increasingly been recognized to be due to the proarrhythmic effects of antiarrhythmic drug therapy.[16] So-called Vaughan Williams class Ia (e.g. quinidine, disopyramide) and class III (e.g. amiodarone, sotalol) agents are common causes of QT_c prolongation. Prolongation of the QT interval in this context is usually due to inhibition of the HERG-encoded delayed rectifier potassium current I_{Kr}, and the main actions of quinidine are actually due to a class III action.[16] Several 'non-cardiac' drugs used in the intensive care unit have also been implicated in the development of polymorphic VT and/or torsades and also inhibit potassium channel function: the tranquillizers haloperidol and thioridazine, cisapride (now withdrawn from clinical use as an esophagogastric prokinetic agent), and the macrolide antibiotics erythromycin and clarithromycin. (An up-to-date list of drugs that prolong the QT_c interval may be found at http://dml.georgetown.edu/depts/pharmacology/torsades.html.) Other causes of QT_c prolongation include hypokalemia, hypomagnesemia, and the rare congenital long QT syndromes. Management usually consists of the recognition of QT prolongation in conjunction with torsades and the withdrawal of the causative agent.

Management of monomorphic sustained VT following coronary surgery

Other factors are required to act as a trigger for the initiation of VT such as a premature ventricular beat or a change in heart rate. In the setting of cardiac surgery, these triggers may arise from a malpositioned intracardiac catheter, a mediastinal chest drain, or inadvertent VOO pacing after the transfer from the operating room. The outcome of the interaction between substrate and trigger is influenced by other modulating factors such as electrolyte imbalance (hypokalemia, hypomagnesemia), metabolic derangement (hypoxia, acidosis), and the effects of catecholamines (endogenous, as a result of poorly controlled pain or exogenous, resulting from the use of inotropic agents).

Ventricular tachycardia is detrimental because it increases myocardial oxygen demand and opens the risk of deterioration to VF. Prompt treatment is imperative but the priorities depend upon the degree of hemodynamic compromise. A suggested approach to management is illustrated in Figure 27.3. Rapid polymorphic or

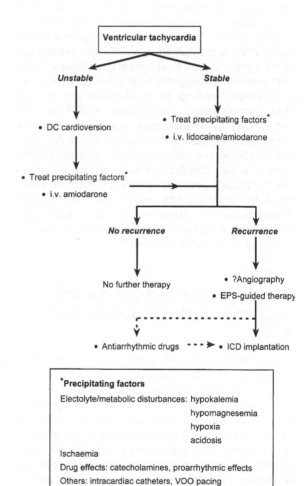

Figure 27.3

Suggested approach to the management of sustained ventricular tachycardia after coronary artery surgery.

'pulseless' VT, usually with a rate greater than 150 bpm, is treated as a cardiac arrest, with a precordial thump, if appropriate, followed by an unsynchronized 200 J DC shock.[17] With lesser degrees of hemodynamic compromise seen with monomorphic VT at rates greater than 150 bpm, accompanied by pulmonary congestion and hypotension, synchronized DC cardioversion is appropriate, starting with a 100 J shock.

For well-tolerated monomorphic VT, usually at rates less than 150 bpm, and after cardioversion, modulating factors such as electrolyte imbalance, hypoxia or severe acidosis should be identified and corrected at the same time as antiarrhythmic therapy is initiated. The plasma potassium concentration should be maintained at levels greater than 4.0–5.0 mmol l^{-1} [18] and magnesium supplementation should be considered, particularly in association with hypokalemia, prior diuretic therapy, or impaired LV function.[19] Concomitant drug therapy should be reviewed: the dosage of intravenous catecholamines should be reduced, if possible, and drugs that might lead to QT_c prolongation substituted or stopped. Although intravenous lidocaine given as a 100 mg bolus (1.0–1.5 mg kg^{-1}) has been widely used for the termination of an acute episode of VT, amiodarone is now the first-line drug (usually given as 300 mg (5 mg kg^{-1}) over 1 hour, followed by 900 mg (15 mg kg^{-1}) over 23 hours). This drug is effective in the treatment of VT in the absence of marked negative inotropic effects and is well tolerated in patients with impaired LV function.[20] We have given doses as high as 1200 mg day^{-1} for 4–5 days without adverse effects.

Overdrive pacing is occasionally useful for the temporary control of persistent, recurrent monomorphic VT, achieved by transvenous placement of a pacing wire in the right ventricle. A burst of pacing at 10–20 bpm faster than the ventricular rate may terminate ventricular tachycardia but there is a risk of acceleration and the precipitation of VF with pacing.[21]

Recurrent VT should prompt evaluation of any other correctable factors such as recurrent ischemia or electrolyte imbalance. Coronary angiography has been recommended if there is ECG evidence of acute ischemia and no identifiable contributing factors such as electrolyte or metabolic abnormalities.[8] Intra-aortic balloon counterpulsation is valuable in the management of the intractable ventricular tachycardia associated with ongoing ischemia, and in extremis re-establishment of CPB has been life-saving for refractory VT/VF.[22]

The in-hospital mortality from postCABG VT is up to 50%.[7, 8, 10, 11] Further investigation following survival of new-onset VT is mandatory since the recurrence rate is estimated to be 30–35% in the first year and 10–15% in the second.[23] Empirical antiarrhythmic drug therapy has been found to be relatively ineffective in the suppression of life-threatening VT induced by programmed electrical stimulation[10] and recurrent VT was observed in 40% of cases with monomorphic VT inducible by programmed stimulation.[24] Management with implantable cardioverter-defibrillators (ICDs) is most effective in preventing late deaths from recurrent VT.[25] Electrophysiological studies to guide management should be performed at least 1 week after surgery to allow transient postoperative electrolyte, metabolic, and hemodynamic disturbances to resolve so that the continuing risk of VT can be best assessed.[26]

Conclusions and learning points

- Broad-complex tachycardia is a rare but potentially life-threatening complication of CABG.
- Examination of the ECG will usually allow differentiation between VT, SVT with aberrant conduction, and antidromic AVRT or pre-excited AF in the setting of the WPW syndrome.
- Adenosine is useful in both the diagnosis and the acute treatment of postCABG broad-complex tachycardia.
- New-onset VT occurs after 3% of CABG cases with a reported in-hospital mortality up to 50%.
- Monomorphic VT is more common in patients with previous myocardial infarction and impaired LV function and probably results from the reperfusion of viable tissue within old infarcts that form a substrate for re-entrant tachycardia. There is a high incidence of recurrence and the consideration of implantable device therapy is indicated in the majority of cases.

• Polymorphic VT is associated with perioperative ischemia or infarction and with transient electrical instability. It is less likely to be inducible by programmed electrical stimulation and the risk of recurrence and the requirement for long-term therapy is less than for monomorphic VT. Torsades de pointes polymorphic VT may be associated with proarrhythmic drugs that prolong the QT interval.

References

1. Antunes E, Brugada J, Steurer G et al. The differential diagnosis of a regular tachycardia with a wide QRS complex on the 12-lead ECG: ventricular tachycardia, supraventricular tachycardia with aberrant intraventricular conduction, and supraventricular tachycardia with anterograde conduction over an accessory pathway. Pacing Clin Electrophysiol 1994;17:1515–24.

2. Waldo AL, MacLean WA, Cooper TB et al. Use of temporarily placed epicardial atrial wire electrodes for the diagnosis and treatment of cardiac arrhythmias following open-heart surgery. J Thorac Cardiovasc Surg 1978;76:500–5.

3. Griffith MJ, Linker NJ, Ward DE, Camm AJ. Adenosine in the diagnosis of broad complex tachycardia. Lancet 1988;i:672–5.

4. Al-Khatib SM, Pritchett EL. Clinical features of Wolff–Parkinson–White syndrome. Am Heart J 1999;138:403–13.

5. Dagres N, Clague JR, Kottkamp H et al. Antidromic atrioventricular reentrant tachycardia mimicking ventricular tachycardia in the setting of previous myocardial infarction. Clin Cardiol 2000;23:63–5.

6. Kunze KP, Schluter M, Kuck KH. Sotalol in patients with Wolff–Parkinson–White syndrome. Circulation 1987;75:1050–7.

7. Kron IL, DiMarco JP, Harman PK et al. Unanticipated postoperative ventricular tachyarrhythmias. Ann Thorac Surg 1984;38:317–22.

8. Topol EJ, Lerman BB, Baughman KL et al. De novo refractory ventricular tachyarrhythmias after coronary revascularization. Am J Cardiol 1986;57:57–9.

9. Sapin PM, Woelfel AK, Foster JR. Unexpected ventricular tachyarrhythmias soon after cardiac surgery. Am J Cardiol 1991;68:1099–100.

10. Tam SK, Miller JM, Edmunds LH Jr. Unexpected, sustained ventricular tachyarrhythmia after cardiac operations. J Thorac Cardiovasc Surg 1991;102:883–9.

11. Steinberg JS, Gaur A, Sciacca R, Tan E. New-onset sustained ventricular tachycardia after cardiac surgery. Circulation 1999;99:903–8.

12. Smith RC, Leung JM, Keith FM et al. Ventricular dysrhythmias in patients undergoing coronary artery bypass graft surgery: incidence, characteristics, and prognostic importance. Study of Perioperative Ischemia (SPI) Research Group. Am Heart J 1992;123:73–81.

13. Janse MJ, Wit AL. Electrophysiological mechanisms of ventricular arrhythmias resulting from myocardial ischemia and infarction. Physiol Rev 1989;69:1049–169.

14. Saxon LA, Wiener I, Natterson PD et al. Monomorphic versus polymorphic ventricular tachycardia after coronary artery bypass grafting. Am J Cardiol 1995;75:403–5.

15. Azar RR, Berns E, Seecharran B et al. De novo monomorphic and polymorphic ventricular tachycardia following coronary artery bypass grafting. Am J Cardiol 1997;80:76–8.

16. Roden DM. Antiarrhythmic drugs: from mechanisms to clinical practice. Heart 2000;84:339–46.

17. Advanced Life Support Working Group of the European Resuscitation Council. The 1998 European Resuscitation Council guidelines for adult advanced life support. BMJ 1998;316:1863–9.

18. Pinski SL. Potassium replacement after cardiac surgery: it is not time to change practice, yet. Crit Care Med 1999;27:2581–2.

19. Sueta CA, Clarke SW, Dunlap SH et al. Effect of acute magnesium administration on the frequency of ventricular arrhythmia in patients with heart failure. Circulation 1994;89:660–6.

20. Schwartz A, Shen E, Morady F et al. Hemodynamic effects of intravenous amiodarone in patients with depressed left ventricular function and recurrent ventricular tachycardia. Am Heart J 1983;106:848–56.

21. Carlson MD, Biblo LA, Waldo AL. Post open heart surgery ventricular arrhythmias. Cardiovasc Clin 1992;22:241–53.

22. Rousou JA, Engelman RM, Flack JE 3rd et al. Emergency cardiopulmonary bypass in the cardiac

surgical unit can be a lifesaving measure in postoperative cardiac arrest. *Circulation* 1994;**90**:II280–4.

23. Willems S, Weiss C, Meinertz T. Tachyarrhythmias following coronary artery bypass graft surgery: epidemiology, mechanisms, and current therapeutic strategies. *Thorac Cardiovasc Surg* 1997;**45**:232–7.

24. Costeas XF, Schoenfeld MH. Usefulness of electrophysiologic studies for new-onset sustained ventricular tachyarrhythmias shortly after coronary artery bypass grafting. *Am J Cardiol* 1993;**72**:1291–4.

25. The Antiarrhythmics versus Implantable Defibrillators (AVID) Investigators. A comparison of antiarrhythmic-drug therapy with implantable defibrillators in patients resuscitated from near-fatal ventricular arrhythmias. *N Engl J Med* 1997;**337**:1576–83.

26. Bhandari AK, Au PK, Rose JS *et al.* Decline in inducibility of sustained ventricular tachycardia from two to twenty weeks after acute myocardial infarction. *Am J Cardiol* 1987;**59**:284–90.

28
Ventricular assist devices

Berend Mets

Introduction

Since the advent of the first heart transplant performed by Barnard in 1967[1] there has been a need for mechanical cardiac assist devices either as a bridge or as an alternative to transplantation.[2] This case report deals with a patient who was successfully bridged to transplantation using a left ventricular assist device (LVAD) placed at the time of cardiac decompensation when a donor heart was not available. Not only does this case report highlight many of the important perioperative management issues but serves to underscore the utility of heart assist devices in maintaining life long enough to allow subsequent transplantation. It is of interest to know that the first successful bridge to transplantation by Oyer was performed in 1985.[3]

Although the cost of LVAD implantation and maintenance is considerable, it remains less than the cost of maintaining a 'status 1' candidate for heart transplantation for 75 days — the median waiting time in 1992.[3] Currently 91% of patients fitted with an assist device for severe cardiac failure can be discharged from the hospital and 74% survive to undergo transplantation.[4] There are indications that LVAD patients subsequently transplanted do better than those not subjected to the LVAD bridge.[5]

Case history

The patient was a 40-year-old black male, awaiting heart transplantation, who had dilated cardiomyopathy with a left ventricular ejection fraction (LVEF) of 12% as well as inducible ventricular tachycardia for which an automatic implantable cardioventor defibrillator (AICD) had been placed 7 months previously. He now presented with worsening cardiac failure, (for which he had been on a continuous infusion of dobutamine 5 µg kg^{-1} min^{-1} for 3 weeks) complicated by the development of intermittent supraventricular tachycardia as well as decreasing renal perfusion/function demonstrated by a rise in serum creatinine from 0.9 to 1.7 mg dl^{-1} (80–150 µmol l^{-1}) over a 2-week period.

Because discontinuation of the dobutamine infusion was associated with a fall in blood pressure from 90/60 to 70/50 mmHg, a dopamine infusion had been started to maintain blood pressure prior to his transfer to our hospital.

The patient gave a previous history (some 15 years earlier) of cocaine, alcohol and tobacco use and was diagnosed as having dilated cardiomyopathy at the age of 27 — his presenting complaint having been 'palpitations'. A cardiac catheterization performed at that time revealed normal coronary arterial anatomy, elevated pulmonary artery pressures (PAP) 55/38 mmHg, a cardiac output (CO) of 4.26 l min^{-1} and LVEF 12%. He was managed medically and at the age of 37, (3 years before the present admission) was evaluated for possible heart transplantation. At this time, cardiac catheterization revealed worsening pulmonary hypertension (PAP 81/28 mmHg), cardiac output (2.8 l min^{-1}) and mixed venous saturation (SvO$_2$ 50%) with significant improvement following the administration of sodium nitroprusside (PAP 51/26 mmHg, CO 6.6 Lmin^{-1}, SvO$_2$ 73%) while calculated pulmonary vascular resistance decreased from 458 to 229 dyne s cm^{-5} (5.7–2.9 Wood units). The patient was not listed for transplantation at this time.

Past medical history	Cocaine, alcohol and tobacco abuse 15 years earlier. Palpitations 13 years earlier leading to a diagnosis of dilated cardiomyopathy. Allergic to penicillin.
Regular medications	Coumadin (warfarin), isordil, furosemide, zaroxylin and aldactone, captopril, digoxin. Dopamine 7 mg kg-1 min-1 via right antecubital PICC.
Examination	Weight 111 kg. Height 1.75 m. BMI 36 kg m^{-2}. Alert and orientated. Temperature 36.7°C. HR 110 bpm. RR 16 bpm. BP 110/60 mmHg. JVP not assessible. Cardiac apex displaced laterally, heart sounds — distant, no murmurs. Bibasal inspiratory crepitations, no wheeze. Abdomen distended, tender liver edge palpable 3–4 inches below costal margin. No peripheral edema. No erythema or induration at PICC entry site. Pulmonary artery catheter in situ.
Investigations	Hb 11.0 g dl^{-1}, WBC 8.8 × 10^9 l^{-1}, platelets 283 × 10^9 l^{-1}, PT 20.9 s (ratio 1.76), PTT 37.7 s. [Na$^+$] 124 mmol l^{-1}, [K$^+$] 4.0 mmol l^{-1}, BUN 32 mg dl^{-1} (11.4 mmol l^{-1}), creatinine 1.7 mg dl^{-1} (150 μmol l^{-1}), glucose 298 mg dl^{-1} (16.5 mmol l^{-1}). Liver function tests — within normal limits. Digoxin level 1.7 ng ml^{-1} (2.18 nmol l^{-1}), troponin I 0.2 ng ml^{-1} (normal <2 ng ml^{-1}), creatine kinase 119 u l^{-1}. **CXR:** Poor inspiratory effort. Heart enlarged. Prominent pulmonary vasculature with mild pulmonary venous congestion. **ECG:** 120 bpm, normal axis with evidence of intraventricular conduction defect. **Right heart catheterization:** RA 10 mmHg, RV 62/12 mmHg, PCWP 40 mmHg, CO 4.79 l min^{-1} (CI 2.18 l min^{-1} m^{-2}).

The patient did well until the beginning of the year of admission when he experienced a decline in his effort tolerance with palpitations and a presyncopal syndrome. At this time he was found to have inducible ventricular tachycardia for which an AICD was placed.

Over the last 7 months the patient experienced increasing shortness of breath, paroxysmal nocturnal dyspnea, three-pillow orthopnea and effort intolerance necessitating 10 admissions over this period to the referring hospital.

Initial management in coronary care unit

The patient was scheduled for heart transplantation pending a suitable donor organ and started on a continuous intravenous infusion of milrinone 0.35 μg kg^{-1} min^{-1} while the dopamine infusion was decreased to a 'renal' dose of 3 μg kg^{-1} min^{-1}. Enalapril 6.25 mg twice daily was

started and captopril stopped. Coumadin was stopped and heparin administered by continuous intravenous infusion.

Four days after admission the patient developed a fever of 38.6°C associated with an increased white cell count (11.2 × 10^9 l^{-1}), increasing shortness of breath and an episode of rigors. Intravenous levofloxacin and vancomycin were commenced to combat *Staphylococcus hemolyticus* cultured from blood taken on the day of admission. The pulmonary artery catheter was replaced and the pulmonary indwelling intravenous catheter (PICC) line removed.

The patient developed recurrent episodes of SVT as well as VT resulting in AICD discharge during this period but the renal status improved: [Na$^+$] 138 mmol^{-1}, [K$^+$] 4.2 mmol^{-1}, blood urea nitrogen (BUN) 18 mg dl^{-1} (6.4 mmol l^{-1}) creatinine 1.2 mg dl^{-1} (106 μmol l^{-1}) 7 days after admission to the CCU. Because of persistent fever and positive blood cultures (initially *Staph. hemolyticus*, subsequently *Staph. epidermidis*) levofloxacillin was replaced with cefotaxime while vancomycin was continued.

Nine days after admission the patient was evaluated for possible LVAD placement at which time the milrinone infusion had been increased from 0.35 to 0.5 µg kg^{-1} min^{-1}. Transesophageal echocardiography revealed severe mitral regurgitation secondary to a prolapsing mitral valve and moderate tricuspid regurgitation. No vegetations suggestive of endocarditis were seen.

The patient deteriorated further over the next 2 days. In response to recurrent episodes of SVT and ventricular tachycardia — resulting in repetitive AICD discharges — the AICD was disabled and the patient loaded with amiodarone and a continuous infusion started. The patient then developed copious diarrhea and was found to be positive for *Clostridium difficile* toxin for which metronidazole was administered.

On the day of surgery, the patient was febrile (39.7°C), hypotensive (90/60 mmHg) and tachycardic (130 bpm). The CVP was 20 mmHg, PAP 64/35 mmHg, CI 1.7 l min^{-1} m^{-2} and SvO$_2$ 48%. His liver function tests, which had previously been within normal limits, now demonstrated elevation of AST to 1172 u l^{-1} (normal <35 u l^{-1}) and ALT to 461 u l^{-1} (normal <35 u l^{-1}) while his serum creatinine had risen from 1.2 to 1.9 mg dl^{-1} (106–168 µmol l^{-1}), his hematocrit had decreased from 30 to 22% and his white cell count was 13.4 × 10^9 l^{-1}. His prothrombin time was 23 s, for which Vitamin K 10mg was administered intravenously prior to surgery.

He deteriorated further and was urgently transferred to the first available operating room where he was found by the author to be in decompensated cardiogenic shock with a heart rate of 143 bpm, a blood pressure of 63/41 and frank pulmonary edema with a respiratory rate of 56 breathing 100% oxygen administered by face-mask.

Preinduction management

The patient was reassured as best as possible, maintained in an upright position and received 100% oxygen by face-mask while the preoperative infusions of amiodarone, milrinone and dopamine were continued. A large bore peripheral intra-

venous catheter, and a radial arterial catheter were sited prior to induction of anesthesia; a second central line for rapid infusion of blood and blood products was established after tracheal intubation. At the same time an infusion of noradrenaline was started and increased to maintain a systolic blood pressure 90–100 mmHg, and baseline urine output was noted. Twelve units of platelets and fresh frozen plasma, and 6 units of packed red blood cells were ordered.

Induction of anesthesia

The patient's labored respiration was assisted by manual face-mask ventilation. Midazolam 1mg was then administered, followed by graded (100 µg) doses of fentanyl while the noradrenaline infusion was steadily increased to 0.16 µg kg^{-1} min^{-1} to maintain systolic blood pressure above 90 mmHg. After 800 µg of fentanyl the patient lost consciousness and rocuronium 100 mg was administered, cricoid pressure applied, the trachea intubated and the lungs ventilated with 100% oxygen. Anesthesia was maintained with isoflurane (0.3% inspired) and incremental doses of midazolam and fentanyl. Arterial blood gas analysis following induction revealed: pH:7.20, PaCO$_2$ 61 mmHg (8.1 kPa), PaO$_2$ 131 mmHg (17.5 kPa), SBC 24 mmol l^{-1}, base excess −4 mmol l^{-1}.

Maintenance of anesthesia and transesophageal echocardiography

A median sternotomy was performed and a preperitoneal pouch fashioned for placement of a TCI Heartmate LVAD[6] (Thermo Cardiosystems Inc; Woburn, MA, USA; Figures 28.1 and 28.2). After this heparin 32 000 units was administered in preparation for cardiopulmonary bypass aiming to achieve an ACT of ≥480 seconds. This dose achieved an ACT of 312 s. As a further dose of heparin 15 000 units failed to produce adequate prolongation of the ACT, antithrombin III 540 units was administered resulting in an ACT of 549 s.

When adequate ACT levels had been achieved and the aorta cannulated a test dose of aprotinin

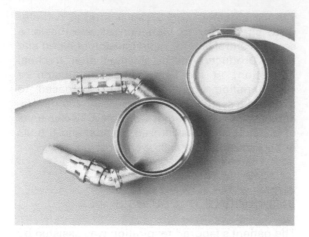

Figure 28.1

Photograph of TCI-Heartmate LVAD showing a cross-section and the location of unidirectional porcine xenografts in the device in and outflows. (Reproduced with permission of Thermo Cardiosystems Inc.)

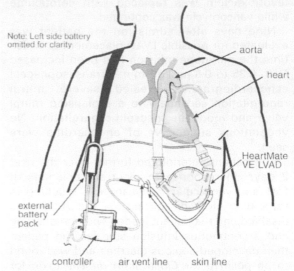

Note: Left side battery omitted for clarity

aorta

heart

HeartMate VE LVAD

external battery pack

controller   air vent line   skin line

Figure 28.2

Schematic of a TCI-Heartmate LVAD 'plugged' into the left ventricular apex, located in a preperitoneal pocket and connected to the ascending aorta. The diagram demonstrates the use of a battery pack containing rechargeable batteries (worn as a shoulder holster) providing 4–6 hours of charge. (Reproduced with permission of Thermo Cardiosystems Inc.)

1 ml (1.4 mg / 10 000 kiu) was administered. This was followed a few minutes later by a further bolus of 199 ml (total loading dose 280 mg / 2 Mkiu) and then a continuous infusion (70 mg h^{-1} /0.5 Mkiu h^{-1}) until the end of surgery. In addition, aprotinin 280 mg was added to the extracorporeal circuit prime.

A multiplane TEE probe was placed in the esophagus and the heart was examined to exclude a patent foramen ovale (PFO), significant aortic regurgitation, and mitral or tricuspid stenosis. In addition, the extent of right ventricular compromise was ascertained by determining the extent of tricuspid regurgitation and right ventricular dilatation.[7, 8] The patient was found to have both severe mitral and tricuspid regurgitation.

A left ventricular vent was placed through the right superior pulmonary vein and cardiopulmonary bypass (CPB) established between the right atrium and ascending aorta. Then without the use of cardioplegia or the application of an aortic cross-clamp, the LVAD inflow cannula was advanced through the diaphragm and 'plugged' into a Teflon cuff sewn onto the epicardium the left ventricular apex (Figure 28.2).[6] The LVAD outflow cannula was anastomosed to the right lateral aspect of the ascending aorta. Prior to weaning from CPB the LVAD was hand-cranked using a manual device with the patient in a head-down position to assure deairing of the LVAD and thereby minimizing the potential for cerebral air embolism.[6]

At this time TEE evaluation was performed to ensure that the LVAD inflow cannula was directed towards the mitral valve and away from the interventricular septum for fear of inflow occlusion as well as to assess the extent of deairing (Figure 28.3). Further, because when the LVAD is operational, the left atrium (LA) and left ventricle (LV) act as conduits for blood that drains via the ventricular apex into the LVAD pump it is important to use TEE to ensure that the LA and LV are decompressed. In addition, aortic regurgitation and PFO were again excluded as these lesions may only be manifest at this time because of the altered pressure relationships that occur once the LVAD is functioning.[2]

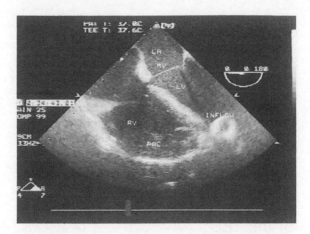

Figure 28.3

Intraoperative echocardiogram in the patient described in this case report demonstrating the LVAD inflow cannulae (INFLOW) at the left ventricular apex sited towards the mitral valve (MV) and away from the septum. A dilated right ventricle (RV) is demonstrated. The left atrium (LA) and left ventricle (LV) are decompressed and the intra-atrial septum shifted to the left suggesting appropriate functioning of the LVAD device. An echogenic pulmonary artery catheter (PAC) is demonstrated.

Weaning from bypass

During CPB, the infusions of dopamine, milrinone, amiodarone and noradrenaline were continued. Because of the preoperative elevation of pulmonary artery pressures and continued severe tricuspid regurgitation and right ventricular failure, nitric oxide 20 ppm was added to the fresh gas mixture, and an infusion of dobutamine 2.5 μg kg^{-1} min^{-1} commenced.

The patient was weaned of CPB and after administration of protamine had a blood pressure 120/50 mmHg, PAP 39/24 mmHg, CVP 18 mmHg with an LVAD flow of 5.2 l min^{-1} and a thermodilution cardiac output of 4.57 l min^{-1}. Initial arterial blood gas analysis indicated adequate oxygenation and mild hypercarbia.

To ensure hemostasis and achieve a hematocrit of ≥23%, 2 units of packed red blood cells, 6 units of platelets, 6 units of fresh frozen plasma and 3 units of 'cell saved' blood were administered. The patient was transferred to the ICU where coagulation studies revealed PT 21 s (INR 1.77) and PTT 85 s, which required further blood product transfusion to assure hemostasis.

ICU Follow-up

The patient was gradually weaned off nitric oxide over the next 24 hours and extubated 36 hours after arrival in the ICU at which time he still required milrinone 0.4 μg kg^{-1} min^{-1}, dopamine 1.2 μg kg^{-1} min^{-1}, and dobutamine 5 μg kg^{-1} min^{-1} to maintain LVAD flows at 5.7 l min^{-1}. At this time his coagulation profile was near normal and his serum creatinine was 1.0 mg dl^{-1} (88 μmol l^{-1}). By the fifth postoperative day, all vasopressors and inotropes had been weaned and a slow wean of milrinone was started when acute dehiscence of the sternum occurred (postoperative day 6), requiring a return to theatre to rewire the sternum. The patient was weaned from mechanical ventilation and extubated a day later when the milrinone wean had been completed and LVAD flows remained at 5 l min^{-1}.

Twelve days after LVAD implantation, while the patient was still being treated with intravenous vancomycin and cefotaxime as well as oral vancomycin for *Clostridum difficile*, a suitable heart donor was identified and a successful LVAD explant and heart transplant were performed. The patient was extubated within 24 hours of surgery but his posttransplant course was complicated by mild renal insufficiency (BUN 39 mg dl^{-1} (13.9 mmol l^{-1}), creatinine 3.4 mg dl^{-1} (300 μmol l^{-1})) as well as a second occurrence of sternal wound dehiscence. *Candida albicans* infection of the sternal bone was found and the dehisced sternum required debridement and interposition of a pectoralis major flap as well as intravenous fluconazole therapy for 4 weeks.

The patient was discharged home on intravenous fluconazole 6 weeks after the date of LVAD placement.

Discussion

This case report demonstrates some of the key points that are relevant to the management of these challenging patients, which have been extensively reviewed elsewhere.[8]

Induction of anesthesia

Firstly it demonstrates that so often, while discussion about placing an LVAD is elective, (for which criteria have been established[9] the final decision to operate is often made when the patient is near terminal, as in the case presented. Thus the anesthetist is faced with a patient with cardiac decompensation who invariably is coagulopathic (secondary to liver decompensation), may have impaired renal function and may be infected.[10, 11]

While the hepatic and renal impairment may have an impact on anesthetic drug choice[12] another important consideration is the maintenenace of hemodynamic stability during induction. It should be remembered that these patients are often taking angiotensin-converting enzyme (ACE) inhibitors and amiodarone[13, 14] and that patients with cardiac failure have high circulating levels of endogenous catecholamines.[15] The anesthetist should be aware of the potential for adverse interactions when patients taking ACE inhibitors[16] and/or amiodarone[17] are subjected to surgical stress and anesthesia. This should not be surprising when it is appreciated that amiodarone causes a non-competitive α and β adrenergic blockade,[18, 19] while angiotensin II is a potent vasoconstrictor whose formation is blocked by ACE inhibitors.[20] Thus to avoid the inevitable problem of hypotension due to the sympatholysis associated with anesthetic induction and possibly enhanced due to amiodarone, noradrenaline was administered to compensate for this sympatholytic effect.

Another key concern is the need to be prepared for massive transfusion during and after surgery by having sufficient intravenous access, as well as having ordered sufficient blood products in advance as was done in the case presented. Further, it has been demonstrated that administration of intravenous vitamin K may be beneficial.[21] The use of aprotonin in LVAD patients has been associated with decreased chest tube drainage, decreased red cell administration and a reduction in the total units of blood product needed to achieve similar postoperative hemoglobin levels.[22] An important finding was the fact that LVAD patients not receiving aprotonin had an increased incidence of right-sided circulatory failure (18 versus 9.5%) defined by the authors as the need

for right ventricular assist device placement. Twenty-one of the 22 (95%) patients who suffered right-sided circulatory failure died.

The patient presented here showed signs of heparin resistance, which is not uncommon after continuous heparin infusion and is probably due to a decrease in plasma antithrombin III levels.[23] Antithrombin III therapy, as used in this case, has been shown to speed the onset of adequate anticoagulation.[24]

Maintenance of anesthesia and use of the TEE

A major concern in all cardiac patients is the potential for awareness, especially when the administration of anesthetics may lead to enhanced hypotension. To avoid this, the author uses a vasoconstrictor so creating 'room' for the administration of adequate anesthetic and administers isoflurane 0.4% throughout the operation. This low concentration of isoflurane is associated with loss of implicit and explicit memory[25] and is unlikely to have significant hemodynamic impact as these effects are dose dependent. Furthermore, isoflurane maintains cardiac output better than halothane, enflurane,[26] sevoflurane or desflurane.[27] A further important aspect of the anesthetic management of these patients is to assess the native heart using TEE to exclude lesions that must be addressed surgically on CPB such as a PFO, aortic regurgitation, or mitral stenosis.[11] The reasons are; (1) PFO will result in significant right to left shunting postoperatively when the LVAD is activated, as LA pressure will be less than RA pressure. (2) Aortic insufficiency will result in blood ejected by the LVAD into the aorta, refluxing back through the incompetent valve into the left ventricle. This anomalous flow of blood results in a decrease in systemic output[2] and would cause a discrepancy between cardiac output measured by thermodilution and the flow measured by the LVAD pump displayed on its digital monitor. (3) Mitral stenosis would impair blood flow to the LVAD and this lesion needs to be addressed.

TEE evaluation is also key in assessing the extent of tricuspid regurgitation as an indicator of right ventricular failure. Both TEE and pre- and intraoperative pulmonary artery pressure monitoring are used to guide the decision to institute further inotrope therapy or add inhaled nitric oxide. In this case report, both severe tricuspid regurgitation and elevated pulmonary artery pressures were evident and so nitric oxide and dobutamine were started electively just prior to first separation from CPB.

Nitric oxide (NO) administration (20 ppm) in six LVAD patients has been shown to decrease mean PAP from 35 ±6 to 24 ±4 mmHg and increase LVAD flow, from 1.9 ±0.2 to 2.7 ±0.4 l min^{-1} m^{-2} in under 10 minutes.[28] Wagner et al[29] demonstrated similar beneficial effects on hemodynamic parameters in eight male LVAD patients with right ventricular dysfunction treated with NO (25–40 ppm). Prostaglandin E$_1$ infusion has also been used to treat pulmonary hypertension in LVAD patients.[3]

CPB and weaning from CPB

The operation, especially in expert hands is of short duration, so the anesthetist has very little time to prepare to manage significant bleeding, possible vasodilatation and certain right-sided cardiac failure post bypass.[2, 30]

Right-sided cardiac failure usually occurs in the setting of severe postoperative bleeding because excessive bleeding and resuscitation may result in cytokine-mediated pulmonary vasoconstriction.[2] A further contributor to impaired right ventricular function postoperatively is that the LVAD decreases right ventricular contractility while compliance is increased and impairment of septal function occurs.[31] Thus pre-existing right ventricular impairment may be further exacerbated by LVAD placement.

A further problem in the postoperative period is resistant hypotension, which we encountered to a lesser degree in the present patient. We use noradrenaline to maintain systemic vascular resistance and add vasopressin if required.[30] The administration of vasopressin 0.1 u min^{-1} has been shown to be effective in combating a vasodilatory state in LVAD patients. Argenziano et al[30] have demonstrated, in five patients who were receiving > 8 µg min^{-1} of noradrenaline and had mean arterial pressures <70 mmHg, despite LVAD flows of 2.5 l min^{-1} m^{-2} postCPB, that in

less than 15 minutes increases in MAP (57 ±4 to 84 ±2 mmHg) and systemic vascular resistance (813 ±113 to 1188 ±87 dyne s cm^{-5}) occurred without a significant change in cardiac index. This improvement was associated with a decreased requirement for noradrenaline administration (26.6–10.7 µg min^{-1}).[30] We find that occasionally in severe refractory vasodilatory states the addition of an infusion of metaraminol and/or epinephrine is necessary.

Postoperative management

The postoperative management, as was in the case presented, can be complex, which is not surprising considering that the patients are often in a near terminal state before surgery, have multiple organ impairment and are infected.[10, 11]

Key learning points

- Patients have cardiovascular decompensation and invariably present in a near terminal state with multiple organ impairment and sepsis.
- Due cognisance has to be taken of the potential effects of drug therapy on hemodynamic stability during induction and anesthetic maintenance.
- Vitamin K therapy and aprotonin administration have been shown to have benefit in combating the inevitable postoperative coagulopathy experienced in these patients.
- The anesthetist should be adequately prepared for significant hemorrhage and the need for massive transfusion.
- TEE evaluation of the heart is crucial for monitoring right ventricular function and excluding PFO, aortic regurgitation and mitral stenosis.
- Inotropic infusions should probably be maintained during CPB
- Nitric oxide has been shown to be useful in improving LVAD flow and decreasing pulmonary artery pressures postoperatively.
- Vasopressin has been shown to be a useful adjunct in vasodilatory shock in LVAD recipients.

References

1. Barnard CN. The operation. A human cardiac transplant: an interim report of a successful operation performed at Groote Schuur Hospital, Cape Town. *S Afr Med J* 1967;**41**:1271–4.

2. Goldstein DJ, Oz MC, Rose EA. Implantable left ventricular assist devices. *N Engl J Med* 1998;**339**:1522–33.

3. Frazier OH. The development of an implantable, portable, electrically powered left ventricular assist device. *Semin Thorac Cardiovasc Surg* 1994;**6**:181–7.

4. Mehta SM, Aufiero TX, Pae WE *et al*. Combined registry for the clinical use of mechanical ventricular assist pumps and the total artificial teart in conjunction with heart transplantation: sixth official report—1994. *J Heart Lung Transplant* 1995;**14**:585–93.

5. Frazier OH, Rose EA, Macmanus Q *et al*. Multicenter clinical evaluation of the HeartMate 1000 IP left ventricular assist device. *Ann Thorac Surg* 1992;**53**:1080–90.

6. Oz MC, Goldstein DJ, Rose EA. Preperitoneal placement of ventricular assist devices: an illustrated stepwise approach. *J Card Surg* 1995;**10**:288–94.

7. George SJ, Black JJ, Boscoe MJ. Intraoperative transoesophageal echocardiography for implantation of a pulsatile left ventricular assist device. *Br J Anaesth* 1995;**75**:794–7.

8. Mets B. Anesthesia for left ventricular assist device placement. *J Cardiothorac Vasc Anesth* 2000;**14**:316–26.

9. Oz MC, Goldstein DJ, Pepino P *et al*. Screening scale predicts patients successfully receiving long-term implantable left ventricular assist devices. *Circulation* 1995;**92**:II169–73.

10. McCarthy PM, Schmitt SK, Vargo RL *et al*. Implantable LVAD infections: implications for permanent use of the device. *Ann Thorac Surg* 1996;**61**:359–65.

11. Oz MC, Rose EA, Levin HR. Selection criteria for placement of left ventricular assist devices. *Am Heart J* 1995;**129**:173–7.

12. Mets B. The pharmacokinetics of anesthetic drugs and adjuvants during cardiopulmonary bypass. *Acta Anaesthesiol Scand* 2000;**44**:261–73.

13. Mets B, Michler RE, Delphin ED *et al*. Refractory vasodilation after cardiopulmonary bypass for heart transplantation in recipients on combined amiodarone and angiotensin-converting enzyme inhibitor therapy: a role for vasopressin administration. *J Cardiothorac Vasc Anesth* 1998;**12**:326–9.

14. Stevenson WG, Stevenson LW, Middlekauff HR *et al*. Improving survival for patients with advanced heart failure: a study of 737 consecutive patients. *J Am Coll Cardiol* 1995;**26**:1417–23.

15. Thomas JA, Marks BH. Plasma norepinephrine in congestive heart failure. *Am J Cardiol* 1978;**41**:233–43.

16. Colson P, Saussine M, Seguin JR *et al*. Hemodynamic effects of anesthesia in patients chronically treated with angiotensin-converting enzyme inhibitors. *Anesth Analg* 1992;**74**:805–8.

17. Perkins MW, Dasta JF, Reilley TE, Halpern P. Intraoperative complications in patients receiving amiodarone: characteristics and risk factors. *DICP* 1989;**23**:757–63.

18. Liberman BA, Teasdale SJ. Anaesthesia and amiodarone. *Can Anaesth Soc J* 1985;**32**:629–38.

19. Charlier R. Cardiac actions in the dog of a new antagonist of adrenergic excitation which does not produce competitive blockade of adrenoceptors. *Br J Pharmacol* 1970;**39**:668–74.

20. Licker M, Neidhart P, Lustenberger S *et al*. Long-term angiotensin-converting enzyme inhibitor treatment attenuates adrenergic responsiveness without altering hemodynamic control in patients undergoing cardiac surgery. *Anesthesiology* 1996;**84**:789–800.

21. Kaplon RJ, Gillinov AM, Smedira NG *et al*. Vitamin K reduces bleeding in left ventricular assist device recipients. *J Heart Lung Transplant* 1999;**18**:346–50.

22. Goldstein DJ, Seldomridge JA, Chen JM *et al*. Use of aprotinin in LVAD recipients reduces blood loss, blood use, and perioperative mortality. *Ann Thorac Surg* 1995;**59**:1063–7.

23. Dietrich W, Spannagl M, Schramm W *et al*. The influence of preoperative anticoagulation on heparin response during cardiopulmonary bypass. *J Thorac Cardiovasc Surg* 1991;**102**:505–14.

24. Williams MR, D'Ambra AB, Beck JR *et al*. A randomized trial of antithrombin concentrate for treatment of heparin resistance. *Ann Thorac Surg* 2000;**70**:873–7.

25. Ghoneim MM, Block RI. Learning and memory during general anesthesia: an update. *Anesthesiology* 1997;**87**:387–410.

26. Eger EI. Isoflurane: a review. *Anesthesiology* 1981;**55**:559–76.

27. Weiskopf RB. Cardiovascular effects of desflurane in experimental animals and volunteers. *Anaesthesia* 1995;**50 (Suppl)**:14–7.

28. Argenziano M, Choudhri AF, Moazami N *et al.* Randomized, double-blind trial of inhaled nitric oxide in LVAD recipients with pulmonary hypertension. *Ann Thorac Surg* 1998;**65**:340–5.

29. Wagner F, Dandel M, Gunther G *et al.* Nitric oxide inhalation in the treatment of right ventricular dysfunction following left ventricular assist device implantation. *Circulation* 1997;**96**:II291–6.

30. Argenziano M, Choudhri AF, Oz MC *et al.* A prospective randomized trial of arginine vasopressin in the treatment of vasodilatory shock after left ventricular assist device placement. *Circulation* 1997;**96**:II286–90.

31. Santamore WP, Gray LA Jr. Left ventricular contributions to right ventricular systolic function during LVAD support. *Ann Thorac Surg* 1996;**61**:350–6.

29

Cardiac surgery for Jehovah's Witness patients

Martin J Platt, Christopher J Broomhead and Avinash C Shukla

Introduction

There are nearly 4 million Jehovah's witnesses world-wide, of which approximately 140 000 reside in the United Kingdom.[1] An offshot of a fundamentalist Christian sect, originating in the late nineteenth century in the USA, key to their beliefs is the literal interpretation of the bible and the absolute authority of God. From this stems a belief that the end of the world is imminent, leading to the creation of a new world, in which the faithful will enjoy eternal life. Only by breaking the rules laid down in the bible, would the believer be prevented from entering this Utopia.

The *Watchtower* is the monthly journal of the Jehovah's witnesses. In 1945 an article quoted several passages of the bible which were said to support the belief that blood transfusion violated God's law.[2] Although these passages relate to the oral ingestion of blood or meat, which has not been exsanguinated, this has been extrapolated to include receiving blood or its constituents by the intravenous route. Since breaking God's law represents a fate worse than death, Jehovah's witnesses have since this time refused transfusion of blood or blood products, even if the end result may be death itself.

The legal situation has recently been reviewed.[1] For elective surgery, anesthetists who feel they can not comply with the wishes of the patient are entitled to refuse to be involved. In the case of emergency surgery, doctors are bound morally and ethically to do their best for the patient, whilst taking account of their wishes. Giving blood against the expressed wish of the patient, even as a life saving procedure, represents the tort of battery.

The extracorporeal circulation of blood is generally permitted, on the understanding that the blood does not lose continuity with the patient's circulation. Once continuity is lost, the blood may no longer be retransfused. Therefore cardiopulmonary bypass (CPB) is accepted, whilst autologous predonation of blood is not. Other areas are not as clear-cut — some Jehovah's witnesses will accept the use of 'cell-savers' whilst others will not. It is therefore important to clearly establish on a case-by-case basis what is acceptable. We outline below the case history of a patient who presented for revision coronary artery bypass grafting, and discuss the points it highlights in the management of Jehovah's witness patients.

Case history

A 52-year-old male Caucasian Jehovah's Witness was referred to the cardiac department by his general practitioner with a history of increasing angina and decreasing exercise tolerance. Eight years previously he had been admitted with an inferior myocardial infarction, from which he had made a good recovery. Before discharge, an exercise tolerance test had been positive for inferior ischemia. Subsequent coronary angiography demonstrated a critical lesion in the proximal right coronary artery (RCA), which was bypassed with a single saphenous vein graft with good effect. Since that time he had been pain free with a good exercise tolerance and had been back at work. Treatment had been limited to atenolol and simvastatin. He had no other significant medical history.

Over the last 6 months he had again developed angina. His exercise tolerance had gradually reduced, and was now limited to 200 meters by the onset of angina. A resting ECG showed Q waves in the inferior leads, but was otherwise normal. An exercise tolerance test demonstrated ischemia in the anterior leads. A transthoracic echocardiogram (TTE) demonstrated normal intracardiac anatomy and good left ventricular function. A repeat angiogram confirmed good left ventricular function, a patent vein graft to the RCA with no distal disease in the native vessel, a normal left main stem but severe proximal lesions in both the left anterior descending (LAD) and circumflex vessels and minor distal disease. Unfortunately the angiogram was complicated by significant blood loss and a large groin hematoma. The hemoglobin concentration fell from 12.2 g dl^{-1} on admission to 9.8 g dl^{-1} the day after the procedure. However, his angina was not aggravated by this anemia.

Whilst still an inpatient he was referred for consideration for surgical revascularization. Apart from his cardiac history and symptoms, he was otherwise well. The only medications he was currently taking were atenolol, simvastatin and ferrous sulfate. He had no allergies. Examination of the cardiac and respiratory systems was unremarkable. He was normotensive, with a sinus

bradycardia and, apart from his anemia, all other preoperative investigations were normal.

Discussion about his beliefs as a Jehovah's witness confirmed that he would not agree to blood transfusion, nor to the administration of blood products such as FFP or platelets, even as a life-saving treatment. Although autologous predonation was unacceptable, and not a satisfactory option given the urgent need for surgery, he would agree to pre-bypass autologous donation via a central venous line. He also deemed the use of the 'cell saver' to be acceptable.

Discussion between the surgeon and the anesthetist allowed a plan to be formulated. Treatment was commenced with iron, folate, vitamin B$_{12}$ and erythropoeitin. Assuming that his cardiac status remained stable, this would be continued until the hemoglobin concentration rose to >12 g dl^{-1}, and could be continued into the postoperative period. High-dose aprotinin would be used over the perioperative period. Since only two bypass grafts were required — a single vein graft and the left internal mammary artery — a beating heart technique would be used to avoid the problems of CPB. A 'cell saver' would be used during the surgical procedure.

Approximately 2 weeks later the hemoglobin concentration had reached the target level of 12 g dl^{-1}. Premedication with temazepam 30 mg was administered by mouth 90 minutes prior to induction. Routine induction and maintenance of anesthesia was undertaken. The patient was kept

Past medical history	Coronary artery disease. Previous myocardial infarction and CABG. Recurrent angina.
Regular medications	Atenolol 100 mg OD, simvastatin 10 mg OD, ferrous sulfate 200 mg TDS, enoxaparin 20 mg SC OD.
Examination	Unremarkable. Weight 72 kg. BP 145/80 mmHg.
Investigations	Hb 12.2 g dl^{-1}, WBC 7.2 × 10^9 l^{-1}, platelets 240 × 10^9 l^{-1}. Urea, electrolytes, creatinine, glucose, liver function tests — all normal **CXR:** Heart size normal, lung fields clear. **ECG:** Sinus rhythm, 60 beats per minute, old inferior infarct. **TTE:** Good left ventricular function, no structural abnormality. **Coronary angiogram:** Mild inferior hypokinesia but good overall left ventricular function, patent vein graft to right coronary artery, critical disease in the proximal LAD and circumflex vessels.

warm by using a heating mattress, a hot-air convection heater placed over the lower body after the saphenous vein had been harvested, a fluid warmer and by maintaning the ambient temperature in the operating room higher than normal. Aprotinin was administered as a loading dose (2×10^6 kiu), followed by an infusion (0.5×10^6 kiu h^{-1}). Full heparinization with the standard dose of heparin (300 mg kg^{-1}) was undertaken, to achieve an ACT >450 seconds. Two bypass grafts were fashioned without CPB without event. Reversal of anticoagulation to a normal ACT with protamine was ensured at the end of the procedure. Although the 'cell saver' was used, blood loss was so minimal that there was insufficient to retransfuse. Low-dose noradrenaline (0.005–0.01 µg kg^{-1} min^{-1}) was infused throughout the procedure to minimize fluid administration.

On admission to the ICU, the aprotinin infusion was continued for a further 4 hours even though chest tube drainage was less than 50 ml $hour^{-1}$. The patient was weaned from mechanical ventilation and extubated 2 hours after the end of surgery and made good progress. Four hours later, the noradrenaline infusion was discontinued and the patient was discharged to the high dependency unit. By the following morning total volume lost into the drains was 450 ml and the chest drains were removed. The postoperative hemoglobin concentration was 10.6 g dl^{-1}. The patient made an unremarkable recovery, and was discharged home pain free 6 days later.

Discussion

Although 30–70% of patients undergoing primary coronary artery bypass graft (CABG) procedures receive homologous blood transfusions during the perioperative period, the transfusion rate varies widely between institutions. A recent audit of 18 centers demonstrated a mean allogeneic red blood cell transfusion requirement for adult patients undergoing simple, first-time CABG of 2.9 ±0.1 units per patient but the range varied from as low as 0.4 ±0.2 to as high as 6.3 ±0.6 units per patient.[3] It has been concluded that a substantial number of blood components are transfused inappropriately[4] and the development of rational guidelines for

transfusion has recently been the subject of considerable debate.[5]

Transfusion of blood products carries significant risks, including: (1) transmission of infectious diseases; (2) immunosuppresion; (3) transfusion-related acute lung injury; and (4) transfusion reactions.[6] Acute intravascular hemolysis following the administration of mismatched red blood cells is reported to occur in about 1:24 000 units transfused, but data are limited.[7] The mortality associated with this complication is approximately 10%, and is invariably secondary to disseminated intravascular coagulation (DIC) and renal failure. A significant proportion of fatal transfusion reactions occur during general anesthesia, when the reaction may be difficult to diagnose because symptoms such as pain at the infusion site may be masked, and complications such as hypotension, tachycardia and DIC are often attributed to other causes.[8] Infective shock due to bacterial contamination of red cells or platelets is also rare (1:500 000 units transfused) but has a very high mortality.[9] Anaphylaxis is very rare, generally occurring in patients with IgA deficiency who have developed antibodies to IgA that react with IgA-contaminated transfused blood. The treatment is as for other causes of anaphylaxis, and outcome is generally successful. High profile complications, such as transmission of human immunodeficiency virus and hepatitis B and C virus, have decreased dramatically in recent years. The estimated frequency of transmission is 2 per million transfusions for HIV, 16 per million transfusions for hepatitis B and 10 per million transfusions for hepatitis C.[10] However, the discovery of new viruses in healthy, unpaid blood donors, such as hepatitis G virus,[11, 12] human herpes virus 8 (associated with Kaposi's sarcoma),[13, 14] and the possible transmission of new-variant Creutzfeld–Jacob disease[15] via blood transfusion, continue to elicit both professional and public concern.

One of the most important effects of allogeneic red blood cell transfusions is the immunomodulation induced in the recipient.[16, 17] Numerous studies have demonstrated an increase in postoperative infections, prolonging both ICU and total hospital stay.[18, 20] It was hoped that transfusion-induced immunosuppression would be attenuated by the use of leukocyte-depleted blood, but the results have so far been equivocal.

Brand *et al* reported reduced mortality in cardiac surgical patients who had received greater than 3 units of leukocyte-depleted blood compared to patients who received 'normal' blood.[21] Of the three randomized studies comparing leukocyte-depleted blood with routine blood transfusion, two have demonstrated a reduced risk of infection[22, 23] whilst the third did not.[24] The risk of infection with allogeneic blood transfusion remains uncertain, but appears to be an important cause of mortality and morbidity in surgical patients.[25] Two studies comparing autologous with allogeneic blood transfusion in colorectal cancer surgery reached different conclusions; one reporting a lower infection rate in patients receiving autologous blood,[26] while the other found no difference.[27]

The complications of blood transfusion remain legion, and although this chapter focuses on the management of Jehovah's witness patients, the principles should apply equally to all patients undergoing cardiac surgery.

Physiology of hemorrhage

Perioperative blood loss leads to anemia in association with hypovolemia, which rapidly leads to inadequate tissue oxygen delivery as a result of both inadequate cardiac output and inadequate blood oxygen content. However, if normovolemia is maintained the outcome is very different, since the decrease in blood viscosity results in a decreased systemic vascular resistance and increased venous return, which in combination with increased sympathetic stimulation of the heart, leads to an increased cardiac output. This improved cardiac output, along with the improved rheology of the blood, and the compensatory increase in peripheral oxygen extraction, ensures more than adequate tissue oxygen delivery. A decrease in the affinity of hemoglobin for oxygen appears to be a late compensatory mechanism, which is only of relevance in chronic anemia. In acute anemia, it has only been shown to be significant when the hematocrit reaches 0.8%.[28] In the context of controlled blood loss, more emphasis should be placed on a critical value for oxygen delivery, and on the balance between oxygen delivery and oxygen demand, rather than an absolute hemoglobin level.

Our present understanding of the effects of hemorrhage in humans is based on a surprisingly small volume of work. Frequently cited is a paper by Van Woerkens *et al*, published in 1992, that presented the physiological changes following hemorrhage in an 84-year-old male Jehovah's witness undergoing total gastrectomy, who had refused homologous blood products and any form of autologous transfusion.[29] The patient suffered major blood loss totalling 4500 ml and died 12 hours after surgery. During this period, acute hemodilution from a haematocrit of 31 to 20% induced a 53% decrease in systemic vascular resistance and a 54% increase in cardiac output. The critical oxygen delivery index — when oxygen consumption becomes limited by oxygen supply — was reported as 184 ml min^{-1} m^{-2}, corresponding to a hemoglobin concentration of 4 g dl^{-1}. At this point, the oxygen extraction ratio was 0.44 (mixed venous PO_2 34 mmHg (4.5 kPa), mixed venous oxygen saturation 56%). In summary as the hemoglobin concentration decreases, cardiac output increases due to a reduction in systemic vascular resistance.[30] Oxygen transport capacity reaches a maximum at a haematocrit of 30–33%.[31] After this point, further reductions in hematocrit reduce oxygen carrying capacity, and global oxygen delivery is maintained by an increase in heart rate. These compensatory changes increase myocardial oxygen requirements at a time when myocardial oxygen delivery is decreased. Whilst providing an excellent model of the physiological effects of acute hemodilution, care must be taken in translating assumptions derived from this case to the care of perioperative cardiac surgical patients, who cannot be assumed to have a normal coronary circulation.

The myocardium has limited ability to compensate for a reduction in oxygen supply because the heart is virtually aerobic, has limited metabolic reserve and has a resting oxygen extraction ratio of 90% of its maximum.[32] However, increases in local oxygen demand produce marked reductions in coronary vascular resistance, greatly increasing coronary blood flow. Therefore patients without coronary artery disease can compensate well for a reduction in oxygen delivery. By contrast, stenotic coronary arteries dilate distal to the stenosis to maintain distal flow. Critical stenoses (generally regarded as >70% stenosis) require maximal dilatation distal to the stenosis even at rest, just to maintain basal oxygen delivery.[32] The blood flow to areas distal to critical stenoses cannot be increased and any increase in oxygen requirement will precipitate myocardial ischemia. Patients with coronary artery disease have limited ability to tolerate changes in myocardial oxygen delivery. There is little clinical evidence to predict the critical hematocrit or hemoglobin concentration at which ischemia will develop in any particular patient.[33]

The minimal clinical data available from studies of healthy humans suggests that a low hematocrit is well tolerated. A study of Jehovah's witnesses showed that a blood loss of >500 ml during surgery was a more important predictor of death than the preoperative hemoglobin concentration, suggesting that preoperative anemia may be tolerated so long as further blood loss did not occur.[34] A recent study of hemodilution in elderly patients without known cardiac disease using isovolemic hemodilution from a mean hemoglobin concentration of 11.6–8.8 g dl[-1] was not associated with myocardial ischemia or adverse cardiac events.[35] In a study of Jehovah's witness children undergoing pediatric cardiac surgery, extreme intraoperative hemodilution to a hemoglobin concentration of 3 g dl[-1] was not associated with an increase in mortality or morbidity.[36] Moreover, a recent clinical study found no differences in hemodynamic compensatory mechanisms between young and elderly patients during hemodilution,[37] suggesting that extreme hemodilution might be better tolerated in healthy adults than previously assumed.

Animal models have shown that the presence of restricted coronary flow leads to myocardial dysfunction in the region distal to the stenosis under conditions of acute hemodilution. Whilst these studies suggest that hemodilution to a hematocrit of 22% is well tolerated in the presence of single vessel coronary disease, this may not be directly relevant to humans.[38] The threshold hematocrit for the development of myocardial ischemia in the presence of coronary heart disease in humans has not been established. Variation in factors such as myocardial oxygen consumption, severity of coronary occlusion, and presence of collateral flow, means that the hemoglobin concentration below which myocardial ischemia appears is unpredictable and varies from individual to individual. Although the complexity of the contributing factors may prevent the exact hematocrit from being defined, recent clinical studies in patients with cardiac disease suggest that anemia is poorly tolerated. A study of 2000 Jehovah's witness patients undergoing surgery showed marked differences in outcome between those with and those without cardiac disease.[39] The risk of death started to rise sharply in patients with cardiac disease when the preoperative hemoglobin concentration fell below 10 g dl[-1]. Lower pre- and postoperative hemoglobin concentrations were associated with increasing morbidity and mortality. The effect of blood loss was greater the lower the preoperative hemoglobin concentration. The TRICC (Transfusion Requirements In Critical Care) study of nearly 5000 patients in critical care found that survivors had significantly a higher hemoglobin concentration than those who died.[40] In those patients with cardiac disease, increasing the hemoglobin concentration in anemic patients was associated with improved survival, leading to the conclusion that anemia increased the risk of death in patients with cardiac disease.[40] A detailed study of patients undergoing peripheral vascular surgery demonstrated that a hematocrit of 28% was a threshold for adverse cardiac events.[41] Although these studies are small, they do support the maintenance of a higher hematocrit in patients with risk factors for cardiac disease undergoing noncardiac surgery.[41] What these studies demonstrate is the natural history of anemia, they do not however, demonstrate whether or not transfusion modifies the risks associated with anemia.[42] Only large randomized clinical studies will be able to define the efficacy of different transfusion protocols. It has been estimated that 12 000 patients would need to be randomized in order to have 90% power to detect a 25% difference in 30-day mortality between two transfusion strategies.[42] As yet no trials of this magnitude have been performed. Nevertheless it has been suggested that 'patients aged over 40 years of age should not, as an elective procedure, be subjected to a hemoglobin concentration <10 g dl[-1], without prior exclusion of silent myocardial ischemia'.[43]

Perioperative management

Good clinical studies of the minimum safe hematocrit for CPB are rare. Some authors quote hematocrit and others hemoglobin concentration, further confusing the reader. Indeed many authors jump from one measurement to the other without stating the correlation. Despite minimization of prime volume, the hematocrit falls on initiation of CPB by approximately one-third to half of its initial value.[44, 45] Although the minimum safe hematocrit for CPB has not been defined, and will vary according to temperature, many small studies have suggested limits. In a randomized study of hemodilution prior to CPB, patients in the intervention group had a mean hematocrit of 15% at the onset of CPB. The authors concluded that this led to the development of myocardial ischemia, demonstrated by reductions in coronary sinus oxygen tension.[46] A large study of hemodilution showed that dilution to a hemoglobin concentration of 10 g dl[-1] pre-CPB was well tolerated.[47] One study demonstrated that a hemoglobin concentration of 5 g dl[-1] was safe during hypothermic CPB,[44] whilst another study by Rosengart et al demonstrated no postoperative neurological defects in patients subjected to a hematocrit of 18%.[45] Assuming this to be true, then working backwards suggests a preoperative hematocrit of at least 27% is required prior to onset of CPB. To permit acute isovolemic hemodilution, the minimum hematocrit required in order that 500 ml blood may be removed prior to CPB is approximately 30%. To ensure a margin for error, it has been suggested that the hematocrit should be >36% (or hemoglobin concentration >12.5 g dl[-1]) prior to surgery. Should the initial hematocrit be significantly greater, then more blood could be removed preCPB, with the proviso that aliquots of autologous blood are returned to the circulation should the hematocrit fall below 18% during CPB.

Strategies to maintain tissue oxygen delivery can be undertaken before, during and after surgery. The preoperative phase should aim to increase red cell mass prior to surgery in order to minimize transfusion requirements. Anemia should be investigated and treated. Coagulation defects should be corrected if possible and patients on warfarin should be converted to heparin, whose shorter half-life will enable greater control of anticoagulation. Ideally aspirin and any other non-steroidal anti-inflammatory drugs should be stopped 2 weeks prior to surgery.

If the patient remains anemic despite routine investigation and treatment, then the use of erythropoietin (EPO) may be considered. Erythropoiesis is stimulated by EPO, a 34 kDa glycoprotein hormone that is principally produced by the peritubular cells of the cortex and outer medulla of the kidney, although the liver also contributes approximately 15% of EPO production.[48] EPO production is stimulated by hypoxia and reduced red cell mass, — that is, by a lowered hemoglobin concentration and reduced oxygen transport. There is an inverse relationship between hemoglobin concentration and serum EPO concentration. EPO stimulates production of erythroid progenitor cells early in their differentiation from the pluripotent hematopoietic stem cell in combination with other hemopoietic growth factors, such as interleukin-3. More importantly the maturation of the late progenitor cells is entirely dependent on EPO, giving rise to erythroblast colonies within 7 days of stimulation.[49] The maximum bone marrow response in EPO-treated iron replete patients is approximately four times basal marrow red blood cell production.[50] After blood loss, even normal individuals have difficulty providing sufficient iron to support this rate of erythropoiesis.[51] The loss of a single unit of blood (450 ml) results in the loss of approximately 250 mg of iron in males or 210 mg of iron in females, representing 6 and 9% of total body iron respectively.[52] The term 'relative iron deficiency' has been used to describe this situation, when there is a limiting relationship between stored iron and the marrow response in patients receiving EPO therapy.[53] Although iron supplementation with at least 100 mg elemental iron per day can provide the increased iron requirements for autologous blood donation, much higher levels may be needed during EPO therapy for acute anemia.[50]

Inflammation is a potent inhibitor of EPO-induced erythropoiesis. Firstly, iron metabolism is impaired because iron release from the mononuclear phagocytic system is blocked. Activated macrophages produce interleukin-1 which stimulates ferritin production, further reducing iron release. Cytokines reduce the production of EPO, and reduce its stimulatory action on erythroid progenitors. However, these effects can be overcome by pharmocological doses of recombinant human EPO. Although there is considerable debate regarding safety concerns and the ideal dosing regimen, Sowade *et al* suggest a regime involving five 500 u kg^{-1} doses of EPO in combination with supplementary iron 300 mg day^{-1} over 14 days to increase the hemoglobin concentration by 1.6g dl^{-1} and the hematocrit by 6%.[54] In a study of high-risk cardiac surgical patients, this treatment strategy reduced the requirement for red cell transfusion from 53 to 11%.[55]

Intraoperative management should minimize blood loss through the use of hemodilution, pharmacological therapy, autotransfusion of shed blood and modification of surgical technique. Acute isovolemic hemodilution is only acceptable to Jehovah's witnesses if the withdrawn blood remains in continuity with the circulation and stasis is prevented. This can be achieved using an arterial cannula for collecting blood into a plasmapheresis bag, which is connected to a large bore venous cannula for reinfusion when operative bleeding has ceased.[56] The blood is replaced with 2–3 ml crystalloid for every milliliter of blood withdrawn, and a loop diuretic may be administered to stimulate hemoconcentration.

Pharmacological strategies to reduce intra operative bleeding currently involve the serine protease inhibitors, aprotinin or nafamostat; or the lysine analogs, tranexamic acid or epsilon aminocaproic acid. The high-dose aprotinin regime (280 mg loading dose, 280 mg added to the prime, followed by 70 mg h^{-1} by infusion) has been shown to decrease both blood loss and blood transfusion requirements in cardiac surgical patients.[57,58] Proposed mechanisms include; decreasing the contact phase activation of coagulation, 'platelet sparing' through attenuation of plasmin-mediated glycoprotein-1b platelet receptor dysfunction, preservation of glycoprotein-IIb/IIIa receptor populations and reduction in fibrinolysis. The antifibrinolytic, tranexamic acid has also been shown to reduce bleeding and blood transfusions following cardiac surgery when administered as a 10 mg kg^{-1} bolus followed by 1 mg kg^{-1} h^{-1} infusion.[59] Although the lysine analogs have not been shown to be as efficacious as aprotinin, a study by Nuttall *et al* suggests that intraoperative

predonation followed by postCPB reinfusion in combination with tranexamic acid therapy may be as efficacious as aprotinin.[60] A recent meta-analysis of studies examining pharmacological strategies to reduce blood loss in cardiac surgery suggested a significant increase in perioperative infarction associated with the use of desmopressin. This vasopressin analog, which is used in many centers, increases the content of factor VIII and von Willebrand factor in the bloodstream with an associated improvement in primary hemostasis.[61]

Intraoperative recovery of blood involves the collection and reinfusion of autologous red cells shed during surgery. While this reduces the need for intraoperative blood transfusion in cardiac surgery,[62] simple re-infusion of shed mediastinal blood has been shown to increase the frequency of wound infection.[63] In addition, reinfusion of large quantities may have an adverse effect on coagulation and lead to increased postoperative blood losses.[64] Newer systems, such as the Continuous AutoTransfusion System (CATS; Fresenius, Bad Homburg, Germany), wash the shed mediastinal blood prior to reinfusion. Washing removes >93% of activated mediators from shed mediastinal blood compared to unwashed blood, which, it is hoped, should reduce the incidence of coagulopathy following reinfusion.[65] Even though this system appears to be approved for use in Jehovah's witnesses,[65] it is always worth ensuring that the patient has a clear understanding of the processes involved.

Current interest in the use of off-bypass techniques may further improve the outlook for Jehovah's witnesses. Nader *et al* compared equal numbers of patients undergoing conventional revascularization with CPB with those operated upon using an off-pump technique. Patients in the off-pump group had less peri operative bleeding and a lower requirement for blood products.[66] In the future off-pump surgery may be of significant benefit to Jehovah's witness patients, even though at the present time not all revascularization procedures lend themselves to this technique.

The basic premise of maintaining oxygen supply in excess of demand should be continued into the postoperative period. Autotransfusion of processed shed mediastinal blood should be continued. A hematocrit of 22% might be acceptable postoperatively without increased risk of morbidity.[67] If the hematocrit is critical, further measures including active cooling, sedation, and mechanical ventilation with paralysis may be required to minimize oxygen consumption. The use of EPO in the postoperative period may also help restore hematocrit more quickly in patients with severe anemia.[68]

In recent years, there has been increasing interest in the development of red cell substitutes. The two forms presently under investigation include: cell-free hemoglobin solutions, developed to mimic the oxygen carrying and oxygen delivery characteristics of intracellular hemoglobin, and perfluorocarbons as simple synthetic oxygen carriers. It is suggested that the use of acute isovolemic hemodilution in combination with these artificial oxygen carriers may permit lower intraoperative hemoglobin concentrations to be tolerated (oxygen delivery maintained using these novel solutions), with the autologous blood retransfused at the end of the procedure.

Conclusions and learning points

- The management of Jehovah's witnesses undergoing surgery continues to pose significant problems.
- The principles involved are applicable to all patients.
- Future developments such as off-pump surgery, oxygen carrying molecules and newer blood conservation technology is likely to make transfusion-free cardiac surgery much safer. Until then it is important to plan the operation carefully to minimize anemia and to ensure that all blood-related procedures are carefully discussed with each Jehovah's witness to ensure informed consent.

References

1. Cox M, Lumley J. No blood or blood products. *Anaesthesia* 1995;**50**:583–5.

2. Immovable for the right worship. *Watchtower* 1945;**66**:195–204.

3. Goodnough LT, Johnston MF, Toy PT. The variability of transfusion practice in coronary artery bypass surgery. Transfusion Medicine Academic Award Group. *JAMA* 1991;**265**:86–90.

4. Goodnough LT, Soegiarso RW, Geha AS. Blood lost and blood transfused in coronary artery bypass graft operation as implications for blood transfusion and blood conservation strategies. *Surg Gynecol Obstet* 1993;**177**:345–51.

5. Goodnough LT, Despotis GJ, Hogue CW Jr, Ferguson TB Jr. On the need for improved transfusion indicators in cardiac surgery. *Ann Thorac Surg* 1995;**60**:473–80.

6. Goodnough LT, Brecher ME, Kanter MH, AuBuchon JP. Transfusion medicine. First of two parts—blood transfusion. *N Engl J Med* 1999;**340**:438–47.

7. AuBuchon JP, Littenberg B. A cost-effectiveness analysis of the use of a mechanical barrier system to reduce the risk of mistransfusion. *Transfusion* 1996;**36**:222–6.

8. Practice guidelines for blood component therapy: a report by the American Society of Anesthesiologists Task Force on Blood Component Therapy. *Anesthesiology* 1996;**84**:732–47.

9. Dodd RY. The risk of transfusion-transmitted infection. *N Engl J Med* 1992;**327**:419–21.

10. Schreiber GB, Busch MP, Kleinman SH, Korelitz JJ. The risk of transfusion-transmitted viral infections. The Retrovirus Epidemiology Donor Study. *N Engl J Med* 1996;**334**:1685–90.

11. Cantaloube JF, Gallian P, Biagini P et al. Prevalence of GB virus type C/hepatitis G virus RNA and anti-E2 among blood donors in Southeastern France. *Transfusion* 1999;**39**:95–102.

12. Lefrere JJ, Roudot-Thoraval F, Morand-Joubert L et al. Prevalence of GB virus type C/hepatitis G virus RNA and of anti-E2 in individuals at high or low risk for blood-borne or sexually transmitted viruses: evidence of sexual and parenteral transmission. *Transfusion* 1999;**39**:83–94.

13. Blackbourn DJ, Ambroziak J, Lennette E et al. Infectious human herpesvirus 8 in a healthy North American blood donor. *Lancet* 1997;**349**:609–11.

14. Fransen E, Maessen J, Dentener M et al. Impact of blood transfusions on inflammatory mediator release in patients undergoing cardiac surgery. *Chest* 1999;**116**:1233–9.

15. Turner ML, Ironside JW. New-variant Creutzfeldt–Jakob disease: the risk of transmission by blood transfusion. *Blood Rev* 1998;**12**:255–68.

16. Blumberg N, Heal JM. Blood transfusion immunomodulation: the silent epidemic. *Arch Pathol Lab Med* 1998;**122**:117–9.

17. Vamvakas EC. Transfusion-associated cancer recurrence and postoperative infection: meta-analysis of randomized, controlled clinical trials. *Transfusion* 1996;**36**:175–86.

18. El Oakley R, Paul E, Wong PS *et al.* Mediastinitis in patients undergoing cardiopulmonary bypass: risk analysis and midterm results. *J Cardiovasc Surg (Torino)* 1997;**38**:595–600.

19. Ryan T, McCarthy JF, Rady MY *et al.* Early bloodstream infection after cardiopulmonary bypass: frequency rate, risk factors, and implications. *Crit Care Med* 1997;**25**:2009–14.

20. Murphy PJ, Connery C, Hicks GL Jr, Blumberg N. Homologous blood transfusion as a risk factor for postoperative infection after coronary artery bypass graft operations. *J Thorac Cardiovasc Surg* 1992;**104**:1092–9.

21. van de Watering LM, Hermans J, Houbiers JG *et al.* Beneficial effects of leukocyte depletion of transfused blood on postoperative complications in patients undergoing cardiac surgery: a randomized clinical trial. *Circulation* 1998;**97**:562–8.

22. Jensen LS, Andersen AJ, Christiansen PM *et al.* Postoperative infection and natural killer cell function following blood transfusion in patients undergoing elective colorectal surgery. *Br J Surg* 1992;**79**:513–6.

23. Jensen LS, Kissmeyer-Nielsen P, Wolff B, Qvist N. Randomised comparison of leucocyte-depleted versus buffy-coat-poor blood transfusion and complications after colorectal surgery. *Lancet* 1996;**348**:841–5.

24. Houbiers JG, Brand A, van de Watering LM *et al.* Randomised controlled trial comparing transfusion of leucocyte-depleted or buffy-coat-depleted blood in surgery for colorectal cancer. *Lancet* 1994;**344**:573–8.

25. Blajchman MA. Allogeneic blood transfusions, immunomodulation, and postoperative bacterial infection: do we have the answers yet? *Transfusion* 1997;**37**:121–5.

26. Heiss MM, Mempel W, Jauch KW *et al.* Beneficial effect of autologous blood transfusion on infectious complications after colorectal cancer surgery. *Lancet* 1993;**342**:1328–33. (Erratum in *Lancet* 1994;**343**:64).

27. Busch OR, Hop WC, Hoynck van Papendrecht MA *et al.* Blood transfusions and prognosis in colorectal cancer. *N Engl J Med* 1993;**328**:1372–6.

28. Dupuis JF, Nguyen DT. Anesthetic management of the patient who refuses blood transfusions. *Int Anesthesiol Clin* 1998;**36**:117–31.

29. van Woerkens EC, Trouwborst A, van Lanschot JJ. Profound hemodilution: what is the critical level of hemodilution at which oxygen delivery-dependent oxygen consumption starts in an anesthetized human? *Anesth Analg* 1992;**75**:818–21.

30. Laks H, Pilon RN, Anderson W, O'Connor NE. Acute normovolemic hemodilution with crystalloid vs colloid replacement. *Surg Forum* 1974;**25**:21–2.

31. Wood JH, Kee DB Jr. Hemorheology of the cerebral circulation in stroke. *Stroke* 1985;**16**:765–72.

32. Hoffman JI. Determinants and prediction of transmural myocardial perfusion. *Circulation* 1978;**58**:381–91.

33. Wahr JA. Myocardial ischaemia in anaemic patients. *Br J Anaesth* 1998;**81 (Suppl 1)**:10–5.

34. Spence RK, Carson JA, Poses R *et al.* Elective surgery without transfusion: influence of preoperative hemoglobin level and blood loss on mortality. *Am J Surg* 1990;**159**:320–4.

35. Spahn DR, Zollinger A, Schlumpf RB *et al.* Hemodilution tolerance in elderly patients without known cardiac disease. *Anesth Analg* 1996;**82**:681–6.

36. Henling CE, Carmichael MJ, Keats AS, Cooley DA. Cardiac operation for congenital heart disease in children of Jehovah's Witnesses. *J Thorac Cardiovasc Surg* 1985;**89**:914–20.

37. Vara-Thorbeck R, Guerrero-Fernandez Marcote JA. Hemodynamic response of elderly patients undergoing major surgery under moderate normovolemic hemodilution. *Eur Surg Res* 1985;**17**:372–6.

38. Spahn DR, Smith LR, Veronee CD *et al.* Acute isovolemic hemodilution and blood transfusion. Effects on regional function and metabolism in myocardium with compromised coronary blood flow. *J Thorac Cardiovasc Surg* 1993;**105**:694–704.

39. Carson JL, Duff A, Poses RM *et al.* Effect of anaemia and cardiovascular disease on surgical mortality and morbidity. *Lancet* 1996;**348**:1055–60.

40. Hebert PC, Wells G, Tweeddale M *et al.* Does transfusion practice affect mortality in critically ill patients? Transfusion Requirements in Critical Care (TRICC) Investigators and the Canadian Critical Care Trials Group. *Am J Respir Crit Care Med* 1997;**155**:1618–23.

41. Nelson AH, Fleisher LA, Rosenbaum SH. Relationship between postoperative anemia and cardiac morbidity in high-risk vascular patients in the intensive care unit. *Crit Care Med* 1993;**21**:860–6.

42. Chen AY, Carson JL. Perioperative management of anaemia. *Br J Anaesth* 1998;**81 (Suppl 1)**:20–4.

43. Lundsgaard-Hansen P. Safe hemoglobin or hematocrit levels in surgical patients. *World J Surg* 1996;**20**:1182–8.

44. Cook DJ, Oliver WC Jr, Orszulak TA *et al.* Cardiopulmonary bypass temperature, hematocrit, and cerebral oxygen delivery in humans. *Ann Thorac Surg* 1995;**60**:1671–7.

45. Rosengart TK, Helm RE, DeBois WJ *et al.* Open heart operations without transfusion using a multimodality blood conservation strategy in 50 Jehovah's Witness patients: implications for a 'bloodless' surgical technique. *J Am Coll Surg* 1997;**184**:618–29.

46. Jalonen J, Meretoja O, Laaksonen V *et al.* Myocardial oxygen balance during hemodilution in patients undergoing coronary artery bypass grafting. *Eur Surg Res* 1984;**16**:141–7.

47. Spahn DR, Schmid ER, Seifert B, Pasch T. Hemodilution tolerance in patients with coronary artery disease who are receiving chronic beta-adrenergic blocker therapy. *Anesth Analg* 1996;**82**:687–94.

48. van Iperen CE, Biesma DH, van de Wiel A, Marx JJ. Erythropoietic response to acute and chronic anaemia: focus on postoperative anaemia. *Br J Anaesth* 1998;**81 (Suppl 1)**:2–5.

49. Tepperman AD, Curtis JE, McCulloch EA. Erythropietic colonies in cultures of human marrow. *Blood* 1974;**44**:659–69.

50. Goodnough LT, Marcus RE. Erythropoiesis in patients stimulated with erythropoietin: the relevance of storage iron. *Vox Sang* 1998;**75**:128–33.

51. Coleman P, Stevens A, Dodge H, Finch C. Rate of blood regeneration after blood loss. *Ann Intern Med* 1953;**92**:341–8.

52. Finch CA, Cook JD, Labbe RF, Culala M. Effect of blood donation on iron stores as evaluated by serum ferritin. *Blood* 1977;**50**:441–7.

53. Goodnough LT. Controversies in autologous blood procurement. *Br J Anaesth* 1998;**81 Suppl 1**:67–72.

54. Sowade O, Messinger D, Franke W *et al.* The estimation of efficacy of oral iron supplementation during treatment with epoetin beta (recombinant human erythropoietin) in patients undergoing cardiac surgery. *Eur J Haematol* 1998;**60**:252–9.

55. Spahn DR, Casutt M. Eliminating blood transfusions: new aspects and perspectives. *Anesthesiology* 2000;**93**:242–55.

56. Ashley E. Anaesthesia for Jehovah's Witnesses. *Br J Hosp Med* 1997;**58**:375–80.

57. Davis R, Whittington R. Aprotinin. A review of its pharmacology and therapeutic efficacy in reducing blood loss associated with cardiac surgery. *Drugs* 1995;**49**:954–83.

58. Royston D. Aprotinin prevents bleeding and has effects on platelets and fibrinolysis. *J Cardiothorac Vasc Anesth* 1991;**5**:18–23.

59. Pugh SC, Wielogorski AK. A comparison of the effects of tranexamic acid and low-dose aprotinin on blood loss and homologous blood usage in patients undergoing cardiac surgery. *J Cardiothorac Vasc Anesth* 1995;**9**:240–4.

60. Nuttall GA, Oliver WC, Ereth MH *et al.* Comparison of blood-conservation strategies in cardiac surgery patients at high risk for bleeding. *Anesthesiology* 2000;**92**:674–82.

61. Levi M, Cromheecke ME, de Jonge E *et al.* Pharmacological strategies to decrease excessive blood loss in cardiac surgery: a meta-analysis of clinically relevant endpoints. *Lancet* 1999;**354**:1940–7.

62. Dalrymple-Hay MJ, Pack L, Deakin CD *et al.* Autotransfusion of washed shed mediastinal fluid decreases the requirement for autologous blood transfusion following cardiac surgery: a prospective randomized trial. *Eur J Cardiothorac Surg* 1999;**15**:830–4.

63. Body SC, Birmingham J, Parks R *et al.* Safety and efficacy of shed mediastinal blood transfusion after

cardiac surgery: a multicenter observational study. Multicenter Study of Perioperative Ischemia Research Group. *J Cardiothorac Vasc Anesth* 1999;**13**:410–6.

64. Schonberger JP, van Oeveren W, Bredee JJ *et al.* Systemic blood activation during and after autotransfusion. *Ann Thorac Surg* 1994;**57**:1256–62.

65. Walpoth BH, Eggensperger N, Hauser SP *et al.* Effects of unprocessed and processed cardiopulmonary bypass blood retransfused into patients after cardiac surgery. *Int J Artif Organs* 1999;**22**:210–6.

66. Nader ND, Khadra WZ, Reich NT *et al.* Blood product use in cardiac revascularization: comparison of on- and off-pump techniques. *Ann Thorac Surg* 1999;**68**:1640–3.

67. Cosgrove DM, Loop FD, Lytle BW *et al.* Determinants of blood utilization during myocardial revascularization. *Ann Thorac Surg* 1985;**40**:380–4.

68. Levine EA, Rosen AL, Sehgal LR *et al.* Erythropoietin deficiency after coronary artery bypass procedures. *Ann Thorac Surg* 1991;**51**:764–6.

30
Anesthesia for pulmonary thromboendarterectomy

Andrew I Gardner, John Dunning and Alain Vuylsteke

Introduction

Acute pulmonary embolism (PE) is frequently unrecognized and is a major cause of mortality in adults. Chronic thromboembolic pulmonary hypertension (CTEPH) is believed to occur after PE as a result of incomplete clot lysis, and subsequent reorganization of the clot resulting in adherence to the vessel wall and endothelialization of the surface. Without treatment, the natural history is of worsening pulmonary hypertension, right heart failure, and subsequent death. Medical treatment may produce brief symptomatic relief but makes no impact on the universally poor prognosis. Until recently transplantation provided the only therapeutic option to improve survival from this disease process. The popularization of pulmonary thromboendarterectomy (PTE) by Jamieson and colleagues offers a potentially curative procedure without the attendant complications of life-long immunosuppression.

Case history

A 32-year-old male was admitted for elective PTE. He had a history of recurrent venous thrombosis over a period of 6 years, and a 6-month history of recurrent pulmonary embolism. A diagnosis of protein C deficiency had been made and he was identified as factor V Leiden heterozygote.[1] A Greenfield filter had been inserted, via the right femoral vein, in the inferior vena cava to protect the lungs from further episodes of embolism.

He was referred to our center with worsening exertional (NYHA class III/IV) dyspnea. He was not receiving domicilary oxygen therapy at this time. A right heart cardiac catheter study revealed pulmonary hypertension and a cardiac index of 1.83 l min^{-1} m^{-2}. Transthoracic echocardiography showed a small left ventricle with good function, right ventricular dilatation with moderate function and mild tricuspid regurgitation. The left atrium was not dilated. A high resolution CT scan demonstrated areas of mosaic perfusion (Figure

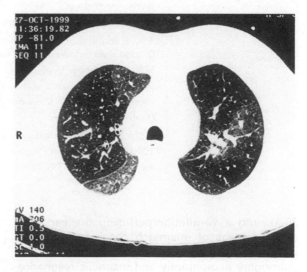

Figure 30.1

High resolution, contrast-enhanced computed tomogram of the chest showing mosaic perfusion of lung parenchyma. Darker areas are relatively underperfused tissue.

Past medical history	Recurrent deep vein thromboses. Lower limb ulcers. No family history.
Regular medications	Warfarin.
Examination	Weight 74 kg. Height 1.68 m. BMI 26 kg.m^{-2}. HR 80 bpm. BP 140/80 mmHg. JVP elevated. No hepatomegaly. No ascites or peripheral edema.
Investigations	Hb 14.8 g dl^{-1}, WBC 7.1 × 10^9 l^{-1}, platelets 189 × 10^9 l^{-1}, [Na$^+$] 142 mmol l^{-1}, [K$^+$] 4.6 mmol l^{-1}, BUN 16.2 mg dl^{-1} (5.8 mmol l^{-1}), creatinine 1.3 mg dl^{-1} (112 µmol l^{-1}), glucose 83 mg dl^{-1} (4.6 mmol l^{-1}). Lipid profile — normal. Liver function tests: within normal limits. PT 15 s (ratio 1.76), PTT 29.9 s, fibrinogen 2.96 g.l^{-1}. Lupus anticoagulant/anticardiolipin antibodies — negative Antithrombin III / factor II — normal. Factor V Q$_{506}$ mutation — heterozygote. Protein C 0.6 iu ml^{-1} (normal 0.7 — 1.4), Protein S 123% (normal 60–140%) **CXR:** Unremarkable except for dilated azygous vein. **ECG:** Sinus rhythm — S$_1$Q$_3$ pattern. Atrial hypertrophy. T wave inversion in V$_{1-5}$. **Lung function (predicted):** FEV$_1$ 2.45 l (64%), FVC 3.0 l (67%), PEFR 450 l min^{-1} (83%), TLC 5.44 l (86%), FRC 2.80 l (89%), residual volume 2.44 l (146%), TL$_{CO}$ 9.09 mmol kPa^{-1} min^{-1} (86%). **12-minute walk :** HR 135 min^{-1}; SaO$_2$ 91% (min) – 94% (max) (distance 560 m **Static exercise:** HR 188 (max). VO$_2$ max 39.4 ml kg^{-1} min^{-1}. **TTE:** Small left ventricle with good systolic function and diastolic septal flattening. LA normal. RA dilated. RV dilated with moderate function. **VQ scan :** Ventilated perfusion defects in the apical segment of the right lobe and basal segment of the left lower lobe. **Pulmonary angiogram:** Multiple arterial occlusions. Tight stenosis left basal pulmonary artery. **High resolution CT pulmonary angiogram:** Laminated thrombus extending into the left lower lober pulmonary artery and into the right upper lobe pulmonary artery. Dilated right-sided cardiac chambers noted. **MR angiography:** Dilated right-sided chambers with right ventricular hypertrophy. Segmental occlusions at the right base and widespread segmental and subsegmental irregular pruning at the left base consistent with chronic thromboembolic disease. Dilated azygous vein. **Right heart catheterization:** Pulsus alternans. RA 19 mmHg, RV 100/24 mmHg, PA 100/40 mmHg (mean PA 60 mmHg), PCWP 32 mmHg, SvO$_2$ 54%, CO 3.4 l min^{-1} (CI 1.83 l min^{-1} m^{-2}), TPG 32 mmHg, PVR 9.38 Wood units (750 dyne s cm^{-5}).

30.1), and a ventilation/perfusion nuclear scan showed areas of mismatch consistent with the anatomical distribution of thrombus. CT pulmonary angiography and magnetic resonance imaging (Figure 30.2) revealed laminated thrombus extending into the left lower lobe pulmonary artery and into the right upper lobe pulmonary artery. Spirometry revealed FEV$_1$ and FVC at 65% of predicted values.

On the day of surgery the patient was given oral diazepam 5 mg 1 hour preoperatively. On arrival in the operating suite, ECG and pulse oximetry monitoring were established. A 14G venous cannula was inserted peripherally, and a cannula was inserted in the left radial artery for invasive monitoring of blood pressure. An infusion of dopamine 5 µg kg^{-1} min^{-1} was commenced via a peripheral vein and continued

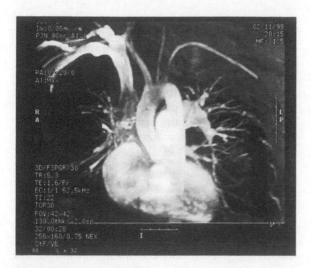

Figure 30.2

Preoperative magnetic resonance angiogram showing an enlarged left main pulmonary artery with abrupt cut-offs of segmental vessels, and a poorly filled right main pulmonary artery.

until the onset of cardiopulmonary bypass (CPB).

Anesthesia was induced with midazolam 0.1 mg kg^{-1}, fentanyl 15 µg kg^{-1} and maintained with an infusion of propofol 3.5 mg kg^{-1} hr^{-1}. Following the administration of pancuronium 0.16 mg kg^{-1}, the trachea was intubated with a single-lumen endotracheal tube and the lungs ventilated with oxygen-enriched air (FiO$_2$ 0.6). Flucloxacillin 1 g and gentamicin 140 mg were given as antimicrobial prophylaxis. A multilumen central venous cannula and pulmonary artery flotation catheter were inserted via the right internal jugular vein. A second arterial cannula was inserted in the left femoral artery to monitor arterial pressure. Body temperature was monitored using a nasopharyngeal probe and a bladder probe combined with the urinary catheter.

Transesophageal echocardiography (TEE) at this time confirmed the preoperative findings of tricuspid regurgitation, and dilated right-sided chambers. In view of the potential for paradoxical embolism, the inter-atrial septum was examined for the presence of a patent foramen ovale.

Full anticoagulation was achieved with heparin 300 iu kg^{-1} and, following bicaval and ascending aortic cannulation, CPB was instituted, and the patient was cooled to 18°C. Once CPB had been established vents were placed in the pulmonary trunk and the left ventricle via the right superior pulmonary vein. Venesection and isovolemic hemodilution was performed at the initiation of CPB to reduce the hematocrit to 18% to improve rheology at deep hypothermia. Prior to the first period of deep hypothermic circulatory arrest the aorta was cross-clamped and 1000 ml of St Thomas' I crystalloid cardioplegia administered into the aortic root. Phenytoin 15 mg kg^{-1} and thiopental 30mg kg^{-1} were administered and the head was packed in ice. After circulatory arrest, the lungs were inflated briefly with room air to expel residual blood from the pulmonary and bronchial vessels in order to produce a bloodless surgical field. Periods of circulatory arrest were limited to 20 minutes, with intermittent reperfusion for ten minutes between each arrest. A total circulatory arrest time of 60 minutes was required to complete the dissection.

After the endarterectomy had been completed the aortic cross-clamp was removed and full CPB reinstituted. Mechanical ventilation was recommenced at this point. Tidal volumes were increased by 20% to account for the paradoxically increased physiological dead space that occurs in the immediate postoperative period. In addition, positive end expiratory pressure (PEEP; 10 cmH$_2$O) was applied. The pulmonary arteriotomies were closed and systemic rewarming commenced. A maximum of 10°C core–peripheral temperature differential was maintained during rewarming. Methylprednisolone 500 mg was administered to decrease reperfusion pulmonary edema, and mannitol 12.5 g was administered to promote diuresis and for its putative free radical scavenging properties. The dopamine infusion was recommenced at 3.5 µg kg^{-1} min^{-1}. An infusion of sodium nitroprusside (SNP) 0.2 mg h^{-1} was commenced to promote uniform rewarming, and a forced air warmer was applied to the lower half of the body. Prior to the termination of CPB the infusion of SNP was stopped in order to avoid potential intrapulmonary shunting. Spontaneous defibrillation of the heart occurred producing sinus bradycardia when the systemic temperature was only 24°C. With further rewarming the cardiac rate increased to around 70 beats per minute. Temporary epicardial pacing wires were applied to the right atrium and right ventricle and atrial pacing was commenced at 110 beats per minute. Once the core temperature had been at 37°C for 30 minutes, and metabolic equilibrium had been restored without the addition of sodium bicarbonate the patient was easily weaned from CPB using TEE to assess cardiac function and guide left-sided cardiac filling. The anticoagulant effect of heparin was reversed with protamine 210 mg.

The patient was transferred to the ICU where he was sedated, and remained intubated and ventilated for 48 hours, prior to extubation. Hemodynamic variables on admission were: HR 74 bpm; BP 97/68 mmHg, CVP 10 mmHg, PAP 33/15 mmHg (mean 24 mmHg), CO 3.2 l min^{-1} (CI 2.7 l min^{-1} m^{-2}). Arterial blood gas (ABG) analysis revealed: [H$^+$] 41.5 nmol l^{-1} (pH 7.38), PaCO$_2$ 36 mmHg (4.8 kPa), PaO$_2$ 254 mmHg (33.8 kPa), SaO$_2$ 99% (PEEP 8 cmH$_2$O, FiO$_2$ 0.65). Serial ABG analysis and chest radiographs suggested the development of only mild reperfusion pulmonary edema. The patient was transferred to the ward on the third postoperative day, and made an uneventful recovery. Subcutaneous tinzaparin 13 000 iu day^{-1} was administered until adequate anticoagulation with warfarin was achieved. He was discharged home 10 days after surgery on warfarin (target INR 2.5–3.5).

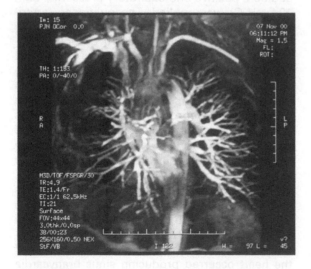

Figure 30.3

Magnetic resonance angiogram 1 year after surgery showing improved pulmonary artery perfusion throughout both lung fields.

Pulmonary artery catheterization 8 weeks after surgery revealed: PA 25/10 mmHg, CI 2.65 l min^{-1} m^{-2}. Transthoracic echocardiography revealed normal sized right-heart chambers, a CT angiogram revealed resolution of the mosaic perfusion pattern, and MR angiography revealed markedly improved pulmonary perfusion (Figure 30.3). At this time the patient had no residual symptoms, and his exercise tolerance was absolutely normal.

Discussion

Thromboembolic pulmonary hypertension is a relatively uncommon condition, although the true incidence remains difficult to estimate with accuracy. Until relatively recently the only surgical therapy for the sequelae of unresolved pulmonary thromboembolism was heart and lung transplantation. However pulmonary endarterectomy provides immediate, effective and long lasting relief of symptoms. It is an uncommon surgical procedure with less than 2000 operations performed world-wide in only a few surgical centers.[2]

Most episodes of PE are undetected, and in patients who subsequently develop pulmonary hypertension, the diagnosis is not made until the onset of the symptoms of right heart failure. Further investigation is then required. The incidence of deep venous thrombosis (DVT) in the USA is estimated to be 2 million cases per year,[3] with approximately 630 000 episodes of acute pulmonary embolism.[4] This conservative estimate means that PE, which has a mortality of approximately 10%, is the third most common cause of death after cardiovascular disease and malignancy.[5] Between 4 and 23% of patients go on to have recurrent PE.[6] Autopsy studies have suggested that pulmonary embolism was clinically unsuspected in 70–80% of patients in whom it was determined to be the major cause of death.[7, 8]

Whilst the incidence of acute PE is difficult to quantify, it is even harder to estimate the true incidence of pulmonary hypertension developing after pulmonary embolism. One suggestion is that 0.1% of all pulmonary embolic events result in CTEPH.[9] Although most patients survive acute PE with apparent resolution of the embolus and no obvious physiological or clinical sequelae, CT scans performed after recovery have demonstrated incomplete reperfusion of pulmonary parenchyma in around half of all patients.[10] It is estimated that 1 in 200 survivors of acute PE go on to develop chronic thromboembolic disease[11, 12] giving an annual incidence of 2500 patients in the USA.

Etiology

It is believed that most patients who develop CTEPH have had unresolved PE from acute embolic episodes. However approximately half of all patients give no clear history of an episode of deep vein thrombosis (DVT) or acute PE. Why some emboli fail to resolve is unclear but a variety of factors may be involved.

It is possible that the volume of embolic material may be such that normal lytic mechanisms are overwhelmed, or that occlusion of a major arterial branch prevents lytic enzymes reaching and dissolving the embolic material. Lytic mechanisms may also be overwhelmed in the presence of a hypercoagulable or prothrombotic state. In some cases the embolic material (e.g. osteosarcoma, choriocarcinoma, renal cell carcinoma, amniotic fluid, medullar fat) is not amenable to lysis by normal mechanisms, and sometimes the lytic pathways are themselves defective.

Once a clot has become lodged at a branch point in a vessel it may undergo one of two fates. The clot may become organized and recanalized, producing multiple small endothelialized channels separated by fibrous septa causing webs and bands to become established within the arterial lumen, or it may undergo fibrous organization with the formation of a solid fibrin plug that occludes the vessel.[13]

Virchow[14] proposed a mechanism whereby the stagnant column of blood distal to the clot would become organized into propagated thrombus adherent to the original lodged embolic material, whilst proximal to the clot laminar thrombus would accumulate back to the previous branch point. The whole surface may then become endothelialized.

Prothrombotic states may lead to in situ thrombosis within the pulmonary vascular bed,

encourage embolization or be responsible for proximal propagation of thrombus after embolus.[15] The common conditions identified in patients with CTEPH are the presence of lupus anticoagulant in 11%,[16] and inherited deficiencies of antithrombin III, protein C, and protein S in 5% patients, and other uncommon abnormalities of the coagulation and/or fibrinolytic pathways such as the presence of factor V Leiden[1] as in the case above.

It is believed that the development of CTEPH is a complex process since it is possible to tolerate pneumonectomy without the development of pulmonary hypertension, but the loss of less than 50% of the pulmonary vascular bed with thromboembolic disease may result in greatly elevated pressures. It has been speculated that a vasculopathy similar to that seen in Eisenmenger's syndrome develops in the precapillary arterioles. This may ultimately result in irreversible pulmonary hypertension even after removal of the thrombotic material. In addition, neuronal or humoral factors such as endothelin may be responsible for producing reflex vasoconstriction in unaffected vascular segments of both the ipsilateral and contralateral lung.

Prognosis

Patients with pulmonary hypertension have a poor prognosis.[17] Death occurs as a result of right ventricular hypertrophy leading to arrhythmias, systemic venous congestion and heart failure. In patients with CTEPH, survival is inversely proportional to pulmonary artery pressure. Reidel and colleagues have shown that 5-year survival for patients with a mean PA pressure >30 mmHg is only 30%, falling to a 2-year survival of only 20% once the mean PA pressure exceeds 50 mmHg.[18]

The principles of medical management are: the prevention of further thromboembolic episodes, and offloading the right ventricle. Long-term anticoagulation is used to prevent further embolic episodes, and may limit the extension of in situ thrombosis in vessels with low flow and stasis. Embolism may also be prevented by the placement of IVC filters. Although useful in the setting of acute PE, thrombolytic therapy has no role to play in the management of chronic thromboembolism.

Right ventricular failure is typically treated with a combination of diuretics and vasodilators (e.g. diltiazem), producing short-lived symptom relief but making no impact on prognosis since the vascular obstruction is still present.[19, 20] In advanced cases continuous central venous administration of prostacyclin, a potent pulmonary vasodilator, may be necessary to stabilize a patient's condition.

Although transplantation has been used to treat CTEPH it should no longer be considered as the first surgical option. PTE carries a lower 1-year mortality than transplantation, avoids the morbidity and mortality associated with the transplant waiting list, and offers a permanent cure without the complications of immunosuppression, rejection and infection.

The first surgical approach to the management of acute PE was described by Trendelenburg in 1908.[21] However, it was not until 1957 that Hurwitt and colleagues performed the first elective pulmonary endarterectomy, using inflow occlusion and systemic hypothermia.[22] Circulatory arrest has proved to be essential for the complete removal of occlusive material and this has only been achieved safely with the development of CPB technology. The technique in common use today was developed at the University of California, San Diego[23, 24] and is suitable for patients with incapacitating symptoms and no life-threatening comorbidity who have CTEPH with PVR >3.75 Wood units (300 dyne s cm^{-5}).[24] The operative mortality for the procedure is approximately 7%, which compares favorably with the alternative of lung transplantation.[6] Long-term follow-up demonstrates a sustained reduction in PVR, an improved ventilation/perfusion ratio, marked remodelling of the right ventricle, resolution of tricuspid regurgitation and right heart failure, and a dramatic improvement in functional status.[25]

The surgical management of these patients presents the cardiothoracic anesthetist with a number of problems. It should be borne in mind that patients with right ventricular dysfunction (i.e. RVEDP >15 mmHg) may not tolerate induction of general anesthesia without inotropic support.[26] If adequate systemic perfusion pressures cannot be maintained with pharmaco-

logical support an intra-aortic balloon pump (IABP) is often the best way to maintain coronary artery perfusion.

The surgical procedure is lengthy with CPB times in the order of 300 minutes, and total deep hypothermic circulatory arrest (DHCA) times around 40 minutes. Significant dysrhythmias are uncommon and spontaneous defibrillation to sinus rhythm typically occurs during reperfusion and rewarming. Temporary epicardial pacing is employed routinely to achieve a satisfactory heart rate. Weaning from CPB may be hampered by persistently elevated PVR and poor RV performance, resulting in relative underfilling of the left heart, and a low cardiac output state. TEE may prove useful in this situation.

If the patient cannot be separated from CPB with low-dose dopamine (5-10 µg kg^{-1} min^{-1}), it is our practice to insert an IABP and thereafter to escalate inotropic support using enoximone, epinephrine and noradrenaline as necessary. Inhaled nitric oxide is also used in the presence of poor gas exchange in an attempt to improve ventilation/perfusion matching. If these measures do not produce adequate left atrial filling an atrial septostomy is then considered.[27]

A pulmonary artery flotation catheter is used routinely in the postoperative period. Inflation of the balloon within the pulmonary artery, however, is contraindicated as it may rupture the endarterectomized vessel. Following deep hypothermia and prolonged CPB a coagulopathy may develop requiring correction with blood products, if there is clinically significant bleeding.

With correct preoperative diagnosis and careful surgery an immediate fall in PVR, and thus in pulmonary artery pressures, is the rule, accompanied by a marked increase in cardiac output. In some patients the fall in pulmonary artery pressure is less dramatic but continues over several days and even weeks. There are some patients in whom the pulmonary artery pressure does not improve substantially, perhaps because the underlying lesion is a pulmonary vasculopathy such as in primary pulmonary hypertension (PPH) or pulmonary veno-occlusive disease with superimposed in situ thrombosis. The differentiation may be difficult to make preoperatively and as many as a third of perioperative deaths may be related to insufficient relief of obstruction resulting from diagnostic inaccuracy. Reinstitution of medical therapy may be used in these cases in an attempt to reduce PAP, but they will not produce long-term benefit.

Many factors are thought to contribute to postoperative pulmonary hypertension. These include anatomical factors such as the hypertrophied vascular smooth muscles in the areas of reperfused lungs; and factors relating to CPB, including heparin/protamine administration, hypoxic vasoconstriction, microemboli, and endothelial dysfunction.

Reperfusion pulmonary edema (RPE) was first defined by Levinson et al in 1986.[28] RPE is limited to lung regions supplied by pulmonary arteries opened at the time of the PTE and there appears to be no correlation between preoperative clinical or laboratory data and the severity and duration of RPE.[29] It occurs to some degree in all patients after thromboendarterectomy, and typically occurs within the first 24 hours, although it may occur up to 72 hours after the procedure.[9, 29] The severity may range from mild to fulminant. It is associated with hypoxemia, hypercarbia, and pulmonary vasoconstriction due to ventilation/perfusion mismatch, and may produce a clinical picture indistinguishable from acute lung injury/ARDS. Alterations in lung lymph flow, and extravascular lung water occur. Various mechanisms have been suggested for this process, including alterations in surfactant distal to pulmonary artery occlusion, pulmonary sequestration of leukocytes and release of oxygen radicals, luxuriant bronchial artery collateral flow, and the activation of the complement which occurs as a result of exposure of medial layers of the arterial wall.[24]

Prevention and treatment of RPE is still a matter of debate and subject to empirical management.There have been several case reports describing the use of NO in the treatment of post-PTE reperfusion edema, at doses between 10 and 30 parts per million.[30] These doses are associated with selective pulmonary vasodilatation, without causing systemic or toxic side-effects. Gerlach et al[31] have suggested that NO causes an increase in oxygenation by redistribution of blood flow towards regions with normal ventilation/perfusion ratios and without a reduction in pulmonary vascular resistance while Snow et al[32] propose that NO recruits vessels with dysfunctional endothelium.

After PTE, perfusion lung scans have disclosed new perfusion defects in segments served by normal arteries (pulmonary vascular steal).[33] Whether the cause is due to inability of the newly endarterectomized segments to autoregulate, or whether there are secondary small vessel changes in the previously open segments has not been clarified. However, long-term follow-up in the majority of patients suggests a remodelling process of the pulmonary vascular bed.

Postoperative delirium may be seen and in common with other units where the service has been developed the incidence of delirium seen in our own unit was higher early in the experience. Although there has been no great change in the conduct of the operation the incidence of delirium is now much lower and is thought to correlate with the reduction in duration of total circulatory arrest times during the dissection[24] and the incidence is around 10%. Focal deficits are uncommon.

Conclusions and learning points

- Chronic thromboembolic pulmonary hypertension (CTEPH) is a potentially curable condition.
- Although significant, the mortality associated with the procedure compares favourably with alternatives.
- Patients generally have right ventricular dysfunction, but normal left ventricular function.
- The surgical procedure requires the use of CPB and DHCA.
- Reperfusion pulmonary edema is inevitable, and both preventive and treatment modalities should be employed.
- Nitric oxide may be of benefit in treating reperfusion pulmonary edema
- Patients who do not undergo PTE have a uniformly poor prognosis with the only alternative being lung transplantation.
- Compared to lung transplantation, PTE offers a lower surgical mortality rate, better long-term survival, and fewer chronic complications.
- The key to successful outcomes from surgery is the appropriate selection of patients with CTEPH.

References

1. Major DA, Sane DC, Herrington DM. Cardiovascular implications of the factor V Leiden mutation. *Am Heart J* 2000;**140**:189–95.

2. Jamieson SW, Kapelanski DP. Pulmonary endarterectomy. *Curr Probl Surg* 2000;**37**:165–252.

3. Hirsh J, Hoak J. Management of deep vein thrombosis and pulmonary embolism. A statement for healthcare professionals. Council on Thrombosis (in consultation with the Council on Cardiovascular Radiology), American Heart Association. *Circulation* 1996;**93**:2212–45.

4. Dalen JE, Alpert JS. Natural history of pulmonary embolism. *Prog Cardiovasc Dis* 1975;**17**:257–70.

5. Gillum RF. Pulmonary embolism and thrombophlebitis in the United States, 1970-1985. *Am Heart J* 1987;**114**:1262–4.

6. Dunning J, McNeil K. Pulmonary thromboendarterectomy for chronic thromboembolic pulmonary hypertension. *Thorax* 1999;**54**:755–6.

7. Rubinstein I, Murray D, Hoffstein V. Fatal pulmonary emboli in hospitalized patients. An autopsy study. *Arch Intern Med* 1988;**148**:1425–6.

8. Goldhaber SZ, Hennekens CH, Evans DA *et al.* Factors associated with correct antemortem diagnosis of major pulmonary embolism. *Am J Med* 1982;**73**:822–6.

9. Moser KM. Pulmonary embolism. In: Murray JF, Nadel JA (eds) *Textbook of respiratory medicine.* 2nd edn. Philadelphia: WB Saunders, 1994.

10. Remy-Jardin M, Louvegny S, Remy J *et al.* Acute central thromboembolic disease: posttherapeutic follow-up with spiral CT angiography. *Radiology* 1997;**203**:173–80.

11. Benotti JR, Ockene IS, Alpert JS, Dalen JE. The clinical profile of unresolved pulmonary embolism. *Chest* 1983;**84**:669–78.

12. Dalen JE, Banas JS, Brooks HL *et al.* Resolution rate of acute pulmonary embolism in man. *N Engl J Med* 1969;**280**:1194–9.

13. Dibble JH. Organization and canalisation in arterial thrombosis. *J Pathol Bacteriol* 1958;**75**:1–4.

14. Virchow R. Uber die Verstopfung der Lungenarterie. *Reue Notizen auf Geb d Natur u Heilk* 1846;**37**:26–31.

15. Fleischner FG. Unilateral pulmonary embolism with increased compensatory circulation through unoccluded lung: Roentgen observations. *Radiology* 1959;**73**:591–7.

16. Auger WR, Permpikul P, Moser KM. Lupus anticoagulant, heparin use, and thrombocytopenia in patients with chronic thromboembolic pulmonary hypertension: a preliminary report. *Am J Med* 1995;**99**:392–6.

17. Ledingham JGG, Weatherall DJ. Pulmonary embolism. In: Weatherall DJ, Ledingham JGG, Warrell DA (eds) *Oxford textbook of medicine.* 3rd edn. Oxford: Oxford Medical Publications, 1996.

18. Riedel M, Stanek V, Widimsky J, Prerovsky I. Longterm follow-up of patients with pulmonary thromboembolism. Late prognosis and evolution of hemodynamic and respiratory data. *Chest* 1982;**81**:151–8.

19. Dantzker DR, Bower JS. Partial reversibility of chronic pulmonary hypertension caused by pulmonary thromboembolic disease. *Am Rev Respir Dis* 1981;**124**:129–31.

20. Dash H, Ballentine N, Zelis R. Vasodilators ineffective in secondary pulmonary hypertension. *N Engl J Med* 1980;**303**:1062–3.

21. Trendelenburg F. Uber die operative behandlung der embolie derlungarterie. *Arch Klin Chir* 1908;**86**:686–700.

22. Hurwitt ES, Schein CJ, Rifkin H, Lebendiger A. A surgical approach to the problem of chronic pulmonary artery obstruction due to thrombosis or stenosis. *Ann Surg* 1958;**147**:157–65.

23. Daily PO, Johnston GG, Simmons CJ, Moser KM. Surgical management of chronic pulmonary embolism: surgical treatment and late results. *J Thorac Cardiovasc Surg* 1980;**79**:523–31.

24. Jamieson SW, Auger WR, Fedullo PF *et al.* Experience and results with 150 pulmonary thromboendarterectomy operations over a 29-month period. *J Thorac Cardiovasc Surg* 1993;**106**:116–26.

25. Kapitan KS, Clausen JL, Moser KM. Gas exchange in chronic thromboembolism after pulmonary thromboendarterectomy. *Chest* 1990;**98**:14–9.

26. Wilson WC, Vuylsteke A. Anaesthesia for pulmonary thrombo-endarterectomy. In: Ghosh S, Latimer RD (eds) *Thoracic anaesthesia: principles*

and practice. Oxford: Butterworth Heinemann, 1999; 223-34.

27. Rothman A, Beltran D, Kriett JM *et al*. Graded balloon dilation atrial septostomy as a bridge to lung transplantation in pulmonary hypertension. *Am Heart J* 1993;**125**:1763–6.

28. Levinson RM, Shure D, Moser KM. Reperfusion pulmonary edema after pulmonary artery thromboendarterectomy. *Am Rev Respir Dis* 1986;**134**:1241–5.

29. Loubser PG. CASE 3—1998. Pulmonary reperfusion edema associated with pulmonary thromboendarterectomy. *J Cardiothorac Vasc Anesth* 1998;**12**:353–7.

30. Gardeback M, Larsen FF, Radegran K. Nitric oxide improves hypoxaemia following reperfusion oedema after pulmonary thromboendarterectomy. *Br J Anaesth* 1995;**75**:798–800.

31. Gerlach H, Pappert D, Lewandowski K *et al*. Long-term inhalation with evaluated low doses of nitric oxide for selective improvement of oxygenation in patients with adult respiratory distress syndrome. *Intensive Care Med* 1993;**19**:443–9.

32. Snow DJ, Gray SJ, Ghosh S *et al*. Inhaled nitric oxide in patients with normal and increased pulmonary vascular resistance after cardiac surgery. *Br J Anaesth* 1994;**72**:185–9.

33. Olman MA, Auger WR, Fedullo PF, Moser KM. Pulmonary vascular steal in chronic thromboembolic pulmonary hypertension. *Chest* 1990;**98**:1430–4.

31
Chronic pain following cardiac and thoracic surgery

Andrew I Gardner and Ian Hardy

Introduction

Patients undergoing cardiac and thoracic surgical procedures may suffer a significant incidence of chronic postoperative pain. Because of the severe and incapacitating nature of the disease necessitating surgery, postoperative pain symptoms may wrongly be attributed to the underlying disease rather than to any postoperative complications.

Case history 1

A 65-year-old woman was referred to the Pain Clinic 5 years after redo sternotomy. She had undergone coronary artery bypass graft (CABG) surgery 9 years previously with harvesting of both internal mammary arteries (IMA). She had suffered some mild postoperative sternal pain, but this was exacerbated following redo CABG performed 4 years later using saphenous vein grafts. In an attempt to reduce her pain, she had undergone removal of sternal wires and bilateral breast reduction surgery, but these had been unsuccessful.

She described a deep-seated aching pain with shooting/stabbing and tingling elements, which had become worse during the previous 12 months. Her pain was related to movement. There was no other significant medical history, other medical problems, or allergies to prescribed drugs. Investigation by a rheumatologist had excluded a rheumatological cause for her pain and she had been prescribed amitriptyline. Unfortunately drowsiness and a persistent dry mouth had caused her to discontinue the drug.

On examination she was tender over the caudal end of her sternotomy scar, with associated hyperesthesia. A diagnosis of neuropathic pain was made, presumed to be due to nerve damage or entrapment at the time of sternotomy, or following IMA harvesting. A combined treatment regime was instituted. She was started on a nocturnal dose of amitriptyline 10 mg and sodium valproate 100 mg TDS. She underwent injections of the tenderest areas with a local anaesthetic (lidocaine) and a corticosteroid (triamcinolone) and was instructed in the use of a transcutaneous electrical nerve stimulator (TENS).

At review 1 month later she was still complaining of pain on movement, because she was not suffering any side-effects of her medications, the dose of amitriptyline was increased to 20 mg and that of sodium valproate to 200 mg TDS. The injections of lidocaine and triamcinolone were repeated.

Over the following 3 months the dose of amitriptyline was gradually increased to 50 mg. In combination with sodium valproate 200 mg TDS, regular use of TENS and repeat parasternal injections, she reported a 90% resolution of her symptoms, with no rest pain. She was able to return to her normal activities without excessive discomfort. After approximately 9 months she was weaned off most of her neuropathic pain medication leaving her on a small dose of amitriptyline 10 mg and very occasional use of the TENS.

Case history 2

A 30-year-old man presented with chronic chest pain. Three years previously he had presented with intermittent right-sided chest pain, which had been diagnosed as 'slipping rib syndrome'. He underwent resection of his right ninth rib via thoracotomy, which resulted in an improvement in his pain. Five months later he developed a continuous chest pain, which gradually increased in severity such that he had become bed bound by the pain and suffered a pulmonary embolism. During this time he had been treated with oral slow release morphine sulfate. There were no other medical problems, no allergies and all routine laboratory investigations revealed no abnormalities.

Three years later he underwent excision of the right lower costochondral cartilages and the two lowest neurovascular bundles after which he had an immediate and complete resolution of his pain and symptoms. After an uneventful postoperative recovery he was discharged from hospital on no prescription analgesics. Ten days later he complained of a recurrence of his pain. When he was reviewed 12 weeks after surgery, he described sharp, stabbing, right-sided chest pain which radiated around towards the back. He complained of tenderness over the area and of having to hold a car seat belt away from his chest. At this stage he was taking oral slow release morphine 90 mg daily.

On examination there was tenderness along the scar line but there was no specific area of hypersensitivity noted and no trigger points could be identified. A provisional diagnosis of neuropathic/neurogenic pain secondary to nerve entrapment was made and the scar was infiltrated with 0.5% prilocaine 15 ml. In addition, he was started on amitriptyline 10 mg at night and sodium valproate 100 mg TDS.

On review 1 month later the pain had reduced significantly and he had been able to reduce his oral morphine dose to 60 mg daily. The scar was once again injected with prilocaine, his amitriptyline dose was increased to 20 mg and his sodium valproate increased to 200 mg TDS. This treatment plan produced a further decrease in his oral morphine requirements as the neuropathic pain medication controlled the neuropathic component of his pain.

Discussion

Reiz and Nath have indicated that chronic pain following CABG surgery is relatively common.[1] However the diagnosis of chronic pain following cardiac surgery may be difficult. In the differential diagnosis of persistent pain following presumed union of the sternum (approximately 6 weeks postsurgery) after CABG surgery, a diagnosis of persistent angina due to inadequate coronary revascularization or early occlusion of a graft must be excluded first. Therefore appropriate investigations for any suspected continuing ischemia must be considered (Figure 31.1).

Non-ischemic poststernotomy pain is usually related to one of two causes: neuropathic pain or musculoskeletal pain. Neuropathic pain may occur as a result of damage to the brachial plexus, to the intercostal nerves, either at the level of the sternotomy, or in the internal mammary artery bed.[2, 3]

Injury to peripheral nerves in cardiac surgery occurs relatively frequently, with one prospective study suggesting that 13.5% of patients may have postoperative peripheral nerve problems.[1] Different types of sternal retractors used to facilitate IMA harvesting are associated with different rates of postoperative brachial plexus pain. To minimize injury during IMA harvesting it is suggested that a sternal retractor that produces minimal chest asymmetry be used and that the patient's arms are placed alongside the body and internally rotated.[1]

Injury or entrapment of intercostal nerves may occur during IMA harvesting. The use of diathermy or hemostatic clips during the dissection of the IMA may cause direct injury to the nerves immediately or the subsequent development of scar tissue may cause problems in the longer term.[4] Sternal wires may entrap or injure nerves and the bony overgrowth that may occur following sternotomy also has the potential to entrap nerves. Neuropathic pain felt immediately in the postoperative period is likely to be caused by the sternal wires or direct injury, whereas that developing later is presumed to be due to scar tissue, scar-entrapped neuromas or the abnormal recovery of damaged nerve tissue.[5] The incidence of nerve entrapment following sternotomy reported in one series was 8%.[1]

As in the first case presented, treatment consists of the injection of both local anesthetic

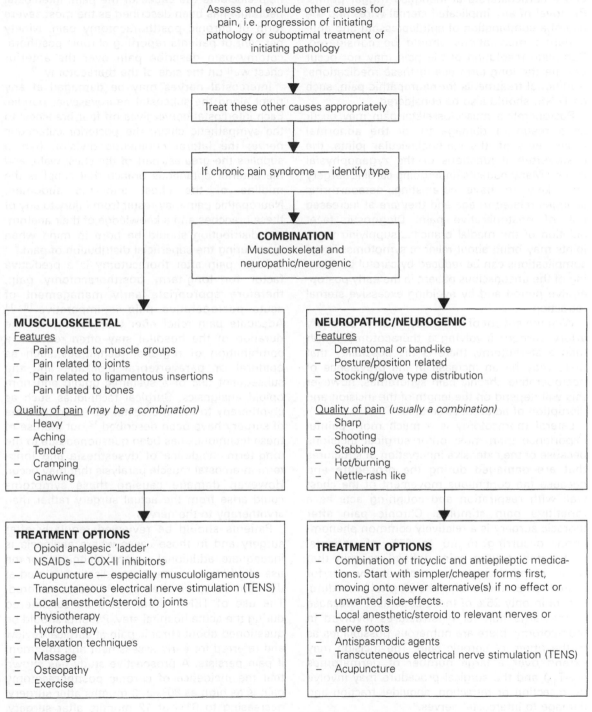

Figure 31.1

Suggested management algorithm for the diagnosis and treatment of chronic pain following thoracic and/or cardiac surgery.

and a corticosteroid at identified trigger points. Removal of any implicated sternal wires and the use of a combination of antidepressant and antiepileptic medications should be considered. Complete resolution of the pain may not occur despite the long-term use of these medications. Additional treatments for neuropathic pain, such as TENS, should also be considered.

Postoperative musculoskeletal pain may occur as a result of damage to, or the abnormal movements of, the sternoclavicular joints, the costovertebral junctions or the zygapophysial joints.[6] Many patients undergoing cardiac surgery are likely to have co-existing osteoarthritic changes related to age and they are at increased risk of postoperative pain. Diagnostic facet ablation of the medial branches supplying these joints may bring about relief of symptoms. These complications can be reduced by careful positioning of the unconscious patient in the early postoperative period and by avoiding excessive sternal retraction.

With the advent of minimally invasive coronary artery surgery involving a thoracotomy rather than a sternotomy, there is the possibility that there may be an increase in the prevalence of postoperative chronic pain syndromes; however this will depend on the length of the incision and disruption of adjacent structures.

Lateral thoracotomy is a much more painful experience than most other surgical incisions because of the extensive innervation of structures that are damaged during the procedure and because the continuous movement of the chest wall with respiration and coughing acts as a repetitive pain stimulus. Chronic pain after thoracic surgery is a relatively common phenomenon, occurring in up to 67% of patients. Fortunately severe pain, defined as pain that recurs or persists along a thoracotomy scar for more than 2 months after the surgical procedure, occurs in only 25% of these patients.[7, 8] Because of the large number of structures involved in thoracotomy, there are numerous possibilities as to the origin of chronic pain. The incision may extend over a large number of dermatomes (T_2-T_{10}) and the surgical procedure may involve rib resection or retraction, shoulder traction and damage to intercostal nerves.[9]

A careful history of the pain — its character, site, radiation, relieving or exacerbating factors and response to medication — is required to help elucidate the cause of the pain. Intercostal neuralgia has been described as the most severe form of chronic postthoracotomy pain. Ninety per cent of patients reporting chronic postthoracotomy pain describe pain over the anterior chest wall on the side of the thoracotomy.[10]

Intercostal nerves may be damaged at any point along the subcostal neurovascular bundle. Each intercostal nerve gives off four branches: to the sympathetic chain; the posterior cutaneous nerve; the lateral cutaneous division (which supplies the greatest part of the chest wall); and the anterior cutaneous branch that supplies the midline of the chest and the abdomen. Neuropathic pain may result from injury to any of these branches and a knowledge of their anatomical distribution should be born in mind when considering the superficial distribution of pain.[9]

Acute pain after thoracotomy is a predictive factor for long-term postthoracotomy pain, therefore appropriate early management of acute postoperative pain is imperative.[10, 11] Adequate pain relief after thoracotomy for the duration of the hospital stay often requires a combination of regional techniques such as epidural or paravertebral blockade and the subsequent use of a systemic opioid and nonopioid analgesics. Surgical techniques such as cryotherapy to the intercostal nerves at the time of surgery have been described,[12] but the use of these techniques has been questioned due to the long-term incidence of dysesthesia and long-term intercostal muscle paralysis that may occur. However, damage causing these symptoms could arise from the actual surgery rather than cryotherapy to the nerves.

Patients should be reviewed regularly after surgery and in those cases where analgesia is inadequate, additional regional techniques or the use of additional systemic medications aimed at different receptor sites should be considered. The use of TENS should also be considered during the acute hospital stay. Patients should be questioned about chronic pain at surgical review and referred for early assessment and treatment if pain persists. A prospective study has shown that the incidence of chronic postthoracotomy pain is as high as 80% at 3 months after surgery, decreasing to 61% at 12 months after surgery. Severe pain may be present in 3–5% of patients. A high consumption of analgesic drugs in the first postoperative week has been shown to be associated with a higher risk of chronic postthoracotomy pain. In one prospective study, patients who developed long-term pain had significantly greater pain 24 hours after surgery.[10]

Previously it had been recognized that patients who are undergoing thoracotomy for malignant disease are more likely to experience postoperative pain than those patients undergoing thoracotomy for non-malignant conditions. However, a recently published study of follow-up after thoracic surgery has contradicted this.[10] Progression of malignant disease, with compression or invasion of neural structures, should always be included in the differential diagnosis of chronic pain, as should the present and prior history of infection at the operative site.

Neuropathic pain may be caused by a crushing injury to a nerve, following the use of certain rib spreaders, or as a result of neuroma formation. As in the first case presented, a combination of antidepressants and aneleptic medications may bring about significant improvement. If no improvement occurs in the presence of adequate serum levels of aneleptic medication, then an alternative aneleptic medication may be tried.

Carbamazepine and gabapentin have both been used successfully in the management of neuropathic pain. Gabapentin is now licensed for the treatment of neuropathic pain. The antispasmodic, baclofen, has also been used in treatment. Surgical ablation or cryotherapy of the intercostal nerve may be considered in persistent pain unresponsive to other measures.

As with patients undergoing cardiac surgery, many patients undergoing thoracotomy will be from older population groups and have coexisting degenerative bone disease. Retraction of the scapula and distraction of costovertebral joints may occur. As such, chronic pain after thoracotomy may not be directly related to the site of incision.

Alternative management strategies should be considered in the absence of response to standard management. Anecdotal reports of successful outcomes following posturing therapy and chiropractic treatments have been described.[13, 14] In the event of failure to completely improve the pain, a multidisciplinary approach involving a psychologist, physiotherapist and occupational therapist may be successful in developing coping

Table 30.1 Summary of drugs and suggested dosages for use in chronic pain following cardiac and thoracic surgery. It is recommended that manufacturer data sheets and local/national formularies are consulted before prescribing.

Antidepressants	Amitriptylline 10–50 mg daily at night for maximum therapeutic effect Dothiepin 25–100 mg daily Imipramine 20–100 mg daily Paroxetine 40 mg daily Citalopram 40 mg daily
Antiepileptics/anticonvulsants	Sodium valproate 100 mg TDS increasing to a maximum of 2400 mg daily in divided doses although maximum therapeutic effect probably achieved at 200 mg TDS Carbamazepine 200 mg TDS increasing to 400 mg TDS Maximum recommended daily dose: 1600 mg Gabapentin 100 mg TDS increasing to a maximum of 3600 mg daily in divided doses although maximum therapeutic effect probably achieved at 400 mg TDS Lamotrigine 20–400 mg daily in divided doses
Antidysrhythmics	Mexilitine 450–600 mg daily in divided doses
NSAIDs	Ibuprofen 400 mg QDS Diclofenac 150 mg daily (maximum dose recommended) as slow release preparation. Mefanamic acid 500 mg TDS
Opioids	Codeine 100–200 mg QDS Dihydrocodeine 60–120 mg QDS Dextropropoxyphene 65 mg QDS Morphine (slow release) 1–30 mg BD
Others	Tramadol 50–100 mg BD increasing to a maximum of 100 mg QDS Capsaicin 0.075% cream applied topically.

and management strategies. These should allow the patient to reach their highest level of functioning in the continuing presence of pain.[15] As with all chronic pain situations, a search for a treatable cause is essential and the inappropriate use of opioid analgesics avoided (Table 31.1).[16]

Conclusions and learning points

- Chronic pain syndromes are quite common after both cardiac and thoracic surgery.
- Good, early postoperative pain management can significantly reduce the incidence of chronic pain following cardiac and thoracic surgery.
- It is important to exclude progression of the initiating pathology or its suboptimal treatment.
- If there is evidence of neuralgia-like symptoms, appropriate medication should be commenced.
- Opioids have a limited role in the treatment of non-malignant chronic pain.
- A combination of treatment regimes is likely to be required to achieve good pain control.

References

1. Vahl CF, Carl I, Muller-Vahl H, Struck E. Brachial plexus injury after cardiac surgery. The role of internal mammary artery preparation: a prospective study on 1000 consecutive patients. *J Thorac Cardiovasc Surg* 1991;**102**:724–9.

2. Stangl R, Altendorf-Hofmann A, von der Emde J. Brachial plexus lesions following median sternotomy in cardiac surgery. *Thorac Cardiovasc Surg* 1991;**39**:360–4.

3. Reiz S, Nath S. Chronic pain after coronary bypass surgery. In: van Zundert A (ed) *Highlights in pain therapy and regional anaesthesia VII*. Proceedings of the XVIIth annual European Society for Regional Anaesthesia (ESRA) congress, Geneva. Cyprus: Hadjigeorgian Printing, 1998: 204–7.

4. Mailis A, Chan J, Basinski A *et al.* Chest wall pain after aortocoronary bypass surgery using internal mammary artery graft: a new pain syndrome? *Heart Lung* 1989;**18**:553–8.

5. Defalque RJ, Bromley JJ. Poststernotomy neuralgia: a new pain syndrome. *Anesth Analg* 1989;**69**:81–2.

6. Roy RC, Stafford MA, Charlton JE. Nerve injury and musculoskeletal complaints after cardiac surgery: influence of internal mammary artery dissection and left arm position. *Anesth Analg* 1988;**67**:277–9.

7. Matsunga M, Dan K, Manable FY, Hara F. Residual pain of 90 thoracotomy patients with malignancy and non-malignancy. *Pain* 1990;**5 Suppl**:S148

8. International Association for the Study of Pain. Subcommittee of Taxonomy. Classification of chronic pain. Post-thoracotomy pain syndrome (XVII–14). *Pain* 1986;**3**:S138–9

9. Conacher ID. Pain relief after thoracotomy. *Br J Anaesth* 1990;**65**:806–12.

10. Perttunen K, Tasmuth T, Kalso E. Chronic pain after thoracic surgery: a follow-up study. *Acta Anaesthesiol Scand* 1999;**43**:563–7.

11. Roberts D, Pizzarelli G, Lepore V *et al.* Reduction of post-thoracotomy pain by cryotherapy of intercostal nerves. *Scand J Thorac Cardiovasc Surg* 1988;**22**:127–30.

12. Bachiocco V, Bragaglia R. Antalgic positions in alleviating post-thoracotomy pain. Their introduction in a pain relief program. *Chest* 1994;**105**:1299.

13. Minor AA. Alternative management for post-thoracotomy pain syndrome. *Can J Surg* 1996;**39**:430–1.

14. Nurmikko TJ, Nash TP, Wiles JR. Recent advances: control of chronic pain. *BMJ* 1998;**317**:1438–41.

15. Graziotti PJ, Goucke CR. The use of oral opioids in patients with chronic non-cancer pain. Management strategies. *Med J Aust* 1997;**167**:30–4.

16. Katz J, Jackson M, Kavanagh BP, Sandler AN. Acute pain after thoracic surgery predicts long-term post-thoracotomy pain. *Clin J Pain* 1996;**12**:50–5.

32
Anesthesia for esophageal surgery

Marc de Kock

Introduction

Surgery of the esophagus requiring thoracotomy is often for treatment of neoplastic disease. Anesthesia for this kind of surgery is a challenge because of the preoperative medical condition of the patient (age, vascular disease, smoking, and alcohol abuse), intraoperative circumstances (one lung ventilation and surgical manipulations close to the heart) and finally postoperative morbidity (pain, respiratory insufficiency and sepsis).[1]

Of the various techniques described for surgical excision of the diseased esophagus,[1] the 'en bloc' resection is the most formidable. It consists of a dissection carried as far from the esophageal wall as possible that results in 'skeletonization' of the vital structures of the posterior mediastinum. Proponents of the technique argue that it has the advantage of resulting in the removal of all potentially diseased lymph nodes as well as all soft tissues in the vicinity of the esophageal wall. Although justifiable from an oncological view-point, it is, for the patient, a major and debilitating procedure[2] as the following case illustrates.

Case history

A 68-year-old Causcasian male presented with a 3-month history of progressive dysphagia. Fiberoptic endoscopy revealed a tumor of the mid-third of the esophagus. Tissue biopsy revealed adenocarcinoma. Computed tomography of the chest and abdomen suggested that the mass was relatively independent of adjacent structures and that there were no metastases. On the basis of these findings the tumor was classified as stage T3 N0 (M0) and the patient was scheduled for 'en bloc' esophagectomy and resection of 'loco-regional' lymph nodes followed by interposition of either the stomach or the colon, as second choice.

On the day of surgery the patient was premedicated with lormetazepan 2 mg SL I hour before transfer to the operating theater. On arrival in the theater routine five-lead ECG and non-invasive blood pressure monitoring was established, and a forearm vein was cannulated under local anesthesia and an intravenous infusion of crystalloid commenced. With the patient in a sitting position, the epidural space was identified at the T_{4-5} interspace using the loss of resistance to saline technique and an epidural catheter was advanced 5 cm into this space. The patient was then placed supine. A test dose of 4 ml lidocaine 2% with epinephrine 1:200 000 failed to elicit a significant change (>20%) in either heart rate or blood pressure, thus excluding intravascular placement.

Five minutes after administration of the epidural test dose, general anesthesia was induced with propofol 2 mg kg^{-1} and atracurium 0.5 mg kg^{-1}. Sufentanil 0.1 µg kg^{-1} and lidocaine 1 mg kg^{-1} were subsequently administered to obtund the autonomic response to direct laryngoscopy. The trachea was intubated with a 41 French Carlens Ruschelit left endobronchial tube with a carinal hook. Placement of the tube proved difficult and fluoroscopy was used to guide the tube into the correct position. The lungs were then ventilated with oxygen in air and anesthesia maintained with propofol 3 mg kg^{-1} hr^{-1} and ketamine 0.5 mg kg^{-1} followed by 0.25 mg kg^{-1} hr^{-1}. A radial arterial

Past medical history	Esophageal reflux. Myocardial infarction. CABG 9 months previously.
	Abdominal aortic aneurysm repair 10 years previously.
	Diverticular disease — right hemicolectomy 15 years previously.
	Tobacco consumption: 40 cigarettes/day.
	Alcohol consumption: >100 units/week.
Regular medications	Omeprazole 20 mg OD, acetylsalicylic acid 80 mg OD.
	No known drug allergies.
Examination	Weight 78 kg BMI 28.7 kg m^{-2}.
	Sternal and abdominal scars consistent with previous cardiac and abdominal surgery.
	Bibasal end expiratory crackles.
Investigations	Hb 15.4 g dl^{-1}, WBC 10.5 × 10^9 l^{-1}, platelets 206 ×10^9 l^{-1}.
	Coagulation screen — within normal limits.
	Serum electrolytes, urea, creatinine — within normal limits.
	CXR: Consistent with previous cardiac surgery. Heart size normal. Prominent pulmonary vascular pattern.
	Fiberoptic bronchoscopy: No endobronchial abnormaility seen. Possible external carinal compression.
	ECG: Normal sinus rhythm and evidence of old transmural anterior myocardial infarction.
	Isotope ventriculography: Good tolerance to exercise without any ischemic changes.

cannula and a pulmonary artery catheter (PAC) were then sited. In an attempt to reduce intraoperative cardiac dysrhythmia magnesium sulfate 3 g (12 mmol) was administered by infusion over 20 minutes. Bupivacaine 0.5% (20 mg), clonidine 2 µg kg^{-1}, and sufentanil 2.5 µg (total volume 5.5 ml) were given epidurally and followed by an infusion of bupivacaine 5 mg hr^{-1}, clonidine 0.2 mg kg^{-1} hr^{-1}, and sufentanil 0.75 µg hr^{-1}.

The patient was moved to the left lateral decubitus position. A heated water mattress, forced air warming blanket, intravenous fluid warming device and airway filter were used to prevent hypothermia. The PAC was used to monitor core (blood) temperature. After isolation of the right lung, the surgeons proceeded with their dissection of the esophagus via a right thoracotomy incision. One-lung ventilation was tolerated well (minimum SpO$_2$ 93%, SvO$_2$ 75%, cardiac index 2.8 l min^{-1} m^{-2}) and there were no major hemodynamic or ST segment changes in response to compression of mediastinal viscera. Dissection of the tumor, however, was very difficult. The tumor could not be easily isolated from adjacent structures, the left main bronchus was disrupted proximal to the endobronchial tube

cuff, and the aorta was torn. Although the aorta and bronchus were repaired without major blood loss, some neoplastic tissue was left in situ.

Following reinflation of the right lung and closure of the thoracotomy, the patient was turned to the supine position and the endobronchial tube exchanged for a single-lumen endotracheal tube. Ketorolac 20 mg was administered as an intravenous bolus. The surgeons then simultaneously began a right cervicotomy and upper midline laparotomy in order to strip the esophagus and to replace it with either stomach or colon. Because the gastroepiploic artery had been used as a conduit for myocardial revascularization, the stomach could not be mobilized to form an esophageal substitute. Over the next 6 hours several attempts were made to mobilize and prepare a segment of colon for interposition. These ultimately proved futile because of previous abdominal vascular surgery and colonic resection. After 10 hours of surgery, the patient was finally left with a feeding jejunostomy and a cervical esophagostomy. At the end of the procedure the patient's core temperature was 36.4°C. Blood gas analysis revealed a hemoglobin concentration of 10.2 g dl^{-1} and normal acid–base status. The patient was awake, cooperative and pain-free within 15 minutes of discontinuation of the propofol infusion, and the trachea was extubated upon return of adequate spontaneous ventilation.

The patient was transferred to the ICU for further observation and returned to the surgical ward 24 hours later. Despite an uncomplicated early postoperative course, at least from the somatic point of view, the patient suffered a rare complication in the postoperative period — Guillain–Barré syndrome. Serial serology later confirmed acute Epstein–Barr virus (EBV) infection. Sixteen days after surgery, this acute demyelinating polyneuropathy was manifest as an areflexic motor palsy of the lower limbs. Two days later, the patient developed respiratory failure necessitating mechanical ventilatory asisstance for a period of several weeks. The patient eventually made a good recovery from his polyneuropathy and was discharged home. He continues to be unable to eat and drink and is sustained by jejunostomy feeding.

Discussion

Patients referred for esophageal surgery frequently have a complicated medical history. The majority are elderly and a considerable number will have a history of significant cardiorespiratory disease and substance abuse. Moreover, patients scheduled for 'en bloc' resection will undergo a major and potentially debilitating procedure. Accordingly anesthetic management must be adapted to reflect the additional physiological 'burden' placed upon the patient.

Independent risk factors for increased postoperative morbidity, length of hospital stay and in-hospital morality include: patient age;[3, 4] pulmonary insufficiency;[3, 5] cardiac dysfunction;[3, 5] hepatic dysfunction;[5] and preoperative radiotherapy.[6] In addition, intraoperative blood loss,[3, 6] the requirement for inotropic support,[3] and postoperative symptomatic supraventricular tachydysrhythmia[4] and vocal cord palsy[7] are associated with increased mortality. As might be expected, mortality is significantly lower in institutions at which a large number of esophagec-

tomies are performed.[8] Interestingly, postoperative management of these patients by a dedicated Acute Pain Service has been shown to significantly reduce both pulmonary and cardiovascular complications as well as in-hospital mortality.[9]

Preoperative assessment must include a thorough evaluation of the pulmonary, cardiovascular and nutritional status of the patient. In addition to a history of tobacco use, a patient with esophageal obstruction may present with recurrent pulmonary infection secondary to chronic aspiration. Physical examination may reveal signs of pulmonary infection and/or airway obstruction. Baseline investigation should include a chest radiograph, spirometry and arterial blood gas analysis. Preoperative measures aimed at improving pulmonary function, such as antibiotics, physical therapy and bronchodilator therapy should be used as necessary. As the majority of patients presenting with esophageal malignancy are elderly, a history of hypertension, dysrhythmia, and peripheral, cerebral and coronary artery disease should be actively sought and appropriately investigated. A resting electrocardiograph should be performed in all patients and, where necessary, exercise electrocardiography, echocardiography and coronary angiography. Malnutrition is a common finding in patients with esophageal malignancy and is associated with an appreciable increase in postoperative morbidity and mortality.[10, 11] In addition to the deleterious effects of dehydration and electrolyte imbalance on cardiovascular and renal function, malnutrition-associated hypoalbuminemia may increase the risk of pulmonary edema and adversely alter the volume of distribution of drugs that are protein bound. Although no single test can identify the 'at-risk' patient the combination of significant (>10%) weight loss, anemia and hypoalbuminemia should alert the anesthetist. Perioperative total parenteral nutrition, commenced 10–15 days *before* surgery, has been shown to significantly reduce complications and mortality in severely malnourished patients undergoing surgery for gastrointestinal malignancy.[11]

While there is no widely accepted 'ideal' technique, many of the general principles that underlie the anesthetic management of patients undergoing esophagectomy have already been alluded to. Invasive hemodynamic monitoring, the facility to respond rapidly to hemodynamic instability, the maintenance of body temperature and measures to prevent pressure sores require careful consideration. The very real risk of regurgitation during induction of anesthesia should prompt consideration of a rapid sequence induction with the application of cricoid pressure. Although high-dose fentanyl (130 µg kg^{-1}) anesthesia has been shown to have a nitrogen-sparing effect,[12] many anesthetists favor a combination of techniques. The potential for myocardial depression and expansion of bowel gas are considered relative contraindications to the use of nitrous oxide.

In the case described, anesthesia was achieved with thoracic epidural anesthesia in combination with propofol-based general anesthesia. Thoracic epidural analgesia has been shown to improve outcome after major surgery, particularly after thoracoabdominal esophagectomy.[9, 13] In our practice, the α_2-adrenoceptor agonist clonidine is routinely added to a 'classical' local anesthetic-opioid mixture. This enhances the analgesic efficacy of the mixture, allowing a significant dose reduction of both the local anesthetic and opioid, preventing tachyphylaxis and respiratory depression, respectively.[14] Clonidine, when administered by the epidural route, has a systemic effect influencing the anesthetic paradigm. It potentiates the effects of hypnotics and thus permits a significant reduction in the dose of agents required to maintain anesthesia.[15] This is particularly useful when rapid emergence is required following a lengthy surgical procedure. The systemic sympatholytic properties of clonidine tend to promote hemodynamically stable anesthesia[15]which is particularly useful when non-cardiac surgeons are working close the heart and great vessels. Of relevance to our patient, clonidine has been used to reduce the symptoms associated with abrupt withdrawal of opiates, benzodiazepines, alcohol[6] and cigarettes.[16, 17] Epidural administration of high doses of clonidine, particularly in the thoracic region, results in marked potentiation of other hypotensive agents (e.g. magnesium sulfate) and, therefore, mandates that these agents be administered by slow infusion. While the risk of excessive hypotension can be reduced by using lower doses of clonidine and hypnotic agents,[14] it is our practice to add a low dose infusion of ketamine to the anesthetic regimen.

In addition to supporting arterial pressure by its sympathomimetic action,[18] ketamine is hypnotic, produces bronchodilatation and reduces postoperative pain by interfering with nociception-induced hyperexcitability in spinal cord neurones.[19] Interestingly, ketamine is also reported to reduce the elaboration of the pro-inflammatory cytokines, interleukin–6[20] and tumour necrosis factor α[21] in the perioperative period. In theory this action may benefit patients genotypically predisposed to developing the postoperative systemic inflammatory response syndrome (SIRS).

The non-steroidal anti-inflammatory drug ketorolac administered immediately prior to the intra-abdominal part of the surgical procedure, was used to reduce the production of 6-keto prostaglandin F_{1a} (6-keto PGF$_{1a}$) in response to mesenteric traction. The rationale for this approach is based upon the known hemodynamic consequences of 6-keto PGF$_{1a}$: vasodilatation, facial flushing, arterial hypotension, tachycardia and increased cardiac output.[22]

In the case described, the trachea was intubated using a left-sided double-lumen tube in order to allow one-lung ventilation during dissection of the esophagus. Although some surgeons are content to operate without isolation of the right lung, our experience indicates that postoperative pulmonary morbidity is reduced if one-lung anaesthesia is utilized. It is likely that a deflated lung is subjected to less contusion from surgical retraction than lung that remains inflated and ventilated. As mentioned, it proved very difficult to place the tip of the endobronchial tube in the left main bronchus. It was later discovered that there was a degree of inflexibility of the left main bronchus secondary to local spread of the esophageal tumor. As tumor invasion of the carina is not an uncommon observation in this group of patients, preoperative investigation should include a diagnostic bronchoscopy. Although fluoroscopy was used to confirm placement of the endobronchial tube, a fiberoptic bronchoscope could have been used as an aid to placement.

Despite undergoing a lengthy surgical procedure, our patient was awakened, weaned from mechanical ventilation and the trachea extubated. This approach was supported by two significant factors: firstly, the routine administration of low molecular weight heparin for thromboembolism prophylaxis in patients receiving epidural analgesia following major surgery, mandates close neurological evaluation, which can only be done when the patient is conscious and able to cooperate. Secondly, the early return of spontaneous ventilation avoids the hemodynamic and neuroendocrine sequelae of prolonged mechanical ventilation, allows closure of an air leak, permits expectoration of bronchial secretions and reduces the incidence of infective complications. With excellent epidural analgesia, the avoidance of inappropriate fluid therapy and close attention to the maintenance of body temperature, rapid recovery and extubation, even after prolonged procedures, is possible.

Acute demyelinating polyneuropathy, the Guillain–Barré syndrome (GBS), is a rare and often fulminant immune-mediated condition that, in the USA, is reported to have an incidence approximately 12 cases per 1 000 000 population per year. Although the precise immunopathology of this condition remains unknown, several so-called trigger factors have been identified. These include; viral infection (herpes, EBV, cytomegalovirus) and a history of trauma or a surgical procedure 1–4 weeks prior to the onset of symptoms.[23] How factors 'trigger' GBS is unknown but the adverse influence of stress and surgical intervention on cell-mediated immunity may be an important factor.[24, 25] In the light of currently available evidence, the combination of major surgery and early postoperative EBV infection seems the most likely cause of GBS in our patient.

Conclusions and learning points

- 'En bloc' resection of the esophagus for neoplastic disease is a major and debilitating procedure.
- Improved perioperative anesthetic management can reduce the incidence of major perioperative complications, allowing older and sicker patients to survive.
- Preoperative assessment should focus particularly on the cardiovascular, respiratory and nutritional status of the patient.
- Pre-operative and early post-operative nutritional support should be considered in all patients.

References

1. Tsui SL. Anesthesia for esophageal surgery. S Afr J Surg 1993;31: 17–8.
2. Collard JM, Otte JB, Reynaert MS et al. Extensive lymph node clearance for cancer of the esophagus or cardia: merits and limits in reference to 5-year absolute survival. Hepatogastroenterology 1995;42:619–27.
3. Ferguson MK, Martin TR, Reeder LB, Olak J. Mortality after esophagectomy: risk factor analysis. World J Surg 1997;21:599–603.
4. Amar D, Burt ME, Bains MS, Leung DH. Symptomatic tachydysrhythmias after esophagectomy: incidence and outcome measures. Ann Thorac Surg 1996;61:1506–9.
5. Bartels H, Stein HJ, Siewert JR. Preoperative risk analysis and postoperative mortality of oesophagectomy for resectable oesophageal cancer. Br J Surg 1998;85:840–4.
6. Tribble CG, Flanagan TL, Christensen CP et al. The influence of preoperative radiation therapy on morbidity and mortality for transhiatal esophagectomy. Am Surg 1991;57:716–9.
7. Nishimaki T, Suzuki T, Suzuki S et al. Outcomes of extended radical esophagectomy for thoracic esophageal cancer. J Am Coll Surg 1998;186:306–12.
8. Swisher SG, Deford L, Merriman KW et al. Effect of operative volume on morbidity, mortality, and hospital use after esophagectomy for cancer. J Thorac Cardiovasc Surg 2000;119:1126–32.
9. Tsui SL, Law S, Fok M et al. Postoperative analgesia reduces mortality and morbidity after esophagectomy. Am J Surg 1997;173:472–8.
10. Daly JM, Redmond HP, Gallagher H. Perioperative nutrition in cancer patients. J Parenter Enteral Nutr 1992;16 (6 Suppl):100S–105S.
11. Bozzetti F, Gavazzi C, Miceli R et al. Perioperative total parenteral nutrition in malnourished, gastrointestinal cancer patients: a randomized, clinical trial. J Parenter Enteral Nutr 2000;24:7–14.
12. Yoshida S, Noake T, Tanaka Y et al. Effect of fentanyl citrate anesthesia on protein turnover in patients with esophagectomy. J Surg Res 1996;64:120–7.

13. Brodner G, Pogatzki E, Van Aken H *et al.* A multi-modal approach to control postoperative patho-physiology and rehabilitation in patients undergoing abdominothoracic esophagectomy. *Anesth Analg* 1998;**86**:228–34.

14. Eisenach JC, De Kock M, Klimscha W. alpha(2)-adrenergic agonists for regional anesthesia. A clinical review of clonidine (1984–1995). *Anesthesiology* 1996;**85**:655–74.

15. Maze M, Tranquilli W. Alpha–2 adrenoceptor agonists: defining the role in clinical anesthesia. *Anesthesiology* 1991;**74**:581–605.

16. Glassman AH, Jackson WK, Walsh BT *et al.* Cigarette craving, smoking withdrawal, and clonidine. *Science* 1984;**226**:864–6.

17. Davison R, Kaplan K, Fintel D *et al.* The effect of clonidine on the cessation of cigarette smoking. *Clin Pharmacol Ther* 1988;**44**:265–7.

18. Kohrs R, Durieux ME. Ketamine: teaching an old drug new tricks. *Anesth Analg* 1998;**87**:1186–93.

19. Chapman V, Dickenson AH. The combination of NMDA antagonism and morphine produces profound antinociception in the rat dorsal horn. *Brain Res* 1992;**573**:321–3.

20. Roytblat L, Talmor D, Rachinsky M *et al.* Ketamine attenuates the interleukin–6 response after cardiopulmonary bypass. *Anesth Analg* 1998;**87**:266–71.

21. Nader D, Ignatowski T, Kurek C *et al.* Clonidine suppresses neuroaxial concentrations of $TNF\alpha$ during perioperative period. *Anesthesiology* 1999;**91**:A219.

22. Hudson JC, Wurm WH, O'Donnel TF Jr *et al.* Ibuprofen pretreatment inhibits prostacyclin release during abdominal exploration in aortic surgery. *Anesthesiology* 1990;**72**:443–9.

23. Asbury AK. Diseases of the peripheral nervous system. In: Isselbacher KJ, Braunwald E, Wilson JD *et al* (eds) *Harrison's principles of internal medicine.* 13th edn. New York: McGraw-Hill, 1994;2372.

24. Salo M. Effects of anaesthesia and surgery on the immune response. *Acta Anaesthesiol Scand* 1992;**36**:201–20.

25. Ben-Eliyahu S, Page GG, Yirmiya R, Shakhar G. Evidence that stress and surgical interventions promote tumor development by suppressing natural killer cell activity. *Int J Cancer* 1999;**80**:880–8.

33
Respiratory syncytial virus in the perioperative period

Roddy O'Donnell and Peter J Murphy

Introduction

Respiratory syncytial virus (RSV) is found world-wide, causes most cases of bronchiolitis, and is the most common reason for a child under 1 year of age to be admitted to hospital. By 3 years of age almost all children have antibodies to RSV. Young children and the elderly are those most likely to have severe illness. Reinfections occur throughout life, in spite of neutralizing serum antibody. RSV causes between 50 and 90% cases of bronchiolitis, 10% cases of croup and up to 25% of pneumonia under 1 year of age.[1-4] In the institutionalized elderly, RSV may account for a quarter of acute respiratory illnesses[1] and has a mortality almost twice that of influenza.[5] Annual outbreaks occur that are usually of abrupt onset and follow regular predictable patterns. In the UK the peak incidence usually occurs between the beginning of January and the end of March.[6] Clinical isolates of RSV are rare in the UK during the summer months and it is not clear where the virus 'goes' or how it re-emerges so rapidly during the next winter season. RSV has shown the most consistent seasonal pattern of the common respiratory viruses.[6] No animal reservoir for human RSV is known to exist. It is believed that primary infections with RSV are always symptomatic but may range from a very mild 'cold' to severe bronchiolitis with respiratory failure.[6] Only a small proportion of RSV-infected infants require admission to hospital: 1–2% infants each year. Despite this it was estimated that RSV accounted for 91 000 admissions to hospital in the USA in 1985 alone, at a cost of $300 000 000.[7] At the New England Medical Center it was calculated that the average cost of hospitalization of a child with RSV was $808 per day in 1991.[8]

Case history

A 5-month-old boy was admitted with severe mitral incompetence and aortic stenosis. He was born by spontaneous vaginal delivery at 40

Past medical history	Spontaneous vaginal delivery at term with no early neonatal problems.
Regular medications	Frusemide 5 mg TDS, captopril 1.5 mg TDS.
Examination	Weight 6.9 kg, BSA 1.7 m². Left parasternal heave. Loud pansystolic murmur radiating to the apex. Hepatomegaly.
Investigations	Blood count, electrolytes, urea, creatinine, coagulation studies — within normal limits. **CXR:** Cardiomegaly. Lung fields clear. **Cardiac catheterization:** Severe mitral incompetence. Aortic stenosis. Good LV function

weeks gestation and required no early neonatal care. His parents noted that he was intermittently wheezy from birth and at 3 months he was hospitalized with respiratory failure that was treated with antibiotics. However an echocardiogram revealed that he had severe mitral incompetence with cardiac failure. He improved markedly with diuretic therapy and was discharged home pending further investigation, including cardiac catheterization, at 5 months of age.

On readmission, he appeared well. Physical examination was consistent with mitral regurgitation and laboratory investigations yielded no significant abnormalities. Cardiac catheterization and transesophageal echocardiography (TEE) confirmed severe mitral regurgitation and revealed good left ventricular function, an aortic pressure gradient of 60 mmHg, and a pulmonary artery wedge pressure of 20 mmHg.

Over the next 24 hours he unexpectedly developed respiratory failure, with falling systemic oxygen saturations and increasing inspired oxygen requirements. On examination he was found to be apyrexial with absent breath sounds on the left side of his chest. A chest radiograph showed collapse-consolidation of the left lung. He was admitted to the pediatric intensive care unit (PICU), intubated, sedated and ventilated. Central venous and arterial cannulae were placed and inotropic support (dopamine 5 µg kg^{-1} min^{-1}) started. The results of a limited septic screen (urine, blood and tracheal aspirate cultures) were all negative. A nasopharyngeal aspirate (NPA) was negative for RSV, adenovirus, parainfluenza, and influenza A and B viruses. It was felt that compression of the left bronchus by a tense left atrium had led to collapse-consolidation of the left lung.

On the following day the patient underwent an aortic valvotomy and debridement, mitral valve repair and ductus arteriosus ligation. An 'on table' postbypass TEE revealed a central mitral jet of mild to moderate regurgitation. Pulmonary artery (PA) and left atrial (LA) cannulae were inserted and he was weaned from cardiopulmonary bypass (CPB) on dopamine 15 µg kg^{-1} min^{-1} and epinephrine 0.15 µg kg^{-1} min^{-1} with PA pressures at 50% of systemic and an LA pressure of 8–10 mmHg. In view of right lung distension, the sternotomy was left unclosed and he was transferred back to PICU on pressure-controlled ventilation.

By the following day his inotrope requirements had fallen and his ventilation was improving (FiO_2 reduced from 1.0 to 0.4). Although the left lung remained collapsed the sternotomy was closed. Ten hours later, however, he deteriorated: his chest compliance decreased and he developed bilateral pneumothoraces, which were drained. At this time his ventilatory parameters were: peak inspiratory pressure (PIP) 30 cmH_2O, positive end expiratory pressure (PEEP) 4 cmH_2O, and FiO_2 1.0.

Although he was apyrexial, blood cultures were taken and broad-spectrum antibiotics (cefotaxime 50 mg kg^{-1} QDS and teicoplanin 10 mg kg^{-1} daily) administered. He continued to deteriorate over the next 24 hours and developed widespread interstitial shadowing on his chest radiograph. Artificial surfactant (Curosurf, Chiesi Farmaceutici SpA, Parma, Italy) was administered without any significant improvement. Similarly, a trial of high-frequency oscillatory ventilation (HFOV) and the addition of inhaled nitric oxide (20 ppm) proved unsuccessful.

On the fifth day after operation the patient developed a fever. Although his chest radiograph showed improved lucency of the left lung, he remained difficult to ventilate despite neuromuscular blockade with vecuronium 100 µg kg^{-1} $hour^{-1}$. Further samples were sent for microbiology. A repeat NPA was positive for RSV. After discussion, he was given human immune globulin (Sandoglobulin, ZLB, Switzerland) 2g and started on intravenous ribavirin.

By the following day he had deteriorated further. He was requiring increasing inotropic support and was becoming even more difficult to oxygenate. At this point his oxygenation index (MAP $\times$ FiO_2 $\times$ 100/post ductal PaO_2) was 46 and it became clear that oxygenation would not be maintained without extracorporeal membrane oxygenation (ECMO). The nearest national centre for ECMO was contacted and preparations for transfer made. Unfortunately a further, rapid deterioration in the patient's condition together with severe local weather conditions precluded safe transfer by either air or road. Therefore, our cardiac surgeons inserted large central cannulae (right internal jugular vein and right common carotid artery). Venoarterial ECMO, using a centrifugal pump (Biomedicus Inc., Eden Prairie, MN) and a membrane oxygenator, was instituted in the PICU with an initial pump flow rate of 600 ml min^{-1}. The ventilator settings were then changed to: PIP 20 cmH$_2$O, PEEP 4 cmH$_2$O, rate 10 min^{-1} and FiO$_2$ 0.21. A chest radiograph shortly after the institution of ECMO revealed complete 'white out' of both lung fields. Heparin was administered to maintain a Celite activated clotting time (ACT) of 180–200 seconds and total parenteral nutrition started. Coagulation and free plasma hemoglobin levels were closely monitored.

During the following week neuromuscular blocking agents were discontinued and sedation maintained with morphine sulfate 40 µg kg^{-1} h^{-1} and midazolam 300 µg kg^{-1} h^{-1}. Regular cranial ultrasonography ruled out intracranial hemorrhage and clinical neurological examination remained reassuring. On the eighth day of ECMO, there was significant bleeding from around the ECMO cannulation sites. Laboratory investigations revealed significant hemolysis and a rise in C-reactive protein (CRP) to 136 mg l^{-1} (normal range <10 mg l^{-1}). Meropenem 20 mg kg^{-1} and teicoplanin 10 mg kg^{-1} daily were started empirically. A 10-day course of teicoplanin had already been administered. Hemolysis and hemoglobinemia (peak concentration 62 mg dl^{-1}) continued until the ECMO pump head was changed. Acute renal failure was treated with peritoneal dialysis (peak creatinine concentration 2.5 mg dl^{-1}/225 µmol l^{-1}).

During the third week of ECMO the patient's pulmonary function improved; there was greatly increased air entry and pulmonary compliance with resolution of radiographic appearances. In view of this improvement, he was weaned from ECMO 30 days after surgery and after 23 days of ECMO. Progress was initially very stormy with an illness consistent with septicemia. All central cannulae were removed and replaced. He was reintubated, his nasotracheal tube being changed from one nostril to the other. Copious quantities of purulent secretions were aspirated from his nose after the removal of the first nasotracheal tube, consistent with ongoing RSV infection. All blood cultures taken during this period remained negative.

Although the patient eventually became more stable, he could not be weaned from mechanical ventilation because of intermittent collapse-consolidation of his left lung. Repeat cardiac catheterization and a bronchogram revealed severe residual mitral valve regurgitation and left atrial compression of the left main bronchus.

Residual aortic stenosis was treated by percutaneous balloon valvotomy. Following this he went back to the operating theatre for a mitral valve replacement (17 mm St Jude) and plication of the left atrium. He received an aprotinin infusion throughout. Following an uneventful procedure he was returned to the PICU with good respiratory indices and minimal inotrope requirements. His postoperative course was uncomplicated and he continued to improve slowly until, after 66 days on PICU, he was weaned from mechanical ventilation and extubated. There was no clinical evidence of neurological injury and transthoracic echocardiography showed excellent left ventricular function.

He was discharged home 3 weeks later and at a recent review was entirely well. He has no evidence of heart failure, has achieved all developmental milestones and has no residual neurological problems.

Discussion

Respiratory syncytial virus is associated with a number of clinical conditions including upper respiratory tract infections (coryza), acute pharyngitis, acute tonsillitis, acute laryngotracheitis (croup), otitis media, bronchitis, viral pneumonia and bronchiolitis. The virus spreads rapidly through susceptible populations such as children in crèches and kindergartens, and elderly people in residential institutions. Almost 100% of infants in childcare during their first RSV 'season' become infected.[9] Spread within families is also common and having older siblings increases the risk of infants developing bronchiolitis.

Children at risk for severe illness include those who were born prematurely, whether or not they have recognized chronic lung disease of prematurity. These infants are increasingly likely to survive the immediate neonatal period because of rapid advances in neonatal intensive care and RSV represents a serious threat to them. Children with congenital cyanotic heart disease are at even more risk. In early studies these infants had up to 44% percent mortality following bronchiolitis where pre-existing pulmonary hypertension was present. Advances in pediatric intensive care, especially in ventilation and fluid balance, have improved the outlook considerably.[10] Today the mortality rate in this group is nearer 9%.[9]

Other groups of special importance are children with congenital or acquired immunodeficiency; in particular those infected with human immunodeficiency virus (HIV), undergoing chemotherapy or with congenital severe combined immunodeficiency. Other risk factors for severe bronchiolitis include: parental smoking; lower socioeconomic status and other causes of lung disease such as cystic fibrosis. Breast-feeding may have a protective influence against severe RSV bronchiolitis[11, 12] but this may be short lived.[13, 14]

Infants with bronchiolitis present with symptoms of a non-specific viral illness: rhinorrhea, cough and sometimes a low-grade fever. Cough is usually, but by no means always, prominent especially in young infants. The child may be irritable, feed less well and may have vomited.[10] The respiratory rate usually exceeds 60 breaths per minute with subcostal, intercostal or suprasternal recession. Inspiratory crackles with or without expiratory crackles and wheezes are usually heard. The child may have signs of mild or moderate dehydration. Pulse oximetry may reveal oxygen desaturation.

Radiographic manifestations of bronchiolitis are non-specific and indeed the chest radiograph may be normal. There is usually diffuse hyperinflation of the lungs with flattening of the diaphragms. Patchy or peribronchial infiltrates suggesting interstitial pneumonia is usually present. Pleural thickening and pleural effusion are very rarely seen and invariably minimal if present.

Pathophysiology of RSV

Airway edema, occlusion and some smooth muscle spasm all result in abnormal respiratory mechanics.[10, 15] Infants with bronchiolitis breathe at high lung volumes and therefore the lungs are stiffer. Pulmonary compliance is decreased because of the inhomogeneous ventilation of different regions of the lung with areas of atelectasis and hyperinflation.[10, 16, 17] Airways resistance is increased both in inspiration and expiration; however, the obstruction is usually more marked during expiration.[16] Ventilation–perfusion mismatch can produce hypoxia. In younger infants hypercarbia may also be present secondary to hypoventilation as a result of the increased work of breathing. Some infants will have evidence of a mild to moderate respiratory acidosis but metabolic acidosis is more commonly seen.[10]

A diagnosis of RSV infection is usually made on the results of direct immunofluorescence of nasopharyngeal aspirates and simultaneous virus culture. Once the diagnosis is confirmed the mainstays of treatment are still supportive: to ensure adequate oxygenation and hydration. In severe cases positive pressure ventilation is often required. Ribavirin, a synthetic nucleoside resembling guanosine, has been shown to be a potent antiviral agent against RSV in vitro. However, studies of the use of small particle ribavirin nebulization in the treatment of bronchiolitis have shown modest benefits and its use is usually reserved for children at very high risk or with severe disease.[18]

Clearance of RSV requires an intact immune system. It is important to note that children with either congenital or acquired immunodeficiency are often unable to terminate the acute infection and can shed high levels of virus for many months.[19–21] It is the immune response to RSV, however, that is probably responsible for much of the pathology of bronchiolitis.

Transmission of RSV

Paramyxoviridae, including RSV, mumps, measles and parainfluenza viruses are transmitted by contact or aerosols. Transmission of RSV is by introduction of infected secretions onto the mucosa of the eyes or nose. Usually this is by self-inoculation with the hands after touching infected secretions or contact with virus on objects such as doors, surfaces or fomites. Aerosolization seems to be a less frequent means of spread. The virus is capable of surviving several hours on inanimate objects.[22, 23] The incubation period between inoculation and disease is 4–5 days in adults. Lower respiratory tract signs appear 1–3 days after the onset of rhinorrhea. Viral antigens have been reported to be present on circulating mononuclear cells in some individuals.[8] More recently viremia has been reported in association with primary infection in children.[13, 24] Virus shedding often occurs for more than 2 weeks, well after the peak of the illness. RSV can be detected by conventional methods even 4 weeks after the onset of bronchiolitis in immunocompetent children.[7]

Enhanced disease due to immunity: lessons from early vaccines

In the 1960s there were trials of vaccines containing formalin-inactivated preparations of RSV precipitated with alum.[5, 15, 25, 26] Vaccinees developed high levels of serum antibody to RSV but were not protected. Alarmingly, when the vaccinees became infected with RSV they experienced augmented pulmonary disease and a number of children died. Work from Openshaw's group[17, 27] and others [28] indicates that different T-helper subsets may be being primed by different RSV proteins leading to either a T_H1 or T_H2 phenotype and enhanced disease.

Cardiopulmonary bypass and SIRS

RSV can cause a severe illness in young infants and present in a similar manner to systemic sepsis. Although interleukin–6 (IL–6) and interferon levels in serum are not measurably increased in RSV bronchiolitis.[29] Peripheral blood monocytes produce cytokines including IL–8, IL–6 and tumor necrosis factor alpha in response to RSV. Plasma IL–8 levels in RSV-infected children requiring ventilation are considerably higher than those who do not need ventilation.[6] Cardiopulmonary bypass also causes a systemic illness that has been compared to the changes associated with sepsis or the systemic inflammatory response syndrome (SIRS). These have been attributed to cellular and humoral activation including increased secretion of cytokines and complement activation.[30] Serum IL–6 concentration has been one indicator of activation of the inflammatory cascade and predictor of subsequent organ dysfunction and death. Prolonged increases in levels of circulating IL–6 are known to be associated with increased morbidity and mortality after cardiac operations.[31]

The combination of CPB and severe RSV infection has been associated with a much worse postoperative course. In our institution this has lead to preoperative testing of all children in the autumn and winter. 'Near-patient' testing for RSV has recently attracted attention as a way of getting rapid bedside confirmation of RSV in hospitals.[32] In adults, nasal brush samples rather than nasopharyngeal aspirates may offer a more consistent result.

Therapies and preventative strategies

Hand washing

The risk of nosocomial RSV infection is very high and hospital staff play a major role in its transmission. The chances of acquiring RSV increase with duration of hospitalization and the number of individuals in a room. Nosocomial infection rates in infants and children vary from 20 to 47%. The risks to children admitted to hospital in the winter with, for example, cyanotic congenital heart disease or immunodeficiency, are therefore immense. Hand washing and cohorting of patients have been shown to be very effective in reducing nosocomial transmission.

Respigam

Hyperimmune immunoglobulin from pooled human donations has been shown to have a role in the prevention of RSV-related illness in high-risk infants. Risks identified with its use include complications of fluid overload and those associated with transfusion. It is very expensive and its use to date in the UK has been very limited. Recently however data about its use in combination with ribavirin in adults undergoing bone marrow transplantation has been published and this approach may substantially reduce mortality.[33, 34]

Palivizumab

Recombinant humanized monoclonal antibody to the F (Fusion) protein of RSV has recently been introduced. Given as an intramuscular injection in high-risk infants it may have a role in the prevention of severe illness. It is very expensive and experience with its use in the UK is limited to date. It is not believed to have a valuable role in the therapy of RSV disease.[35, 36]

Ribavirin

A synthetic antiviral agent that does not induce interferon with activity against both RNA and DNA viruses. It may work by interfering with inosine monophosphate (IMP) dehydrogenase by acting as an IMP-analogue of guanosine monophosphate and inhibiting synthesis of viral ribonucleic acids. Its use in Lassa fever has considerably improved survival.[37, 38] As a therapy in RSV disease however its efficacy has been relatively disappointing.

Vaccines

After the disastrous consequences of the formalin-inactivated vaccine trials of the 1960s, potential RSV vaccines have been subject to even more rigorous investigation. Many subunit vaccines have been shown to produce an antibody response but not perhaps protect. Temperature-sensitive mutants have attracted interest recently and some have been genetically altered to encode cytokines to augment immunogenicity. Vaccination of mothers in the last trimester has been suggested as a means of increasing passively acquired immunity. To date an effective vaccine still seems some years away.

Surfactant

There are attractive reasons for the use of pulmonary surfactant in RSV chest infections. RSV is known to infect and cause the apoptosis of type 2 pneumocytes that produce pulmonary surfactant.[39] RSV infection alters both the level and function of lung surfactant in bronchiolitis.[40, 41] However, from the limited case reports that have been published any improvement in clinical status has been short-lived.

ECMO

Extracorporeal membrane oxygenation now has an established role for respiratory failure that is unresponsive to conventional therapy in children.[42] Its use in viral pneumonia has also been studied and has a survival in RSV bronchiolitis of up to 96%[43, 44] with an excellent neurological outlook.[45] Complications related to cannula insertion and anticoagulation and a relatively prolonged therapeutic course have limited its use to the very sickest children in whom conventional ventilation has failed.

Conclusions and learning points

- The combination of cardiac disease and RSV infection can be devastating.
- In even the sickest patient ECMO is normally associated with a good outcome, even if support has to be maintained for a long time.
- Perioperative RSV infection has serious implications for centers carrying out cardiac operations.
- The pathophysiology of RSV infection and current preventative, diagnostic and therapeutic strategies have been reviewed.

References

1. Chapman RS, Henderson FW, Clyde WA Jr et al. The epidemiology of tracheobronchitis in pediatric practice. Am J Epidemiol 1981;114:786–97.

2. Gardner PS. Respiratory syncytial virus infections. Postgrad Med J 1973;49:788–91.

3. Hall CB. Respiratory syncytial virus. In: Feigin RD, Cherry JD (eds) Textbook of pediatric infectious diseases. Philadelphia: WB Saunders, 1997; 1653–76.

4. Henderson FW, Clyde WA Jr, Collier AM et al. The etiologic and epidemiologic spectrum of bronchiolitis in pediatric practice. J Pediatr 1979;95:183–90.

5. Chin J, Magoffin RL, Shearer LA et al. Field evaluation of a respiratory syncytial virus vaccine and a trivalent parainfluenza virus vaccine in a pediatric population. Am J Epidemiol 1969;89:449–63.

6. Arnold R, Konig B, Galatti H et al. Cytokine (IL-8, IL-6, TNF-alpha) and soluble TNF receptor-I release from human peripheral blood mononuclear cells after respiratory syncytial virus infection. Immunology 1995;85:364–72.

7. Cubie HA, Inglis JM, Leslie EE *et al*. Detection of respiratory syncytial virus in acute bronchiolitis in infants. *J Med Virol* 1992;**38**:283–7.

8. Domurat F, Roberts NJ Jr, Walsh EE, Dagan R. Respiratory syncytial virus infection of human mononuclear leukocytes in vitro and in vivo. *J Infect Dis* 1985;**152**:895–902.

9. Collins PL, McIntosh K, Channock RM. Respiratory syncytial virus. In: Fields BN, Knipe DM, Howley RM *et al*. (eds) *Field's virology*. Philadelphia: Lippincott-Raven, 1996;1313–51.

10. Wohl MEB. Bronchiolitis. In: Chernick V, Kendig EL (eds) *Kendig's disorders of the respiratory tract in children*. Philadelphia: WB Saunders, 1990;360–98.

11. Downham MA, Scott R, Sims DG *et al*. Breast-feeding protects against respiratory syncytial virus infections. *BMJ* 1976;**ii**:274–6.

12. Holberg CJ, Wright AL, Martinez FD *et al*. Risk factors for respiratory syncytial virus-associated lower respiratory illnesses in the first year of life. *Am J Epidemiol* 1991;**133**:1135–51.

13. O'Donnell DR, McGarvey MJ, Tully JM, Balfour-Lynn IM, Openshaw PJ. Respiratory syncytial virus RNA in cells from the peripheral blood during acute infection. *J Pediatr* 1998;**133**:272–4.

14. Wong DT, Ogra PL. Neonatal respiratory syncytial virus infection: role of transplacentally and breast milk-acquired antibodies. *J Virol* 1986;**57**:1203–6.

15. Kim HW, Canchola JG, Brandt CD *et al*. Respiratory syncytial virus disease in infants despite prior administration of antigenic inactivated vaccine. *Am J Epidemiol* 1969;**89**:422–34.

16. Krieger I. Mechanics of respiration in bronchiolitis. *Pediatrics* 1964;**33**:45.

17. Openshaw PJ, O'Donnell DR. Asthma and the common cold: can viruses imitate worms? *Thorax* 1994;**49**:101–3.

18. La Via WV, Grant SW, Stutman HR, Marks MI. Clinical profile of pediatric patients hospitalized with respiratory syncytial virus infection. *Clin Pediatr (Phila)* 1993;**32**:450–4.

19. Chandwani S, Borkowsky W, Krasinski K *et al*. Respiratory syncytial virus infection in human immunodeficiency virus-infected children. *J Pediatr* 1990;**117**:251–4.

20. Fishaut M, Tubergen D, McIntosh K. Cellular response to respiratory viruses with particular reference to children with disorders of cell-mediated immunity. *J Pediatr* 1980;**96**:179–86.

21. Hall CB, Powell KR, MacDonald NE *et al*. Respiratory syncytial viral infection in children with compromised immune function. *N Engl J Med* 1986;**315**:77–81.

22. Hall CB, Douglas RG Jr. Modes of transmission of respiratory syncytial virus. *J Pediatr* 1981;**99**:100–3.

23. Hall CB, Douglas RG Jr, Schnabel KC, Geiman JM. Infectivity of respiratory syncytial virus by various routes of inoculation. *Infect Immun* 1981;**33**:779–83.

24. Rohwedder A, Keminer O, Forster J *et al*. Detection of respiratory syncytial virus RNA in blood of neonates by polymerase chain reaction. *J Med Virol* 1998;**54**:320–7.

25. Fulginiti VA, Eller JJ, Sieber OF *et al*. Respiratory virus immunization. I. A field trial of two inactivated respiratory virus vaccines; an aqueous trivalent parainfluenza virus vaccine and an alum-precipitated respiratory syncytial virus vaccine. *Am J Epidemiol* 1969;**89**:435–48.

26. Kapikian AZ, Mitchell RH, Chanock RM *et al*. An epidemiologic study of altered clinical reactivity to respiratory syncytial (RS) virus infection in children previously vaccinated with an inactivated RS virus vaccine. *Am J Epidemiol* 1969;**89**:405–21.

27. Openshaw PJ. Immunopathological mechanisms in respiratory syncytial virus disease. *Springer Semin Immunopathol* 1995;**17**:187–201.

28. Graham BS, Bunton LA, Wright PF, Karzon DT. Role of T lymphocyte subsets in the pathogenesis of primary infection and rechallenge with respiratory syncytial virus in mice. *J Clin Invest* 1991;**88**:1026–33.

29. Wang CM, Tang RB, Chung RL, Hwang BT. Tumor necrosis factor-alpha and interleukin–6 profiles in children with pneumonia. *J Microbiol Immunol Infect* 1999;**32**:233–8.

30. Duval EL, Kavelaars A, Veenhuizen L *et al*. Pro- and anti-inflammatory cytokine patterns during and after cardiac surgery in young children. *Eur J Pediatr* 1999;**158**:387–93.

31. Roytblat L, Talmor D, Rachinsky M *et al*. Ketamine attenuates the interleukin–6 response after cardiopulmonary bypass. *Anesth Analg* 1998;**87**:266–71.

32. Mackenzie A, Hallam N, Mitchell E, Beattie T. Near patient testing for respiratory syncytial virus in paediatric accident and emergency: prospective pilot study. *BMJ* 1999;**319**:289–90.

33. Englund JA. Prevention strategies for respiratory syncytial virus: passive and active immunization. *J Pediatr* 1999;**135**:38–44.

34. Ghosh S, Champlin RE, Englund J *et al.* Respiratory syncytial virus upper respiratory tract illnesses in adult blood and marrow transplant recipients: combination therapy with aerosolized ribavirin and intravenous immunoglobulin. *Bone Marrow Transplant* 2000;**25**:751–5.

35. The IMpact-RSV Study Group. Palivizumab, a humanized respiratory syncytial virus monoclonal antibody, reduces hospitalization from respiratory syncytial virus infection in high-risk infants. *Pediatrics* 1998;**102**:531–7.

36. Clark SJ, Beresford MW, Subhedar NV, Shaw NJ. Respiratory syncytial virus infection in high risk infants and the potential impact of prophylaxis in a United Kingdom cohort. *Arch Dis Child* 2000;**83**:313–6.

37. Nzerue MC. Lassa fever: review of virology, immunopathogenesis, and algorithms for control and therapy. *Cent Afr J Med* 1992;**38**:247–52.

38. Patterson JL, Fernandez-Larsson R. Molecular mechanisms of action of ribavirin. *Rev Infect Dis* 1990;**12**:1139–46.

39. O'Donnell DR, Milligan L, Stark JM. Induction of CD95 (Fas) and apoptosis in respiratory epithelial cell cultures following respiratory syncytial virus infection. *Virology* 1999;**257**:198–207.

40. Kerr MH, Paton JY. Surfactant protein levels in severe respiratory syncytial virus infection. *Am J Respir Crit Care Med* 1999;**159**:1115–8.

41. Van Schaik SM, Vargas I, Welliver RC, Enhorning G. Surfactant dysfunction develops in BALB/c mice infected with respiratory syncytial virus. *Pediatr Res* 1997;**42**:169–73.

42. Green TP, Moler FW, Goodman DM. Probability of survival after prolonged extracorporeal membrane oxygenation in pediatric patients with acute respiratory failure. Extracorporeal Life Support Organization. *Crit Care Med* 1995;**23**:1132–9.

43. Khan JY, Kerr SJ, Tometzki A *et al.* Role of ECMO in the treatment of respiratory syncytial virus bronchiolitis: a collaborative report. *Arch Dis Child Fetal Neonatal Ed* 1995;**73**:F91–4.

44. Meyer TA, Warner BW. Extracorporeal life support for the treatment of viral pneumonia: collective experience from the ELSO registry. Extracorporeal Life Support Organization. *J Pediatr Surg* 1997;**32**:232–6.

45. Steinhorn RH, Green TP. Use of extracorporeal membrane oxygenation in the treatment of respiratory syncytial virus bronchiolitis: the national experience, 1983 to 1988. *J Pediatr* 1990;**116**:338–42.

34

Complication of a percutaneous tracheostomy in a patient with adult respiratory distress syndrome

Sheena A Millar, Vilas U Navapurkar and Raymond D Latimer

Introduction

Percutaneous dilatational tracheostomy (PDT) is commonly carried out in most general intensive care units.[1, 2] Perforation of the posterior tracheal wall is a complication of PDT that can lead to varying degrees of cardiorespiratory compromise. We describe a patient with pre-existing adult respiratory distress syndrome (ARDS) who had a posterior tracheal wall tear during a PDT and required cardiopulmonary bypass (CPB) to allow surgical repair of the injury. The case highlights many of the problems of managing tracheal injury in the critically ill patient.

Case history

A 33-year-old Caucasian female was involved in a road traffic accident. Examination by an emergency physician, less than 10 minutes after the accident, revealed external evidence of injuries to the right side of the head and left chest. The Glasgow Coma Score was 3/15, and there was partial airway obstruction with tachypnea (SpO_2 85%), anisocoria (right pupil dilated and unresponsive), and crepitus over her left chest. Supplemental oxygen was administered by facemask, intravenous infusions were commenced and the patient was extracted from the vehicle.

Past medical history	Ulcerative colitis.
Medications	No regular medication. Allergic to penicillin.
Examination	Weight 82 kg. GCS 3/15. HR 84 min^{-1}. BP 130/70 mmHg. Right pupil dilated and unresponsive. Spine grossly normal. No obvious limb injuries. Pelvis stable.
Investigations	Hb 8.3 g.dl^{-1}, WBC 12.9 $\times 10^9$ l^{-1}, platelets 230 $\times$ 10^9 l^{-1}. [K$^+$] 2.9 mmol l^{-1}. **ABG:** [H$^+$] 35.7 nmol l^{-1} (pH 7.45), PaO_2 173 mmHg (23 kPa), $PaCO_2$ 24 mmHg (3.2 kPa), base excess –5 mmol l^{-1} (FiO$_2$ 0.5). **Urinalysis:** Microscopic hematuria. **CXR:** 'Normal' — no obvious pneumothorax. **Cervical spine X-rays:** Normal lateral view. **Pelvic X-rays:** Fractures of right superior ramus and left acetabulum. **Cranial CT:** Small brainstem contusion. **CT chest/abdomen/pelvis:** Moderate left pneumothorax, small retroperitoneal hematoma, stable pelvic fractures.

Following a rapid sequence induction with etomidate 10 mg, fentanyl 100 μg and suxamethonium 100 mg, orotracheal intubation was performed and artificial ventilation commenced with cricoid pressure. In view of this a left thoracostomy was performed prior to helicopter transfer to hospital.

On arrival in the emergency department, some 100 minutes after the accident, she was hemodynamically stable. Coma and anisocoria persisted. Following initial investigations she was transferred to the neurosurgical intensive care unit (ICU).

Intermittent positive pressure ventilation was continued. The patient was sedated with propofol 1–4 mg kg^{-1} h^{-1} and fentanyl 0.25–1.5 μg kg^{-1} h^{-1}, and paralyzed with atracurium 0.5 mg kg^{-1} h^{-1}. Cannulation of the right subclavian vein was complicated by a right pneumothorax, which was treated with an intercostal drain, attached to an under-water seal. In view of the low hemoglobin concentration and the presence of abdominal wall bruising, computerized tomographs of the chest, abdomen and pelvis were obtained. Her initial management consisted of general supportive measures (including nasogastric feeding), intracranial pressure (ICP) monitoring with a subdural transducer (initial ICP 17 mmHg) and specific treatment for raised intracranial pressure (i.e. controlled hypertension and mild hypocapnia).

Within 24 hours of admission the ICP became unstable and the patient became hemodynamically unstable. Pulmonary artery catheterization, via the left subclavian vein, revealed a cardiovascular profile consistent with systemic inflammatory response syndrome (SIRS) in a patient with major trauma. Noradrenaline 0.05–0.2 μg kg^{-1} min^{-1} was used to maintain an adequate cerebral perfusion pressure. Over the first 2 days, the leukocyte count rose to 18.8×10^9 l^{-1} and the CRP reached 253 mg dl^{-1}. *Staphylococcus aureus*, isolated from tracheal aspirates on the second day, was treated with vancomycin 1 g BD and meropenem 500 mg TDS. Over the next 8 days pulmonary function deteriorated and the FiO$_2$ had to be increased from 0.4 to 1.0 (lowest PaO$_2$/FiO$_2$ = 92 mmHg (12.2 kPa); normal >450 mmHg (60 kPa)).

The ICP remained unstable throughout this time, peaking at 35 mmHg. A further cranial CT scan 24 hours after admission had shown bilateral loss of sulci suggesting a significantly elevated ICP. The CXR showed increasing alveolar consolidation in all zones in the presence of a low or normal pulmonary artery wedge pressure

consistent with a diagnosis of adult respiratory distress syndrome (ARDS). She was transferred to the general ICU for further management.

Over the next 2 weeks, various ventilatory strategies were used including inverse I:E ventilation, inhaled nitric oxide (5–20 ppm), and ventilation in the prone position. Methylprednisolone 2 mg kg^{-1} was administered followed by a daily dose of 0.0625–0.5 mg kg^{-1}.[3] This may have contributed to the significant improvement in pulmonary compliance and gas exchange such that after 14 days she had stable blood gases on synchronized intermittent mandatory ventilation (SIMV) and pressure support with an FiO$_2$ of 0.5. To facilitate further weaning from ventilatory support a PDT was performed using a modified Ciaglia technique[4] under fiberoptic guidance. At the end of the procedure high airway pressures were observed and a higher FiO$_2$ was required to maintain adequate oxygenation. Five hours later she developed severe pneumoperitoneum accompanied by tachycardia (160–170 min^{-1}), relative hypertension (150/70 mmHg) and a further increase in airway pressure. Associated with this was subcutaneous emphysema most marked around the neck but also extending over the chest and abdominal wall. Arterial blood gas analysis (FiO$_2$ 1.0) results were: [H$^+$] 47 nmol l^{-1} (pH 7.33), PaO$_2$ 74 mmHg (9.9 kPa), PaCO$_2$ 63 mmHg (8.4 kPa). An urgent CT scan confirmed extensive subcutaneous emphysema, pneumomediastinum, retroperitoneal air and a tension pneumoperitoneum. The latter was treated with an intraperitoneal drain. Fiberoptic bronchoscopy confirmed a tear in the posterior wall of the trachea just proximal to the carina. The surgical emphysema in the neck, face and larynx rendered further airway manipulation impossible. The subsequent management of the tracheal tear was discussed with the regional cardiothoracic anesthetic and surgical teams.

The problems presented to the cardiothoracic team were as follows: (1) A large disruption of the posterior wall of the trachea just proximal to the carina requiring surgical repair; (2) a precarious airway, increasing subcutaneous emphysema gradually increasing the distance between the skin and the tracheal stoma with a tracheostomy tube of finite length in place; (3) subcutaneous emphysema around the neck, face and upper airways posing problems for direct laryngoscopy and intubation; (4) high airway pressures and a

FiO$_2$ required to maintain adequate ventilation and oxygenation; (5) recent severe ARDS and therefore pre-existing damaged lung parenchyma.

The patient was scheduled for urgent right thoracotomy with the support of cardiopulmonary bypass. Because the patient was too unstable for interhospital transfer, the cardiothoracic team and their equipment travelled from the regional cardiothoracic unit.

Anesthesia consisted of propofol 3–4 mg kg^{-1} h^{-1}, midazolam 2 mg, fentanyl (total dose 1 mg) and pancuronium 8 mg. The lungs were ventilated with an FiO$_2$ of 1.0 using a Servo (model C, Seimens–Elema AB; Solna, Sweden) ventilator. Methylprednisolone 500 mg was administered because of the recent use of steroids for the treatment of ARDS.

The patient was placed in the supine position, the right femoral vessels were exposed and, following the administration of heparin 35 000 iu, partial (2.8–3.3 l min^{-1}) CPB was insituted. Lung ventilation had to be continued at this stage in order to maintain oxygenation. The surgeon next removed the tracheostomy tube and passed a gum elastic bougie from the tracheal stoma through the vocal cords and into the mouth. The anesthetist then 'railroaded' an uncut cuffed (7 mm) endotracheal tube over the bougie and positioned the tube such that the inflated cuff lay beyond the tracheal tear. With a more secure airway in place the surgeon refashioned the tracheostomy wound and closed the overlying subcutaneous tissue and skin.

The patient was then placed in the left lateral position and the right chest opened through a lateral thoracotomy in the fifth intercostal space. The insertion of a two-stage venous cannula into the right atrium allowed full CPB to be established and lung ventilation to be discontinued, thereby affording better surgical access. The endotracheal tube was withdrawn to allow access to the distal trachea. Surgical findings were of numerous pleural adhesions and lung tissue the consistency of liver. A 3-cm tear in the posterior tracheal wall was associated with fractures of the tracheal cartilages and damage to the esophageal serosa but the mucosa was intact. Following repair of the tracheal tear with an autologous pericardial patch, the endotracheal tube was advanced so that the cuff supported the surgical repair.

Lung ventilation was recommenced with considerable difficulty. Airway pressures remained high and bleeding into the airway necessitated frequent suctioning. After the institution of jet ventilation (frequency 21 min^{-1}) the patient was eventually weaned from CPB (total time 187 minutes), surgical hemostasis was secured and heparin effect was reversed with protamine sulfate 300 mg. Infusions of dopamine 4 µg kg^{-1} min^{-1} and epinephrine 0.1 µg kg^{-1} min^{-1} were started shortly after CPB in order to maintain a mean arterial pressure >70 mmHg. Continued bleeding from the dissected pleural adhesions and the surgical sites in the presence of a coagulopathy (elevated circulating d-dimers, PT 22.2 s, APTT 55 s, platelets 117 × 10^9 l^{-1}), was treated with tranexamic acid 2 g, aprotinin (500,000 kiu followed by 200 000 kiu h^{-1}), fresh frozen plasma (2 units) and packed red blood cells (2 units). After an initial period of cardiovascular instability and poor gas exchange — FiO$_2$ 1.0, [H$^+$] 107 nmol l^{-1} (pH 6.97), PaO$_2$ 56 mmHg (7.4 kPa), PaCO$_2$ 110 mmHg (14.7 kPa) — the patient's condition stabilized and then improved. Sixteen days later she underwent an uneventful and uncomplicated surgical tracheostomy.

Over the next month the patient's condition improved. A right third cranial nerve palsy and weakness presumed secondary to critical illness neuropathy gradually resolved. She was weaned from mechanical ventilatory support and discharged to a neurosurgical ward 61 days after her original injury. A week later she was transferred to a local rehabilitation unit and then to a regional rehabilitation unit closer to her home 5 days later. Eventually she was discharged home being able to care for herself and mobilizing independently. During the latter stages of her recovery it became clear that the patient had persistent cognitive dysfunction characterized by a frivolous manner, poor concentration and indifference to her circumstances. Although formal psychological evaluation did not suggest a cause, it was probably the result of the combination of intracranial trauma, raised ICP, hypoxemia, hypotension, sepsis, cardiopulmonary bypass and sedative drugs.

Discussion

Perforation of the trachea and proximal bronchi may occur as a result of trauma, erosion, and infection or during the course of medical and surgical procedures, (Table 34.1). It is important, therefore for both surgeons and anesthetists to be aware of this hazard and be able to recognize it. The diagnosis should be considered in patients with a precipitating cause who present with dyspnea, hemoptysis, stridor, subcutaneous emphysema, pneumomediastinum, pneumothorax, and/or pneumoperitoneum. The latter two may be under tension. The persistence of an air leak after placement of tube drains should raise the index of suspicion.[5, 6] A radiological sign associated with tracheal injury is reported to be a rounded appearance of the cuff of the endotracheal tube[7] caused by herniation of the cuff through the defect. A surgeon may discover a tracheobronchial injury after endobronchial intubation during the course of a surgical procedure. Alternatively the injury may be manifest as difficulty in maintaining lung isolation necessitating the pressure in the bronchial cuff to be adjusted.[8]. Bronchoscopy is the investigation of choice to confirm the diagnosis but it is important to be aware that an endotracheal tube already in situ may obscure any injury.[9]

The management of tracheal injuries depends upon the type, size and location of the injury. The presence of pre-existing disease and other injuries will also affect the management. Small

Table 34.1 The etiology of tracheobronchial disruption

Trauma	• Penetrating (e.g. stabbing, gunshot)
	• Non-penetrating (e.g. blunt trauma, deceleration injury)
Iatrogenic	• Complication of thoracotomy or thoracoscopy
	• Surgical dehiscence (e.g. following sleeve resection)
	• Endobronchial instrumentation (e.g. endobronchial intubation, rigid bronchoscopy, laser therapy, balloon dilatation, stenting)
	• Complication of (surgical, percutaneous or 'mini') tracheostomy
Erosion	• Chemical (e.g. ingestion of a caustic substance)
	• Tumor (e.g. tracheal, bronchial, esophageal)
	• Aneurysm
Infection	• Empyema discharging through a bronchopleural fistula

wounds with well-apposed edges may be treated conservatively if an endotracheal tube can be placed with the cuff distal to the defect. Preventing air leak through the wound for 48 hours is then usually sufficient to allow the wound to seal. However, larger tracheal injuries, injuries occurring in the distal trachea or injuries involving adjacent structures require surgical exploration and repair.[10] The surgical approach is usually a right lateral thoracotomy unless the injury affects the left bronchus when a left lateral thoracotomy affords better surgical access.

Preoperative assessment should include a careful airway assessment and note any complications of the tracheobronchial disruption. Minimal monitoring standards should be adhered to and additionally invasive blood pressure measurement and if required central venous access secured. Regardless of the technique used, it is vital when planning anesthesia for patients with tracheobronchial disruption that the injury itself and any concomitant air leak are not worsened. The use of a fiberoptic bronchoscope as an aid to intubation allows direct visualization of the airway and provides the safest method of tube placement. Blind endotracheal or endobronchial intubation may convert a small laceration into a much larger disruption. The patient may be intubated awake under local anesthetic or under general anesthetic, either with or without spontaneous ventilation. However, the application of positive pressure ventilation may create tension in a pneumothorax or worsen subcutaneous emphysema. Similarly, the use of nitrous oxide is contraindicated; an air/oxygen mixture appropriate to maintain adequate oxygenation should be used. The site of injury, the surgical procedure to be undertaken and whether lung separation is required will determine the choice of tube. High tracheal injuries may allow a single-lumen tube to be placed in the trachea with the cuff beyond the injury and positive pressure ventilation applied to both lungs. Disruptions at or beyond the carina will require a double-lumen tube to be placed to isolate the disruption before ventilation of the contralateral lung can be safely commenced. Alternatively, in this situation, a small catheter can be passed beyond the disruption and high frequency jet ventilation used to maintain oxygenation although carbon dioxide removal may become a problem. In some cases a tracheostomy, carried out under local anesthesia may be the safest way to maintain the airway. A variety of tracheostomy tubes should be available, ranging from various sizes of standard cuffed tubes to adjustable length tubes and double-lumen tubes. In addition, a selection of sterile endotracheal tubes should be readily available to the surgeon for placement in the airway while the chest is open.[11] Maintenance of anesthesia is unreliable when using inhalation agents in the presence of airway leaks or when high frequency jet ventilation is employed. Total intravenous anesthesia through a reliable intravenous cannula is the preferred method of maintenance of anesthesia. Following surgical repair, the patient should, ideally, be weaned from mechanical ventilatory support and the airway extubated as soon as possible as this gives the best environment for healing of the airway repair. Concomitant injury or illness may necessitate prolonged sedation and ventilation and in that circumstance airway pressures should be minimized.

Tracheobronchial laceration has been described following PDT,[12, 13] open tracheostomy and, less commonly, following tracheal intubation with single- and double-lumen endotracheal tubes.[14] In the case of PDT, a tracheal injury may be recognized, and hopefully avoided, by using fiberoptic bronchoscopic visualization during the procedure. For this reason many operators consider bronchoscopic guidance as mandatory in this situation.[13, 15] However, as in this case, and as previously described by Fish and colleagues,[12] the use of bronchoscopy during the procedure does not always detect injury to the tracheal wall occurring.

The case described presented two further problems for the anesthetists. Firstly, the presence of gross subcutaneous emphysema made it impossible to perform either oral or nasal intubation as neither direct nor fiberoptic laryngoscopy allowed visualization of the glottis. Because we were forced to intubate blindly over a bougie, we chose to use a single lumen tube as a double lumen tube may have been more likely to cause further injury. An alternative strategy would have been to pass a flexible (armored) endotracheal tube through the tracheal stoma and use a fiberoptic laryngoscopy as an aid to endobronchial intubation. Secondly, the presence of severe respiratory failure secondary to ARDS meant that one-lung ventilation would not have been tolerated. The planned use of CPB in this case allowed deflation of the lungs and improved surgical access whilst maintaining adequate gas exchange. As previous authors have indicated, CPB should only be used during tracheal and carinal surgery in exceptional circumstances when ventilatory or circulatory support is not sustainable by other means.[16, 17] The first reported use of extracorporeal support during airway surgery was in 1961[18] and since then there have been several reports of its use in similar situations with some success.[19, 20] None the less, the potential complications associated with CPB require careful consideration of the risks and benefits before its use in this setting. The main concerns about the use of extracorporeal support in this case were hemorrhage and exacerbation of ARDS as a result of the systemic inflammatory response to CPB.[21] Corticosteroid therapy may be useful in the recovery phase of ARDS[3] and since it had been used in this case its administration intraoperatively seemed logical in an attempt to minimize any further pulmonary damage secondary to CPB. It is suggested that serine protease inhibitors, such as aprotinin, may reduce the inflammatory response associated with CPB[22] and, in retrospect, it may have been more beneficial to administer the drug prior to the onset of CPB.

Conclusions and learning points

- Tracheobronchial injury although not common can complicate procedures commonly carried out by anesthetists and so they should be able to recognize the symptoms and signs.
- Bronchoscopy is mandatory if tracheobronchial injury is suspected.
- Site and severity of the injury and any other pre-existing disease will determine the choice of anesthetic and ventilatory strategy.
- Use of CPB should be reserved for exceptional circumstances and its detrimental effects anticipated and ameliorated if possible.

References

1. Simpson TP, Day CJ, Jewkes CF, Manara AR. The impact of percutaneous tracheostomy on intensive care unit practice and training. *Anaesthesia* 1999;**54**:186–9.

2. Cooper RM. Use and safety of percutaneous tracheostomy in intensive care. Report of a postal survey of ICU practice. *Anaesthesia* 1998;**53**:1209–12.

3. Meduri GU, Headley AS, Golden E *et al.* Effect of prolonged methylprednisolone therapy in unresolving acute respiratory distress syndrome: a randomized controlled trial. *JAMA* 1998;**280**:159–65.

4. Ciaglia P, Firsching R, Syniec C. Elective percutaneous dilatational tracheostomy. A new simple bedside procedure; preliminary report. *Chest* 1985;**87**:715–9.

5. Ramzy AI, Rodriguez A, Turney SZ. Management of major tracheobronchial ruptures in patients with multiple system trauma. *J Trauma* 1988;**28**:1353–7.

6. Jones WS, Mavroudis C, Richardson JD *et al.* Management of tracheobronchial disruption resulting from blunt trauma. *Surgery* 1984;**95**:319–23.

7. Millham FH, Rajii-Khorasani A, Birkett DF, Hirsch EF. Carinal injury: diagnosis and treatment — case report. *J Trauma* 1991;**31**:1420–2.

8. Roxburgh JC. Rupture of the tracheobronchial tree. *Thorax* 1987;**42**:681–8.

9. Morelock RJ, Kesler KA, Broderick LR *et al.* A penetrating mediastinal tracheal injury. *J Trauma* 1998;**44**:552–4.

10. Symbas PN, Hatcher CR Jr, Boehm GA. Acute penetrating tracheal trauma. *Ann Thorac Surg* 1976;**22**:473–7.

11. Benumof JL. Anesthesia for emergency thoracic surgery. In: Benumof JL (ed) *Anesthesia for Thoracic Surgery*. Philadelphia: WB Saunders, 1995; 642–4.

12. Fish WH, Boheimer NO, Cadle DR, Sinclair DG. A life-threatening complication following percutaneous tracheostomy. *Clin Intens Care* 1996;**7**;206–8.

13. Trottier SJ, Hazard PB, Sakabu SA *et al.* Posterior tracheal wall perforation during percutaneous dilational tracheostomy: an investigation into its mechanism and prevention. *Chest* 1999;**115**:1383–9.

14. Massard G, Rouge C, Dabbagh A *et al.* Tracheobronchial lacerations after intubation and tracheostomy. *Ann Thorac Surg* 1996;**61**:1483–7.

15. Berrouschot J, Oeken J, Steiniger L, Schneider D. Perioperative complications of percutaneous dilational tracheostomy. *Laryngoscope* 1997;**107**:1538–44.

16. Symbas PN, Justicz AG, Ricketts RR. Rupture of the airways from blunt trauma: treatment of complex injuries. *Ann Thorac Surg* 1992;**54**:177–83.

17. Theman TE, Kerr JH, Nelems JM, Pearson FG. Carinal resection. A report of two cases and a description of the anesthetic technique. *J Thorac Cardiovasc Surg* 1976;**71**:314–20.

18. Woods FM, Neptune WB, Palatchi A. Resection of the carina and mainstem bronchi with the use of extracorporeal circulation. *N Engl J Med* 1961;**264**:492–4.

19. Adkins PC, Izawa EM. Resection of tracheal cylindroma using cardiopulmonary bypass. *Arch Surg* 1964;**88**:405–9.

20. Neville WE, Thomason RD, Peacock H, Colby C. Cardiopulmonary bypass during noncardiac surgery. *Arch Surg* 1966;**92**:576–87.

21. Hall RI, Smith MS, Rocker G. The systemic inflammatory response to cardiopulmonary bypass: pathophysiological, therapeutic, and pharmacological considerations. *Anesth Analg* 1997;**85**:766–82.

22. Murkin JM. Cardiopulmonary bypass and the inflammatory response: a role for serine protease inhibitors? *J Cardiothorac Vasc Anesth* 1997;**11**:19–23.

35

Acute respiratory distress syndrome following cardiac surgery with cardiopulmonary bypass

David P Stansfield and Mark Messent

Introduction

Acute respiratory distress syndrome (ARDS) is an infrequent complication of cardiopulmonary bypass (CPB). Despite recent improvement in survival figures this condition remains difficult to treat and still has a significant mortality.

Case history

A 62-year-old Caucasian male presented for coronary artery bypass grafting. The patient had a 10 year history that consisted mainly of

exertional dyspnea with little classical cardiac chest pain. He had three-pillow orthopnea and an exercise tolerance of 5 m. Risk factors for ischemic heart disease included hypertension, hypercholesterolemia and cigarette smoking.

The patient was premedicated with papaveretum 20 mg and metoclopramide 10 mg 1 hour before transfer to the operating theater. The right radial artery and a peripheral vein were cannulated under local anesthetic. Following preoxygenation, anesthesia was induced with fentanyl 0.5 mg, etomidate 16 mg, and pancuronium 10 mg. Following tracheal intubation the lungs were ventilated with nitrous oxide in oxygen (FiO_2 0.45). A quadruple-lumen catheter was inserted

Past medical history	Bilateral varicose vein surgery, left nephrolithotomy, transurethral resection of prostate. All previous anesthetics were without complication.
Regular medications	Isosorbide mononitrate 60 mg OD, amlodipine 10 mg OD, atenolol 50 mg OD, nicorandil 10 mg BD and simvastatin 20 mg OD. Aspirin 75 mg OD — stopped 5 days prior to admission. No known drug allergies. Alcohol intake 50-units per week.
Examination	Weight 71 kg. BMI 25.8 kg m^{-2}. Alert and orientated. Pulse 60 regular. BP 140/80 mmHg. Bilateral basal inspiratory crepitations — reduced after coughing..
Investigations	Hb 17.2 g dl^{-1}, WBC 11 × 10^9 l^{-1}, platelets 220 × 10^9 l^{-1}, coagulation studies normal. [Na$^+$] 131 mmol l^{-1}, [K$^+$] 4.0 mmol l^{-1}, urea 27 mg dl^{-1} (9.8 mmol l^{-1}), creatinine 1.1 mg dl^{-1} (98 µmol l^{-1}) **CXR:** Patchy reticular nodular shadowing of both bases. **ABG:** (On air) pH 7.44, PaO$_2$ 85 mmHg (11.3 kPa), PaCO$_2$ 33 mmHg (4.4 kPa), bicarbonate 22 mmol.l^{-1}, base excess –0.4 mmol.l^{-1}. **ECG:** Sinus rhythm, right bundle branch block and left axis deviation. **Coronary angiography:** Triple vessel coronary artery disease. Good LV function.

into the right internal jugular vein and the bladder was catheterized per urethra. A nasopharyngeal temperature probe was placed. Anesthesia was maintained with a propofol infusion 6 mg kg^{-1} h^{-1}. Arterial blood gas analysis following induction of anesthesia (FiO$_2$ 0.45) revealed pH 7.38, PaCO$_2$ 37 mmHg (4.9 kPa), and PaO$_2$ 92 mmHg (12.2 kPa). Peak airway pressure was 23 cmH$_2$O.

He was given a bolus dose of gentamicin 80 mg and the first of three doses of flucloxacillin 1 g. The left radial artery and left short saphenous vein were harvested, the left internal mammary artery mobilized and then the patient was fully anticoagulated with heparin sodium 300 iu kg^{-1}. Cardiopulmonary bypass was established between the right atrium and the ascending aorta, and the patient cooled to 28°C. Myocardial protection was achieved with intermittent cold blood cardioplegia administered via an aortic root cannula. Four coronary vessels were grafted with an aortic cross-clamp time of 80 minutes and a total CPB time of 144 minutes. Isoprenaline 2 μg min^{-1} was required to maintain an adequate heart rate after separation from CPB. Closure of the chest was uneventful. The lungs were ventilated with oxygen in air (FiO$_2$ 0.45). Peak airway pressure was unchanged and arterial blood analysis, prior to transfer to the intensive care unit (ICU), revealed pH 7.36, PaCO$_2$ 37 mmHg (4.9 kPa), and PaO$_2$ 103 mmHg (13.7 kPa).

Eleven hours after his return from theater he was awake and cooperative, peripherally warm, cardiovascularly stable, not bleeding and had acceptable arterial blood gases and was therefore extubated. Subsequently, he required FiO$_2$ 0.75 and intermittent CPAP to maintain good oxygenation, but was otherwise well and was transferred to the high dependency unit on the third postoperative day.

Over the next 4 days, his respiratory condition deteriorated. He developed bilateral basal pulmonary collapse, abdominal distension and paroxysmal atrial flutter that precipitated left ventricular failure and pulmonary edema. The chest radiograph showed pulmonary edema and transthoracic echo suggested only moderate left ventricular function. He was started empirically on ceftazidime 1 g BD. His diet was supplemented with high energy supplements because of his poor oral intake (due to CPAP requirement and abdominal distension).

By the tenth postoperative day there were fine inspiratory crackles in both mid zones on auscultation and patchy shadowing and prominent vascular markings on the chest X-ray. Central venous access was re-established to aid optimization and an infusion of dopamine 10 μg kg^{-1} min^{-1} commenced. However, on the following day, his respiratory rate gradually increased to 50 min^{-1}, and the SpO$_2$ fell to 80% on 100% oxygen.

The patient was readmitted to the ICU, sedated, reintubated and mechanically ventilated. Pulmonary artery catherization revealed: CI 4.2 l min^{-1} m^{-2}, PCWP 10 mmHg, SVR 720 dyne s cm^{-5}, PVR 220 dyne s cm^{-5} — consistent with a vasodilated, hyperdynamic circulation. An infusion of norepinephrine 0.28 μg kg^{-1} min^{-1} was started. A repeat transthoracic echocardiogram revealed good biventricular function despite right ventricular dilation. Although blood and sputum cultures were negative, an elevated leukocyte count of 25 × 10^9 l^{-1} prompted the administration of ciprofloxacin 400 mg BD and co-amoxiclav 1.2 g TDS. The patient was placed on a supine rotation bed (Respicair, Hill-Rom Co. Inc., East Batesville, IN, USA) to facilitate lateral and prone ventilation.

Within a short period of time copious quantities of purulent secretions were aspirated from the airways and respiratory function rapidly deteriorated. Respiratory support was escalated to pressure controlled ventilation with a peak inspiratory pressure (PIP) 24 cmH$_2$O, PEEP 12 cmH$_2$O, respiratory rate 15 and inverse inspiratory:expiratory (I:E) ratio 2:1. The patient was paralyzed with atracurium 20–40 mg h^{-1}. Arterial blood gas analysis with FiO$_2$ 0.85 revealed pH 7.37, PaO$_2$ 71 mmHg (9.5 kPa), PaCO$_2$ 57 mmHg (7.6 kPa).

A 24-hour trial of continuous prostacyclin administration 40 μg h^{-1} by nebulizer had no beneficial effect on either oxygenation or PVR. Similarly, a trial of prone ventilation had no effect on oxygenation. An infusion of glyceryl trinitrate 1–5 mg h^{-1} was started and frusemide 10 mg h^{-1} administered to achieve a negative fluid balance. Despite a urine output of 80 to 100 ml h^{-1}, the serum concentrations of urea and creatinine rose to 87 mg dl^{-1} (31 mmol l^{-1}) and 2.5 mg dl^{-1} (220 μmol.l^{-1}) respectively.

Gram-negative organisms were seen on urine microscopy and a single dose of gentamicin 160 mg was recommended by the microbiologists. In view of the absence of any improvement in respiratory function the dose of ceftazidime was increased to 2 g BD. Blood cultures drawn at the end of the first week yielded a mixture of coagulase negative *Staphylococci* and *Streptococci*. All invasive lines were changed and vancomycin 1 g BD started.

At the beginning of the second week in the ICU the patient had become cardiovascularly more stable. The dose of dopamine had been reduced to 3 μg kg^{-1} min^{-1} and the norepinephrine infusion had been stopped. Oxygen requirement had decreased to 60% and peak airway pressures had decreased to a level where it was possible to stop the atracurium infusion. By the end of the second week, however, this improvement had reversed. The patient was reparalyzed, PIP increased to 28 cmH$_2$O and FiO$_2$ to 0.7. Although elevated levels of arterial CO$_2$ had previously been accepted, they now were not allowed to exceed 60 mmHg (8 kPa). The chest radiograph now demonstrated a classical ARDS pattern — bilateral pulmonary infiltrates in all quadrants. A CT scan of the chest showed diffuse ground glass pulmonary opacity, some long-standing fibrosis with areas of potentially reversible inflammation.

Continuing cardiovascular instability necessitated epinephrine 0.1 μg kg^{-1} min^{-1} and the reintroduction of norepinephrine 0.05 μg kg^{-1} min^{-1}. Gentamicin (210 mg loading dose and then dosed according to blood levels) was added to the antibiotic regime because of the persistent sepsis. By the end of the third week, there was little in the way of focal signs of pulmonary infection, although pulmonary compliance and gas exchange remained poor. All antibiotics were stopped and it was decided to administer a course of methylprednisolone 35 mg QDS.

Although some weaning of respiratory support was possible during the following week, he remained on 50% oxygen, PIP 22 cmH$_2$O with PEEP 10 and PaO$_2$ 71 mmHg (9.5 kPa). A percutaneous tracheostomy was performed at the end of the fourth week using a Seldinger technique with fiberoptic confirmation of position.

During the fifth week purulent sputum was produced, and ventilatory requirements increased again. Methicillin-resistant *Staphylococcus aureus* (MRSA) was isolated from the sputum and vancomycin 1 g BD and ceftazidime 2 g BD were restarted. Methylprednisolone was gradually withdrawn over the following week. At the end of the fifth week the sternum became unstable necessitating a return to the operating theater for rewiring.

During the sixth week the patient developed a left-sided simple pneumothorax which was treated with an intercostal tube drain. Ten days later another left sided pneumothorax occurred, which was loculated and required the insertion of two further intercostal tubes.

On day 54 respiratory function abruptly deteriorated — with SpO$_2$ dropping to 60% on 100% oxygen. A chest X-ray revealed a totally opaque left lung field. Urgent rigid bronchoscopy revealed an extensive blood clot occluding the left main bronchus. This was removed manually, but shortly after the procedure the patient developed electromechanical dissociation and could not be resuscitated. A post mortem examination was not performed.

Discussion

Acute respiratory distress syndrome is the most severe manifestation of acute lung injury. The American-European Consensus Conference (AECC) on ARDS defined the spectrum of lung injury to allow consistency in epidemiological and clinical studies. ARDS is diagnosed in a patient with acute onset refractory hypoxemia (PaO$_2$/FiO$_2$ $\leq$200 mmHg/27 kPa) in the presence of bilateral pulmonary infiltrates on the chest radiograph, with no cardiogenic cause (PCWP <18 mmHg). If the hypoxemia is less severe (i.e. PaO$_2$/FiO$_2$ $\leq$300 mmHg/40 kPa) the pulmonary dysfunction is defined as acute lung injury (ALI).[1] Murray and colleagues[2] have expanded this definition taking into account lung compliance, the amount of positive end expiratory pressure (PEEP), the degree of hypoxemia and the number of quadrants involved on chest X-ray. The lung injury score derived indicates whether the patient has: (i) no injury; (ii) mild to moderate injury (ALI); or (iii) severe injury (ARDS).

The incidence of ARDS following CPB in adults is reported to be 0.5–2.5%.[3–5] Mortality in this setting may be dictated by the etiology. ARDS resulting from direct trauma to the lungs may have a better outcome than lung injury that is the pulmonary manifestation of systemic inflammation (e.g. sepsis). Consequently, the mortality from ARDS following CPB has been quoted in the range 28–90%,[3–5] but the latter rate is noted to be in the presence of multiorgan failure.

Etiology

The features of ARDS are due to inflammatory damage to the endothelium of the pulmonary microvasculature. Increased microvascular permeability allows accumulation of interstitial fluid that causes intrapulmonary shunting, hypoxia and respiratory failure. The exact mechanism by which CPB can cause a systemic inflammatory response and ARDS is not fully understood, but is likely to involve a combination of humoral and cellular components.[6–8] The inflammatory response is possibly triggered by a combination of blood coming into contact with foreign surfaces (i.e. elements of the extracorporeal circuit), the development of end-organ (i.e. gut) ischemia and subsequent reperfusion injury, endotoxemia and direct operative trauma.

When blood comes into contact with foreign material it causes activation of complement (via classical and alternate pathways) and neutrophils. C5a attracts neutrophils and promotes their adhesion to vascular endothelium by stimulating expression of P-selectin (an adhesion molecule). The 'primed' neutrophils are sequestered in the pulmonary vasculature where they release inflammatory mediators including interleukins, interferons, colony stimulating factor, tumor necrosis factor (TNF) and leukemia inhibitory factors. These cytokines not only propagate the inflammatory response, but also cause localized tissue damage. Serine proteases, such as elastase and matrix metalloproteinases, are released by the injured tissue leading to a breakdown of components of the extracellular matrix (e.g. elastin and basement membrane collagen type IV). The microvascular endothelium is damaged, manifested as increased permeability. This change is exacerbated by the release of oxygen-derived free radicals by activated neutrophils. These moieties oxidize α_1-antiprotease, which normally inhibits elastase activity.

Endotoxin, a lipopolysaccharide derived from Gram-negative organisms, is a potent trigger of the inflammatory cascade. Levels of endotoxin in the blood are elevated following CPB. This elevation is associated with hemodynamic compromise and aortic cross-clamp (ischemic) time, suggesting that decreased splanchnic blood flow may lead to increased bacterial translocation. Endotoxin also stimulates increased levels of the inducible form of nitric oxide synthase (iNOS).

Nitric oxide, in addition to its role in systemic smooth muscle relaxation and myocardial depression, is implicated in ALI. Increased levels of iNOS have been demonstrated in human lungs following CPB.[9]

As the pathophysiology of ARDS following CPB is elucidated preventative measures against each contributing stage are suggested. Because the inflammatory response may be triggered by contact with components of the extracorporeal circuit, modifications have been tried to minimize this effect. Hemoconcentration filters remove inflammatory cytokines and may modify the response. No difference has been demonstrated between membrane and bubble oxygenators. Heparin-bonded circuits have been shown to decrease cytokine release and neutrophil activation, but there are no outcome studies at present. Pulsatile perfusion flow has not demonstrated any benefit. The outcome studies looking at normothermic and hypothermic bypass have conflicting results.

Modification of the inflammatory process may be targeted at both cellular and humoral components. Because of the difficulties surrounding neutrophil depletion, agents that target neutrophil-specific terminal effectors have been suggested as a strategy to combat the development of ARDS.[10] The effects of matrix metalloproteinases and elastase may be inhibited by a chemically modified tetracycline (CMT–3) which, in a pig model of CPB-induced ARDS, has been shown to prevent the pathological changes associated with ALI. Positive findings in animal models do not necessarily make a significant clinical difference in humans. For example, liposomal prostaglandin E_1 modulates neutrophil activation and decreases neutrophil-mediated inflammation in animal models. When used in humans, however, it had no effect on duration of mechanical ventilation or 28-day survival despite improving indices of oxygenation.[11]

Protease inhibitors such as aprotinin decrease kinin release during cardiac surgery and may decrease neutrophil accumulation in the lungs, but outcome studies are awaited.[12] Drugs that decrease production of TNF or antagonize its effects (antibodies or soluble receptors) have not demonstrated any useful effect. Corticosteroids modify many parts of the inflammatory pathway including decreased release and synthesis of TNFα, decreased expression of endothelial selectins, decreased expression of integrins by neutrophils and decreased nitric oxide production. Despite these effects, outcome studies are needed to demonstrate clinical efficacy. The choice of opioids in anesthesia for cardiac surgery may be based on hemodynamic and analgesic considerations. But the choice of opioids and timing of their administration may affect the inflammatory response.[13]

Investigations

1. Plain chest X-rays are important in the diagnosis and tracking the progression of ARDS, but may miss abscesses, mediastinal emphysema and pneumothorax.
2. CT scans may be useful if the patient's condition does not improve or starts to deteriorate.
3. Bronchoscopy and lavage is useful to determine microbiological sensitivities or absence of infection if steroid use is being considered.[14]
4. Routine 'blood picture'/biochemistry.

Management

Currently, management of ARDS is predominantly supportive. The aims are to maximize gas exchange and minimize pulmonary trauma, which in itself may stimulate a systematic inflammatory response.[15] As with all ventilated patients, it is important to avoid nosocomial infection. Good nutrition must be maintained in this catabolic state and, as there is increased microvascular permeability, a negative fluid balance is desirable.[14]

Ventilatory strategies have been extensively investigated, but whilst many studies have shown improved results in interim outcome (e.g. improved oxygenation and duration of ventilatory support) few have looked at their effect on mortality and hospital discharge. Strategies for avoiding pulmonary trauma (volutrauma and barotrauma) have evolved from CT scan studies demonstrating that in ARDS the lung has normal areas, collapsed areas (available for recruitment) and areas of consolidation and necrosis.[16] Smaller tidal volumes (10 ml kg^{-1}) are advocated to minimize the distending and shearing forces on alveoli by

limiting mean transalveolar pressures to less than 35 cmH_2O.[17–19] A prospective randomized controlled trial by the ARDS Network[20] revealed that using tidal volumes of 6 ml kg^{-1} resulted in a 22% reduction in mortality and a decrease in the number of days ventilated when compared with a control group. Positive end expiratory pressure (PEEP) is used to recruit collapsed areas of lung and this is believed to redistribute the tidal volume leading to an increase in overall lung compliance.[21] The use of permissive hypercapnia (allowing higher than normal $PaCO_2$, provided that acidemia is not excessive) and accepting PaO_2 as low as 60 mmHg (8 kPa) gives greater flexibility in the use of protective ventilatory strategies.

The prone position can improve oxygenation in severe ARDS. This is due to increased regional ventilation without alteration to the distribution of blood flow. It has little affect on hemodynamics and is a safe maneuver providing adequate protocols and safeguards are in place.[22, 23] Unfortunately there is, at present, no way to predict which patients will respond to this stategy, but as non-responders do not seem to be detrimentally affected it may be worth assessing the response in every patient with ARDS and refractory hypoxia. Long-term outcome studies have not been conducted.

Inhaled therapy with nitric oxide or nebulized prostacyclin has been shown to improve oxygenation.[24, 25] These agents dilate the pulmonary vasculature in ventilated areas of lungs and decrease ventilation–perfusion mismatch. Neither has been shown to have long-term benefit. Techniques that have a place in neonatal and pediatric practice, such as high frequency ventilation and extracorporeal membrane oxygenation have not yet been shown to have a beneficial effect in adults.

Conclusions and learning points

- Acute respiratory distress syndrome following CPB in adults occurs in 1–2% patients and has a mortality of up to 90%.
- Patients invariably succumb to multi-organ failure rather than respiratory failure.
- Adoption of the AECC definitions of ARDS and ALI allows data from different studies to be compared.

- Despite over three decades of intense research, protective lung ventilation is the only management strategy shown to decrease mortality from ARDS (Table 35.1).[26]
- Other management strategies may improve intermediate measures of outcome, but have little effect on mortality.

References

1. Bernard GR, Artigas A, Brigham KL et al. The American-European Consensus Conference on ARDS. Definitions, mechanisms, relevant outcomes, and clinical trial coordination. Am J Respir Crit Care Med 1994;149:818–24.

2. Murray JF, Matthay MA, Luce JM, Flick MR. An expanded definition of the adult respiratory distress syndrome. Am Rev Respir Dis 1988;138:720–3 [Erratum in Am Rev Respir Dis 1989;139:65].

3. Kaul TK, Fields BL, Riggins LS et al. Adult respiratory distress syndrome following cardiopulmonary bypass: incidence, prophylaxis and management. J Cardiovasc Surg (Torino) 1998;39:777–81.

4. Asimakopoulos G, Taylor KM, Smith PL, Ratnatunga CP. Prevalence of acute respiratory distress syndrome after cardiac surgery. J Thorac Cardiovasc Surg 1999;117:620–1.

5. Asimakopoulos G, Smith PL, Ratnatunga CP, Taylor KM. Lung injury and acute respiratory distress

Table 35.1 The evidence for various management strategies in ARDS (constructed from McIntyre et al).[26]

Management strategy	Level of evidence	Recommendation
Ventilation		
Non-invasive positive pressure	2,4	C
Lung protective strategies	1,2	B
Inverse ratio	3,4	D
Prone	3	D
Partial liquid	4	E
ECMO	Conflicting results	More studies needed
Fluid restriction ± diuretics	2	C
Pharmacological		
Surfactant	3	C
Non-selective vasodilation	Not stated	Limited use — systemic side effects
Nitric oxide	1	No effect on outcome
Almitrine	3	C
Prostacycline	3	C
Immune modulators		
Prostaglandin E_1	1	No effect on outcome
Ketoconazole	1,2	No effect on outcome
Antioxidants	2	Mixed results
Steroids	2	C

Levels of Evidence
Level 1 Large, randomized, prospective controlled investigations
Level 2 Small, randomized, prospective controlled investigations with uncertain results
Level 3 Non-randomized, concurrent, or historical cohort investigations
Level 4 Peer-reviewed state-of-the-art articles, review articles, editorials or substantial case series
Level 5 Non peer-reviewed published opinions, such as textbook statements or official organizational publications

Recommendations
A. Convincingly justifiable on scientific evidence alone
B. Justifiable by available scientific evidence
C. Reasonably justifiable by available scientific evidence and strongly supported by expert critical care opinion
D. Adequate scientific evidence is lacking but widely supported by available data and expert critical care opinion
E. No scientific data exists to justify support

syndrome after cardiopulmonary bypass. *Ann Thorac Surg* 1999;**68**:1107–15.

6. Miller BE, Levy JH. The inflammatory response to cardiopulmonary bypass. *J Cardiothorac Vasc Anesth* 1997;**11**:355–66.

7. Shah PK. Targeting the proteolytic arsenal of neutrophils. A promising approach for postpump syndrome and ARDS. *Circulation* 1999;**100**:333–4.

8. Hall RI, Smith MS, Rocker G. The systemic inflammatory response to cardiopulmonary bypass: pathophysiological, therapeutic, and pharmacological considerations. *Anesth Analg* 1997;**85**:766–82.

9. Delgado R, Rojas A, Glaria LA *et al.* Ca^{2+}-independent nitric oxide synthase activity in human lung after cardiopulmonary bypass. *Thorax* 1995;**50**:403–4.

10. Carney DE, Lutz CJ, Picone AL *et al.* Matrix metalloproteinase inhibitor prevents acute lung injury after cardiopulmonary bypass. *Circulation* 1999;**100**:400–6.

11. Abraham E, Baughman R, Fletcher E *et al.* Liposomal prostaglandin E1 (TLC C–53) in acute respiratory distress syndrome: a controlled, randomized, double-blind, multicenter clinical trial. TLC C–53 ARDS Study Group. *Crit Care Med* 1999;**27**:1478–85.

12. Hill GE, Pohorecki R, Alonso A *et al.* Aprotinin reduces interleukin-8 production and lung neutrophil accumulation after cardiopulmonary bypass. *Anesth Analg* 1996;**83**:696–700.

13. Scott BH. Opioids in cardiac surgery: cardiopulmonary bypass and inflammatory response. *Int J Cardiol* 1998;**64 (Suppl 1)**:S35–41.

14. Wyncoll DL, Evans TW. Acute respiratory distress syndrome. *Lancet* 1999;**354**:497–501.

15. Berthiaume Y, Lesur O, Dagenais A. Treatment of adult respiratory distress syndrome: plea for rescue therapy of the alveolar epithelium. *Thorax* 1999;**54**:150–60.

16. Gattinoni L, Bombino M, Pelosi P *et al.* Lung structure and function in different stages of severe adult respiratory distress syndrome. *JAMA* 1994;**271**:1772–9.

17. Brower RG, Shanholtz CB, Fessler HE *et al.* Prospective, randomized, controlled clinical trial comparing traditional versus reduced tidal volume ventilation in acute respiratory distress syndrome patients. *Crit Care Med* 1999;**27**:1492–8.

18. Slutsky AS. Consensus conference on mechanical ventilation—January 28–30, 1993 at Northbrook, Illinois, USA. Part 1. European Society of Intensive Care Medicine, the ACCP and the SCCM. *Intensive Care Med* 1994;**20**:64–79 [erratum in *Intensive Care Med* 1994;**20**:378].

19. Slutsky AS. Consensus conference on mechanical ventilation — January 28–30, 1993 at Northbrook, Illinois, USA. Part 2. *Intensive Care Med* 1994;**20**:150–62.

20. The Acute Respiratory Distress Syndrome Network. Ventilation with lower tidal volumes as compared with traditional tidal volumes for acute lung injury and the acute respiratory distress syndrome. *N Engl J Med* 2000;**342**:1301–8.

21. Pesenti A, Fumagalli R. PEEP: blood gas cosmetics or a therapy for ARDS? *Crit Care Med* 1999;**27**:253–4.

22. Trottier SJ. Prone position in acute respiratory distress syndrome: turning over an old idea. *Crit Care Med* 1998;**26**:1934–5.

23. Jolliet P, Bulpa P, Chevrolet JC. Effects of the prone position on gas exchange and hemodynamics in severe acute respiratory distress syndrome. *Crit Care Med* 1998;**26**:1977–85.

24. Lundin S, Mang H, Smithies M *et al.* Inhalation of nitric oxide in acute lung injury: results of a European multicentre study. The European Study Group of Inhaled Nitric Oxide. *Intensive Care Med* 1999;**25**:911–9.

25. Zwissler B, Kemming G, Habler O *et al.* Inhaled prostacyclin (PGI_2) versus inhaled nitric oxide in adult respiratory distress syndrome. *Am J Respir Crit Care Med* 1996;**154**:1671–7.

26. McIntyre RC Jr, Pulido EJ, Bensard DD *et al.* Thirty years of clinical trials in acute respiratory distress syndrome. *Crit Care Med* 2000;**28**:**33**14–31.

Suggested further reading

Ware LB, Matthay MA. Medical progress: the acute respiratory distress syndrome. *N Engl J Med* 2000;**342**:1334–49.

36

High frequency oscillatory ventilation

Heather P Duncan and Andrew R Wolf

Introduction

High frequency oscillatory ventilation (HFOV) is a useful tool in the treatment of respiratory failure in children. A child with tricuspid and pulmonary atresia developed severe hypoxic respiratory failure secondary to infection in the postoperative period following a cavopulmonary shunt. She was successfully treated with HFOV. The discussion that follows explores the role of HFOV in the pediatric age group for respiratory failure and following cardiac surgery.

Case report

A 15-month-old female infant was admitted for an elective right bi-directional cavopulmonary (Glenn) shunt. Following an uneventful term gestation and the spontaneous onset of labor, she had been delivered by ventouse extraction because of fetal distress. At delivery Apgar scores were 8 at 1 minute and 10 at 5 minutes and she required no resuscitation. She remained with her mother on the postnatal ward until her routine first day examination when she was found to be tachypneic and cyanosed with a peripheral oxygen saturation of 40% while breathing 100% oxygen, but clinically not in cardiac failure. She had oligemic lung fields on chest radiograph and a left axis on ECG. Cyanotic congenital heart disease was suspected, an infusion of prostaglandin E_1 10 ng kg^{-1} min^{-1} was started and she was transferred by ambulance to the regional tertiary neonatal intensive care unit (ICU). The diagnosis, confirmed by transthoracic echocardiography, was an atrioseptal defect, with tricuspid and pulmonary atresia. The ventricular septum was intact. She required ventilation because of apnea associated with the prostaglandin infusion but was otherwise stable. A right modified Blalock–Taussig shunt (RMBTS) was performed on day 3 to improve pulmonary blood flow. The modification consisted of a 4 mm Goretex shunt placed between the subclavian and pulmonary arteries in contrast to the original described operation, which connected the subclavian artery directly into the pulmonary artery. The procedure was complicated by a small pericardial effusion, that did not require drainage, and a right Horner's

Past medical history	Term gestation. Ventouse delivery for fetal distress. Cyanosed on day 1. Right modified BT shunt on day 3 complicated by right Horner's syndrome and right pulmonary stenosis. Gastroesophageal reflux. No known drug allergies.
Regular medications	Frusemide 1 mg kg^{-1} BD, Gaviscon QDS, cisapride 0.2 mg kg^{-1} QDS.
Examination	Weight 6 kg. Tachypneic. Jugular veins distended. Hepatomegaly. Widespread bilateral inspiratory crackles.
Investigations	**CXR**: Oligemic lung fields. **Transthoracic Echo**: Atrial septal defect, tricuspid and pulmonary atresia, right pulmonary artery stenosis. **ECG**: Left axis deviation.

syndrome. She recovered well and was discharged home at 27 days old on frusemide 1 mg kg^{-1} BD and treatment for gastroesophageal reflux (GER) that included Gaviscon and cisapride 0.2 mg kg^{-1} QDS. She remained well on the same medication, adjusted for weight, until, at 13 months of age cardiac failure caused failure to thrive. Echocardiography at this time demonstrated a restrictive atrioseptal defect. In addition, cardiac catheterization revealed stenosis of the right pulmonary artery at the shunt anastomosis site. The atrioseptal defect was enlarged by balloon septostomy after which, the cardiac failure resolved. Weight gain remained poor secondary to GER and feeding difficulties.

At 15 months of age, weighing 6 kg, she was admitted for an elective Glenn shunt, left pulmonary artery reconstruction and atrial septectomy. Following an uneventful procedure, she was weaned rapidly from inotropic support (dopamine 5 µg kg^{-1} min^{-1}) and extubated 6 hours after surgery. Right middle lobe collapse-consolidation, diagnosed on the first postoperative day, was treated with physiotherapy and cefuroxime. On the second postoperative day she had good peripheral perfusion with oxygen saturations of 86% in room air and was discharged to the general pediatric ward. Her medication included oral digoxin 30 µg BD, phenoxybenzamine 3 mg TDS, frusemide 6 mg BD, spironolactone 6 mg BD, aspirin 30 mg OD, cisapride 1.5 mg TDS and intravenous cefuroxime 180 mg TDS.

On the fourth postoperative day she developed a fever of 39°C associated with a tonic-clonic, febrile seizure. She was cyanosed with SaO$_2$ 60% in 100% oxygen, not in cardiac failure and had a clearly audible shunt flow murmur. Clinical examination did not reveal an obvious source of infection. The chest radiograph and blood biochemistry were unchanged. A raised C-reactive protein of 85 mg dl^{-1} (normal <10 mg dl^{-1}) and platelet count of 65 × 10^9 l^{-1} supported the diagnosis of infection and intravenous flucloxacillin 180 mg QDS was started.

On the fifth postoperative day she was readmitted to the pediatric ICU following two further seizures and a respiratory arrest. She remained pyrexial and hypoxic (SpO$_2$ 65%; FiO$_2$ 1.0) with a blood pressure of 80/60 mmHg. A prolonged episode of apnea precipitated intubation, pressure cycled ventilation (PCV) and inotropic support with dopamine up to 15 µg kg^{-1} min^{-1} and epinephrine 0.1 µg kg^{-1} min^{-1}. She was sedated with fentanyl 4–8 µg kg^{-1} h^{-1}, paralysed with vecuronium 60 µg kg^{-1} h^{-1} and anticoagulated with heparin 10 iu kg^{-1} h^{-1}. A full septic screen, including full blood count, C-reactive protein, blood cultures, lumbar puncture, virology and microbiology investigation of urine, nasopharyngeal, endotracheal and stool samples, was performed. Computed tomography of her brain was normal. Transthoracic echocardiography demonstrated a patent Glenn shunt, excluded a pericardial effusion and confirmed adequate cardiac function. These findings were confirmed when further marked deterioration in the blood pressure and saturations initiated an emergency sternotomy in pediatric ICU.

Clinically a respiratory infection was the most likely diagnosis despite the normal chest radiograph. Norwalk virus was isolated from the stool. Coagulase-negative staphylococci, *Klebsiella pneumoniae*, and *Neisseria* species were isolated from the nasopharyngeal aspirate necessitating the addition of intravenous gentamicin 15 mg TDS.

Respiratory failure persisted (pH 7.17, PaCO$_2$ 81 mmHg (10.8 kPa), PaO$_2$ 52 mmHg (6.9 kPa)) on PCV despite peak inspiratory pressures of 32 cmH$_2$O and 100% oxygen. She deteriorated further and it was doubtful whether she would survive. A trial of nitric oxide up to 40 ppm was unhelpful. Despite increasing the peak airway pressure up to 40 cmH$_2$O and using a variety of respiratory rates (15–50 breaths per minute) using PCV mechanical and hand ventilation, adequate oxygenation could not be maintained. The best oxygen saturation was eventually achieved by applying rapid hand ventilation approaching 6 Hz with high flow oxygen (15 l min^{-1}) and an Ayre's T-piece. The settings on a high frequency oscillatory ventilator (SensorMedics 3100A SensorMedics Critical Care; Yorba Linda, CA, USA) were carefully adjusted to closely mimic this rapid hand ventilation. She settled on a frequency of 8 Hz, inspiratory time 33% (41 mS), mean airway pressure (MAP) 12 cmH$_2$O and delta pressure (amplitude of oscillation) of 30. Oxygenation improved and the respiratory acidosis corrected over the next 7 hours. HFOV was continued for a further 48 hours before weaning on PCV.

On the eighth day after surgery, left lower lobe pneumonia was evident on the chest radiograph and Influenza A was isolated from the naso pharynx. Amantidine 25 mg day^{-1} replaced the antibiotics. During this time she was fully nasogastrically fed and her infective markers returned to normal.

On the twelfth postoperative day, she had weaned to pressures of 16/4 cmH$_2$O, inspiratory time of 0.7 seconds and a rate of 5 breaths per minute and was successfully extubated. She made a full recovery and was discharged back to her referring district general hospital twenty-nine days after surgery. She has remained well with normal neurodevelopment and growth at follow-up. At age 5 she had a total cavopulmonary shunt (Fontan procedure), which was uneventful.

In summary, a 15-month-old girl with a univentricular heart developed severe respiratory failure secondary to viral pneumonia in the postoperative period following a bidirectional cavopulmonary shunt. Rescue HFOV maintained oxygenation without cardiovascular compromize during recovery.

Discussion

The main challenge in this case was maintaining adequate oxygenation and hemodynamic stability.

Tricuspid and pulmonary atresia produce the pathophysiology of a univentricular heart. A cavopulmonary (Glenn) shunt connects the superior vena cava to the pulmonary artery. A total cavopulmonary shunt (Fontan procedure) connects the inferior vena cava to the pulmonary artery. Pulmonary blood flow is therefore completely dependent on passive venous return through the shunts. Respiratory failure caused by viral pneumonia often requires high inspiratory pressures to maintain adequate oxygenation. However, high intrathoracic pressures in this case following a cavopulmonary shunt decreased venous return, thereby reducing pulmonary arterial blood flow and compromising oxygenation. A balance must be achieved to ensure adequate perfusion of the lungs and alveolar ventilation to ensure oxygenation. HFOV provides a continuous distending airway pressure, avoids the high peak pressures of PCV and reduces pulmonary vascular resistance. This allows adequate venous return and pulmonary perfusion and at the same time maintains alveolar recruitment for gas exchange.

HFOV was required for a period of only 48 hours in this case and the patient could have been weaned directly to continuous positive airway pressure (CPAP) instead of changing back to PCV. The reason for reverting back to conventional ventilation was to improve lung toilet by regular endotracheal suction. More recently, routine in-line suction has decreased the need for weaning on PCV.

This case highlights the key advantages of HFOV providing a useful rescue treatment by avoidance of high peak pressures that compromise venous return and optimization of the ventilation perfusion ratio to improve oxygenation.

High frequency ventilation

High frequency ventilation (HFV) can be delivered by an oscillator that applies positive and negative pressure to the lungs (HFOV); a rapid firing jet of gas at the end of an endotracheal tube (HFJV); or by a high frequency flow interrupter that works like a conventional ventilator but at high speed. It is not clear whether there are any clinical advantages between the types of HFV. A comparative study in piglets showed no hemodynamic difference between conventional mandatory ventilation (CMV), HFOV, HFJV and external negative pressure oscillation combined with pressure support ventilation during induced periods of pulmonary and cardiac failure.[1] During the pulmonary failure period, transpulmonary pressure was higher in the HFOV group than in the other modes of ventilation. There have been concerns about HFJV in premature infants causing neurological damage and increased mortality resulted in the trial being terminated early.[2, 3]

High frequency oscillatory ventilation

HFOV delivers low tidal volumes (1–3.6 ml kg^{-1}) at supraphysiological frequencies. In premature neonates with infant respiratory distress syndrome (IRDS) it has been shown to decrease the incidence of chronic lung disease when compared with conventional ventilation. Clinical trials in neonates show that HFOV produces better oxygenation and fewer complications when a high or optimal volume strategy is used.[4, 5] When initiating HFOV, MAP is usually set 3–5 cmH$_2$O higher than PCV and increased until the optimum lung volume is reached and oxygenation improves. A constant distending pressure promotes alveolar recruitment, improves gas exchange and reduces shearing stresses between expanded and collapsed lung units. In the neonatal age group frequency is usually set between 10 –15 Hz, older children often require 5–10 Hz.

Beyond the neonatal age group there are two groups of pulmonary disease amenable to HFOV: diffuse alveolar disease and air leak syndrome. The initial settings for HFOV are similar in both. In diffuse alveolar disease MAP is increased until optimum lung volume is achieved, FiO$_2$ is then decreased aiming for a reduction from 1.0 to less than 0.6. In 'air-leak syndrome', adequate oxygenation is achieved on regular settings and then the MAP is decreased until the air leak stops. It may be necessary to allow higher inspired oxygen for a period of time.

The principles of HFOV, including the use of a high volume strategy in children, are based on information obtained from animal and neonatal studies. In children and adults HFOV has been used safely and effectively as a rescue treatment.[6–8] A prospective, randomized trial comparing HFOV and CMV in 58 children showed that the HFOV group had improved oxygenation and a decreased requirement for oxygen at 30 days.[9] Initiating HFOV within 24 hours of mechanical ventilation in 26 patients (aged between 1 month and 24 years) appeared to improve survival from 12.5% to 58.8%.[10] Adults with inadequate ventilation on CMV had improved gas exchange without compromising oxygen delivery or cardiac output on HFOV.[11]

A reduction in chronic lung disease following HFOV is attributed to less barotrauma, a reduction in shearing forces and oxygen toxicity. Pressure measured at the airway opening appears to be much lower than that delivered to the alveoli and small airways.[12, 13] A comparison of I:E ratio indicates that this drop-off in pressure occurs with an I:E ratio of 1:2 but not with a ratio of 1:1.[14]

Hemodynamics

There is a concern that the high MAP associated with HFOV could compromise cardiovascular function. Animal and premature infant studies have found that at the same MAP, HFOV improves cardiac output, oxygenation (PaO$_2$/FiO$_2$ ratio) and CO$_2$ elimination when compared to CMV,[15–19] but increasing MAP during HFOV can reduce cardiac output.[17, 18] Studies in children using an optimum volume strategy showed no adverse effects on cardiac index, mean arterial blood pressure, peripheral and systemic vascular resistance.[6, 9, 13, 20, 21, 22] The key is to prevent overdistension by increasing MAP until, but not beyond the optimal volume. The chest radiograph gives guidance on under- or over-inflation of the lungs. Optimal expansion is achieved when eight or nine ribs are visible posteriorly in the absence of intercostal bulging and diaphragmatic flattening. Improved alveolar recruitment improves pulmonary ventilation and reduces pulmonary vascular resistance thereby improving perfusion. This reduces intrapulmonary shunting and improves oxygenation.

HFOV following cardiac surgery

Maintenance of venous return and transpulmonary gradient were critical to oxygenation in this patient and provided a greater challenge than respiratory disease alone. Reports in the literature on HFOV in the postoperative cardiac patient are encouraging.

Hemodynamic responses to flow-interrupted HFOV 2–48 hours following cardiac surgery in six infants (five ventricular septal defect (VSD) closure, one total anomalous pulmonary venous drainage (TAPVD) correction) aged 1–8 months were studied using the same MAP on HFOV and CMV.[13] There were no clinically significant changes in heart rate, systemic and pulmonary artery pressure, cardiac index, or systemic and pulmonary vascular resistance.

The hemodynamic responses in dogs with open and closed chests have been compared during both CMV and HFJV.[23] No clinically significant differences in gas exchange, pulmonary capillary wedge pressure, pulmonary and systemic arterial pressure, vascular resistance and cardiac index were demonstrated. Physiologically, ventilation was adequate and peak and mean airway pressures were similar. There was a decrease in both PaO_2 and $PaCO_2$ when the chest was open that did not cause clinical compromise.

Thirteen children (0.9–8.5 years) were studied prospectively to determine whether HFJV would improve cardiac output after the Fontan procedure.[24] The study succeeded in demonstrating that by reducing intrathoracic pressures, HFJV enhanced pulmonary blood flow and thereby improved hemodynamics. There was no difference in gas exchange and HFJV resulted in a 50% reduction in MAP, 59% reduction in pulmonary vascular resistance and a 25% increase in cardiac index. Unfortunately only a short study period is reported without long-term outcomes.

Case reports show favorable outcome using high volume strategy HFOV in the postoperative period. Two term infants with open chests following arterial switch procedures complicated by pulmonary hemorrhage did not require any additional inotropic or volume support during the transition to HFOV and survived with good outcomes.[25] A 3-month-old infant was successfully treated with HFOV for pneumomediastinum following closure of a persistent ductus arteriosus.[26]

Limitations of HFOV

Gaining familiarity with the equipment and technique takes time and experience.[2, 27] Pneumothoraces are reported but there is no difference in the frequency and grade of a new air leak developing on HFOV and CMV.[4, 7, 9] Limited access to the airway for suctioning can be a problem but the introduction of in-line suction catheters has reduced this problem. Although not universal, neuromuscular blockade is more frequently required in older children. Unlike the early neonatal data using low volume strategies, no adverse neurological events have been reported in children.[9, 18]

HFOV is not the panacea for respiratory failure: not all children respond. In one randomized trial up to 38% of children failed on HFOV, crossed over to CMV and went on to have a mortality rate of 82%.[9] In an adult study only 47% had a 30-day survival.

Most investigators are in agreement that the oxygen index (OI) gives an indication of possible adverse outcome following the transition to HFOV. The OI indicates the pressure and inspired oxygen cost required for oxygenation. An increasing OI over time or an OI that does not continue to decrease after 3 days suggested poor outcome.[9, 18]

HFOV is one of a number of options including HFJV and continuous negative external pressure (CNEP) ventilation that are useful ventilatory modes in patients following cardiac surgery for congenital heart disease. CNEP leads to a reduction in intrathoracic pressure that improves pulmonary blood flow and cardiac output.[28–30]

Conclusions and learning points

- Cardiovascular stability during HFOV is mainly due to two factors:
  1. Avoidance of high peak inspiratory pressures: high peak pressure compromises venous return to the heart and increases intrathoracic pressures. Adequate venous return is imperative for pulmonary blood flow and cardiac output following a cavopulmonary shunt.
  2. Continuous distending pressure: alveolar recruitment is improved and maintained and pulmonary vascular resistance is reduced providing better ventilation–perfusion matching.
- The clinical picture described was hypoxic respiratory failure complicated by sepsis. Decreased venous return and the cavopulmonary shunt circulation, which requires venous blood to flow passively into the pulmonary circulation, made HFOV a more successful form of ventilation. In this circumstance a high intrathoracic pressure caused by high inspiratory pressures of conventional ventilation appeared to compromise cardiovascular stability and, in particular, oxygenation.
- In the vast majority of patients undergoing cardiac surgery CMV is a safe, reliable form of ventilation. Children who have a complicated postoperative course, particularly following cavopulmonary shunts, sometimes require alternative measures and in these circumstances rescue HFOV can be a useful option.

References

1. Zobel G, Dacar D, Rodl S. Hemodynamic effects of different modes of mechanical ventilation in acute cardiac and pulmonary failure: an experimental study. *Crit Care Med* 1994;**22**:1624–30.

2. Marlow N. High frequency ventilation and respiratory distress syndrome: do we have an answer? *Arch Dis Child Fetal Neonatal Ed* 1998;**78**:F1–2.

3. Wiswell TE, Graziani LJ, Kornhauser MS *et al.* High-frequency jet ventilation in the early management of respiratory distress syndrome is associated with a greater risk for adverse outcomes. *Pediatrics* 1996;**98**:1035–43.

4. Gerstmann DR, Minton SD, Stoddard RA *et al.* The Provo multicenter early high-frequency oscillatory ventilation trial: improved pulmonary and clinical outcome in respiratory distress syndrome. *Pediatrics* 1996;**98**:1044–57.

5. Bhuta T, Henderson-Smart DJ. Rescue high frequency oscillatory ventilation versus conventional ventilation for pulmonary dysfunction in preterm infants. *Cochrane Database Syst Rev* 2000;**2**:CD000438.

6. Arnold JH, Truog RD, Thompson JE, Fackler JC. High-frequency oscillatory ventilation in pediatric respiratory failure. *Crit Care Med* 1993;**21**:272–8.

7. Duval EL, Markhorst DG, Gemke RJ, van Vught AJ. High-frequency oscillatory ventilation in pediatric patients. *Neth J Med* 2000;**56**:177–85.

8. Claridge JA, Hostetter RG, Lowson SM, Young JS. High-frequency oscillatory ventilation can be effective as rescue therapy for refractory acute lung dysfunction. *Am Surg* 1999;**65**:1092–6.

9. Arnold JH, Hanson JH, Toro-Figuero LO *et al.* Prospective, randomized comparison of high-frequency oscillatory ventilation and conventional mechanical ventilation in pediatric respiratory failure. *Crit Care Med* 1994;**22**:1530–9.

10. Fedora M, Klimovic M, Seda M *et al.* Effect of early intervention of high-frequency oscillatory ventilation on the outcome in pediatric acute respiratory distress syndrome. *Bratisl Lek Listy* 2000;**101**:8–13.

11. Fort P, Farmer C, Westerman J *et al.* High-frequency oscillatory ventilation for adult respiratory distress syndrome—a pilot study. *Crit Care Med* 1997;**25**:937–47.

12. Gerstmann DR, Fouke JM, Winter DC *et al.* Proximal, tracheal, and alveolar pressures during high-frequency oscillatory ventilation in a normal rabbit model. *Pediatr Res* 1990;**28**:367–73.

13. Vincent RN, Stark AR, Lang P *et al.* Hemodynamic response to high-frequency ventilation in infants following cardiac surgery. *Pediatrics* 1984;**73**:426–30.

14. Pillow JJ, Neil H, Wilkinson MH, Ramsden CA. Effect of I/E ratio on mean alveolar pressure during high-frequency oscillatory ventilation. *J Appl Physiol* 1999;**87**:407–14.

15. Kinsella JP, Gerstmann DR, Clark RH *et al.* High-frequency oscillatory ventilation versus intermittent mandatory ventilation: early hemodynamic effects in the premature baboon with hyaline membrane disease. *Pediatr Res* 1991;**29**:160–6.

16. Mirro R, Tamura M, Kawano T. Systemic cardiac output and distribution during high-frequency oscillation. *Crit Care Med* 1985;**13**:724–7.

17. Mirro R, Busija D, Green R, Leffler C. Relationship between mean airway pressure, cardiac output, and organ blood flow with normal and decreased respiratory compliance. *J Pediatr* 1987;**111**:101–6.

18. Traverse JH, Korvenranta H, Adams EM *et al.* Impairment of hemodynamics with increasing mean airway pressure during high-frequency oscillatory ventilation. *Pediatr Res* 1988;**23**:628–31.

19. Goodman AM, Pollack MM. Hemodynamic effects of high-frequency oscillatory ventilation in children. *Pediatr Pulmonol* 1998;**25**:371–4.

20. Gutierrez JA, Levin DL, Toro-Figueroa LO. Hemodynamic effects of high-frequency oscillatory ventilation in severe pediatric respiratory failure. *Intensive Care Med* 1995;**21**:505–10.

21. Mellema JD, Baden HP, Martin LD, Bratton SL. Severe paroxysmal sinus bradycardia associated with high-frequency oscillatory ventilation. *Chest* 1997;**112**:181–5.

22. Nelle M, Zilow EP, Linderkamp O. Effects of high-frequency oscillatory ventilation on circulation in neonates with pulmonary interstitial emphysema or RDS. *Intensive Care Med* 1997;**23**:671–6.

23. Hoff BH, Smith RB, Bunegin L, Cherry D. High frequency ventilation in dogs with open chests. *Crit Care Med* 1982;**10**:517–21.

24. Shinozaki T, Deane RS, Perkins FM *et al.* Comparison of high-frequency lung ventilation with conventional mechanical lung ventilation. Prospective trial in patients who have undergone cardiac operations. *J Thorac Cardiovasc Surg* 1985;**89**:268–74.

25. Meliones JN, Bove EL, Dekeon MK *et al.* High-frequency jet ventilation improves cardiac function after the Fontan procedure. *Circulation* 1991;**84**:III364–8.

26. Baden HP, Li CM, Hall D *et al.* High-frequency oscillatory ventilation in the management of infants with pulmonary hemorrhage after cardiac surgery. *J Cardiothorac Vasc Anesth* 1995;**9**:578–80.

27. Miyahara K, Ichihara T, Watanabe T. Successful use of high frequency oscillatory ventilation for pneumomediastinum. *Ann Thorac Cardiovasc Surg* 1999;**5**:49–51.

28. Shekerdemian LS, Schulze-Neick I, Redington AN *et al.* Negative pressure ventilation as haemodynamic rescue following surgery for congenital heart disease. *Intensive Care Med* 2000;**26**:93–6.

29. Pierce JM, Jenkins IA, Noyes JP *et al.* The successful use of continuous negative extrathoracic pressure in a child with Glenn shunt and respiratory failure. *Intensive Care Med* 1995;**21**:766–8.

30. Penny DJ, Hayek Z, Redington AN. The effects of positive and negative extrathoracic pressure ventilation on pulmonary blood flow after the total cavopulmonary shunt procedure. *Int J Cardiol* 1991;**30**:128–30.

37
Resuscitation of the multiorgan donor

Christopher J Rozario, M Krishna Prasad and John D Kneeshaw

Introduction

Currently, the demand for donor organs exceeds supply. This has led to a reduction in the number of solid organs transplanted in the United Kingdom.[1] Possible options to ameliorate this situation include the greater use of live donors, changes in legislation to enable greater numbers of organs to be harvested, early donor referral with increased numbers of organs used per donor, a revision of donor acceptance criteria and improved donor management.

This chapter attempts to address the strategies that may be employed to improve the medical management of multiorgan donors in order to increase the number of hearts, lungs and heart lung blocks available for transplantation. A target-directed approach is advocated to optimize donor organ function. Anesthetic physician involvement in managing multiorgan donors may be beneficial in both critical care and operating room environments.

Recognition of the organ donor

The characteristics of an ideal heart donor include a stable cardiac rhythm, maintenance of a good cardiac output with minimal doses of inotropic drugs, and no history of cigarette smoking or ischemic heart disease. For lung donation there should be no chest trauma, minimal bronchial secretions and no radiographic evidence of pulmonary collapse or consolidation. There should be a minimal alveolar to arterial oxygen tension gradient ($D_{A-a}O_2$) and positive pressure lung ventilation should have been used for less than 24 hours. However, not all potential donors are ideal and indicators for poor graft survival have been defined. These include males over 55 years of age, females over 60 years of age, a history of cigarette smoking, hypertension or ischemic heart disease. Other factors predictive of poorer outcome are intuitive: hypoxic episodes; pulmonary aspiration; cardiac arrest; severe metabolic acidosis; significant disparity between right and left atrial filling pressures; left ventricular hypertrophy; and poor hemodynamic performance despite optimization of cardiac filling pressures.

Principles of donor management

Donor organ management cannot begin before confirmation of brain stem death by standardized protocols.[2] Up to 8% of potential donor organs may be lost if the time elapsed between the onset of clinical brain stem death and organ retrieval is protracted.[3, 4]

Once the decision to donate organs has been taken, the emphasis in management changes from intravascular volume contraction, as needed for cerebral protection, to optimal organ perfusion. The need for transfusion should be anticipated since disruption of hemostatic mechanisms occurs as a result of cerebral ischemia. At least 4 units of packed red cells should be available before organ harvesting occurs. After brain stem death, hypothalamic dysfunction results in a poikilothermic state. Cold fluids exacerbate hypothermia and active warming measures are necessary to achieve and maintain a core temperature greater than 35°C.

Cardiovascular management

Hypotension secondary to impaired myocardial function, reduced vascular tone, and dehydration must be reversed to ensure adequate organ perfusion. Multiple electrocardiograph (ECG) abnormalities, which are rarely a cause for concern, occur at the time of brain stem death.[5] However, if these are associated with hemodynamic instability, they should be treated. Hypovolemia is the commonest cause of hypotension and inadequate cardiac output. Adequate intravascular volume replacement should precede the institution of inotropic therapy but a critical balance exists.

In order to prevent intravascular volume overload and achieve target values for organ donation invasive hemodynamic monitoring is required. A pulmonary artery flotation catheter (PAFC) allows quantitative assessment of cardiac function and can be used to monitor the response to therapeutic maneuvers.[6] A mean arterial pressure of 60–70 mmHg should be achieved with a pulmonary artery occlusion pressure of less than 12 mmHg. This should result in a cardiac index of 2.2–2.5 l min^{-1} m^{-2}. A hematocrit of 30% with a hemoglobin concentration of 10 g dl^{-1} is maintained with packed red blood cells and colloid as necessary. In the rare event of volume overload, venesection may be necessary. Dextrose saline (0.18% sodium chloride and 4% dextrose) and potassium chloride are administered to replace normal urinary water and electrolyte losses. In order to maintain a systemic vascular resistance of 800–1200 dyne s cm^{-5} a low-dose, synergistic combination of infusions of antidiuretic hormone (ADH) and epinephrine has been advocated.[7] Early commencement of ADH will prevent excessive diuresis. Some donors will have been treated with desmopressin (I-desamino–8-D-arginine vasopressin, DDAVP), to control diabetes insipidus associated with brain stem death. This has minimal pressor activity and should be replaced by arginine vasopressin (i.e. ADH), which is a potent vasoconstrictor. If optimal adjustment of preload fails to achieve target values then an inotropic agent such as dopamine may be added to the regime.[8] Less favored agents in this setting include dobutamine and isoprenaline since excessive beta adrenergic stimulation may exacerbate peripheral vasodilatation. Noradrenaline causes splanchnic vasoconstriction[9] and its use is not recommended. Some transplant centers have employed cardiopulmonary bypass to facilitate

organ preservation and retrieval. The use of a portable extracorporeal pump, oxygenator and heat exchanger system enables circulatory support at flow rates of up to 1.5 l min^{-1} m^{-2} and allows splanchnic dissection to be undertaken at normothermia.

Respiratory management

Pulmonary gas exchange and ventilation are frequently compromised either by the trauma that resulted in brain stem death or by the sequelae of intermittent positive pressure ventilation. The lungs should be ventilated at the lowest FiO$_2$ compatible with normal oxygenation.

Considerable improvement in lung function may be produced before the donor harvesting operation by endobronchial suctioning, bronchoscopic lavage and manual inflation of the lungs. Normocarbia (PaCO$_2$ 34–41 mmHg/4.5–5.5 kPa) can be achieved with large tidal volumes (12–15 ml kg^{-1}), which help to limit the development of pulmonary atelectasis. Positive end-expiratory pressure (5 cmH$_2$0) may also be added if this does not cause cardiovascular compromise. The minimum acceptable criterion for lung transplantation is that the donor lungs should generate a PaO$_2$ of 225 mmHg (30 kPa) with FiO$_2$ 0.6 (i.e. PaO$_2$:FiO$_2$ ratio >375 mmHg/50 kPa).

Endocrine management

Asystolic cardiac arrest generally follows within 72 hours of the neuroendocrine storm attending brain stem death.[10] Clinical observation and histopathological changes[11] confirm a sequence of events adversely influencing donor heart function[12–14] and pulmonary vascular permeability.[15]

Following the sympathetic nervous system storm, alterations in endocrine function occur. Reductions in circulating tri-iodothyronine (T$_3$), thyroxine (T$_4$), cortisol, insulin and ADH have been noted. It is possible that these endocrine fluctuations both cause and exacerbate hemodynamic instability. Thyroid dysfunction results in normal circulating levels of thyroid stimulating hormone (TSH) and reduced levels of free T$_3$ —

'the sick euthyroid state'.[16] It is postulated that this causes donor myocardial dysfunction, which can be ameliorated by the administration of T_3.[17] A direct relationship exists between the number of unoccupied T_3 nuclear receptors and the extent of donor myocardial cell damage.[18] In addition, animal and human studies reveal a beneficial effect on donor heart function after T_3 replacement.[19–21]

Diabetes insipidus is frequently associated with intracranial catastrophies.[22] The administration of ADH rationalizes subsequent fluid administration and eases donor management[23] whilst excessive use of cold saline infusions exacerbates hypernatremia and hypothermia.

Hyperglycemia and hyperosmolality are associated with a low plasma insulin concentration and an impaired stress response is associated with depressed cortisol levels.[24] When exogenously administered, these hormones can help to maintain the homeostasis required for organ retrieval.[25] The administration of an endocrine package (Table 37.1) has therefore been recommended as early as possible after confirmation of brain stem death. This has been incorporated into the Papworth Hospital protocol following studies in which the recruitment of marginal donors resulted in additional successful cardiac transplant operations.[26–28]

Management of the donor operation

The involvement of several different surgical teams in multiorgan donor harvesting inevitably results in a procedure that will take many hours. Conflicting clinical interests may arise and in an

Table 37.1 Hormone Replacement Package used by Papworth Hospital donor organ retrieval team

T_3	Bolus	4 μg
	Infusion	3 μg h^{-1}
ADH (Pitressin)	Bolus	1 iu
	Infusion	1.5 iu h^{-1}
Soluble Insulin	To maintain blood glucose 109–200 mg dl^{-1} (6–11 mmol l^{-1})	
Methylprednisolone	Bolus	30 mg kg^{-1}

unfamiliar operating environment an air of equanimity is essential to ensure that the function of all the organs recovered for transplantation is optimized. Considerable fluctuations in the hemodynamic and homeostatic status of the donor may arise and anticipatory anesthetic management will help to achieve the best possible organ perfusion and later function. Intraoperative monitoring of systemic arterial and right-sided internal jugular pressures are preferred because of the surgical sequence of ligation of great vessels during cardiopulmonary harvesting procedures. Additional monitoring should include ECG, oximetry, urine output, end tidal CO_2, inspired oxygen concentration and temperature measurement. Arterial blood gas analysis and hemoglobin concentration measurement are performed periodically. Several venous blood samples may also be requested by coordinating members from differing teams. In addition, blood is also required for preparation of pneumoplegic solution if the lungs are to be harvested. Antimicrobial prophylaxis is administered according to institutional protocol.

Traditionally, anesthesia was not administered in the presence of brain stem death.[29] However the possibility of persistent somatic awareness has been raised and this may warrant the use of low concentrations (i.e. 1 minimal alveolar concentration; MAC) of volatile agents.[30] Accurate documentation of intraoperative events and hemodynamic variables as per routine anesthesia is required and prudent practice would include the retention of a separate copy of the record for later perusal. Muscle rigidity hinders surgical access and intact spinal reflexes may cause fluctuations in blood pressure. Neuromuscular blocking agents are therefore administered together with specific antihypertensive agents or increased concentrations of volatile or intravenous anesthetic drugs as necessary. Normocarbia and normal oxygenation (PaO_2 98–113 mmHg/13–15 kPa) are maintained with large tidal volumes (12–15 ml kg^{-1}) using an oxygen/air mixture.

The surgical procedures involved in organ procurement are quite standardized, although some variation may exist in the extent of dissection before cold flushing of the abdominal organs.[31] The standard approach is a long midline incision from suprasternal notch to pubis. Inspection of the thoracic organs follows a median sternotomy. Good ventricular motion, good lung expansion and the absence of coronary artery disease, are confirmed before mobilization of the intra-abdominal organs. After full heparinization (300 units kg^{-1}) the great vessels are cannulated. It is emphasized that aspiration of blood from the central venous line is absolutely essential to confirm systemic heparin administration. Cannulation of the abdominal aorta, portal vein and a femoral vein is then undertaken. If the lungs are to be retrieved, prostacyclin (5–20 ng kg^{-1} min^{-1}) is infused into the pulmonary arteries for 10 minutes. This ensures pulmonary vasodilatation before circulatory arrest. The PAFC is withdrawn before ligation of the superior vena cava. Aortic cross-clamping is followed by aortic root perfusion with cardioplegic solution. Mechanical ventilation and monitoring are then discontinued. If the lungs are to be harvested pneumoplegic solution is then administered via the main pulmonary artery while topical cooling is undertaken. The endotracheal tube is removed after the lungs have been inflated to a volume slightly greater than functional residual capacity (FRC) and the trachea then cross-clamped. The thoracic organs are double wrapped in sterile plastic bags, boxed in a cold container and readied for rapid transportation while the abdominal surgical team continues to operate in circulatory arrest.

Summary

Management of the brain stem dead multiorgan donor is a complex, time consuming, cooperative venture requiring significant input from a large team. A coordinated, protocol-driven approach, helps to ensure the retrieval of good organs for transplantation and may also improve graft survival.

Conclusions and learning points

- The demand for solid donor organs for transplantation exceeds supply.
- Optimal management of potential organ donors after brain stem death can increase organ retrieval rates.

- Operative management requires several teams to work together in unfamiliar surroundings.
- Anesthesia may be advocated due to the possibility of persisting somatic awareness.

References

1. United Kingdom Transplant Services Support Authority (UKTSSA). *Cardiothoracic organ transplant audit December 2000.* http://www.uktransplant.org.uk.

2. Morgan G, Morgan V, Smith M. *Donations of organs for transplantation. The management of the potential organ donor. A manual for the establishment of local guidelines.* Oxford: The Alden Group/Intensive Care Society, 1999.

3. Ihle BU. Management of the multi-organ donor. *Anesth Intens Care* 1993;**21**:710.

4. Nygaard CE, Townsend RN, Diamond DL. Organ donor management and organ outcome: a 6-year review from a level I trauma center. *J Trauma* 1990;**30**:728–32.

5. Logigian EL, Ropper AH. Terminal electrocardiographic changes in brain-dead patients. *Neurology* 1985;**35**:915–8.

6. Pickett JA, Wheeldon D, Oduro A. Multi-organ transplantation: donor management. *Curr Opin Anaesthesiol* 1994;**7**:80–3.

7. Yoshioka T, Sugimoto H, Uenishi M et al. Prolonged hemodynamic maintenance by the combined administration of vasopressin and epinephrine in brain death: a clinical study. *Neurosurgery* 1986;**18**:565–7.

8. Milner QJW, Vuylsteke A, Ismail F et al. ICU resuscitation of the multi-organ donor. *Br J Intensive Care* 1997;**7**:49–54

9. Scheinkestel CD, Tuxen DV, Cooper DJ, Butt W. Medical management of the (potential) organ donor. *Anaesth Intens Care* 1995;**23**:51–9.

10. Powner DJ, Hendrich A, Nyhuis A, Strate R. Changes in serum catecholamine levels in patients who are brain dead. *J Heart Lung Transplant* 1992;**11**:1046–53.

11. Shivalkar B, Van Loon J, Wieland W et al. Variable effects of explosive or gradual increase of intracra-

nial pressure on myocardial structure and function. *Circulation* 1993;**87**:230–9.

12. Szabo G, Sebening C, Hackert T *et al.* Effects of brain death on myocardial function and ischemic tolerance of potential donor hearts. *J Heart Lung Transplant* 1998;**17**:921–30.

13. Szabo G, Sebening C, Hagl C, Tochtermann U *et al.* Right ventricular function after brain death: response to an increased afterload. *Eur J Cardiothorac Surg* 1998;**13**:449–58.

14. Bittner HB, Chen EP, Kendall SW, Van Trigt P. Brain death alters cardiopulmonary hemodynamics and impairs right ventricular power reserve against an elevation of pulmonary vascular resistance. *Chest* 1997;**111**:706–11.

15. Mayer SA, Fink ME, Homma S *et al.* Cardiac injury associated with neurogenic pulmonary edema following subarachnoid hemorrhage. *Neurology* 1994;**44**:815–20.

16. Masson F, Thicoipe M, Latapie MJ, Maurette P. Thyroid function in brain-dead donors. *Transpl Int* 1990;**3**:226–33.

17. Novitzky D, Cooper DK, Morrell D, Isaacs S. Change from aerobic to anaerobic metabolism after brain death, and reversal following triiodothyronine therapy. *Transplantation* 1988;**45**:32–6.

18. Montero JA, Mallol J, Alvarez F *et al.* Biochemical hypothyroidism and myocardial damage in organ donors: are they related? *Transplant Proc* 1988;**20**:746–8.

19. Davis PJ, Davis FB. Acute cellular actions of thyroid hormone and myocardial function. *Ann Thorac Surg* 1993;**56**:S16–23.

20. Novitzky D, Wicomb WN, Cooper DK, Tjaalgard MA. Improved cardiac function following hormonal therapy in brain dead pigs: relevance to organ donation. *Cryobiology* 1987;**24**:1–10.

21. Novitzky D, Cooper DK. Results of hormonal therapy in human brain-dead potential organ donors. *Transplant Proc* 1988;**20**:59–62.

22. Hiatt HH, Lowis S. Diabetes insipidus following head injury. *Arch Intern Med* 1957;**100**:143.

23. Kinoshita Y, Yahata K, Yoshioka T *et al.* Long-term renal preservation after brain death maintained with vasopressin and epinephrine. *Transpl Int* 1990;**3**:15–8.

24. McLean AD, Rosengard BR. Aggressive donor management. *Curr Opin Organ Transplant* 1999;**4**:130–4.

25. Novitzky D, Cooper DK, Reichart B. Hemodynamic and metabolic responses to hormonal therapy in brain-dead potential organ donors. *Transplantation* 1987;**43**:852–4.

26. Wheeldon DR, Potter CD, Jonas M *et al.* Transplantation of 'unsuitable' organs? *Transplant Proc* 1993;**25**:3104–5.

27. Wheeldon DR, Potter CD, Oduro A *et al.* Transforming the 'unacceptable' donor: outcomes from the adoption of a standardized donor management technique. *J Heart Lung Transplant* 1995;**14**:734–42.

28. Wheeldon DR, Potter CD, Jonas M, Wallwork J, Large SR. Using 'unsuitable' hearts for transplantation. *Eur J Cardiothorac Surg* 1994;**8**:7–9.

29. Working Party of the Royal Colleges of Physicians on behalf of the Academy of Medical Royal Colleges. *A code of practice for the diagnosis of brain stem death — including guidelines for the identification and management of potential organ and tissue donors.* London; Department of Health, 1998.

30. Young PJ, Matta BF. Anaesthesia for organ donation in the brainstem dead — why bother? *Anaesthesia* 2000;**55**:105–6.

31. Szmalc FS, Kittur DS. Organ donor maintenance and procurement. *Curr Opin Organ Transplant* 2000;**5**:232–56.

38

Two-stage repair of a stab wound to the heart

Fiona M Gibson

Introduction

A stabbing injury to the heart may present the admitting team with a dead patient or with one of the most challenging emergency management problems in the Accident and Emergency department. There is much debate currently in cardio-thoracic trauma circles as to the optimum management strategy for this type of patient.[1] The case presented demonstrates some of the problems that may occur and will facilitate discussion of the options available to help deliver a successful outcome.

Case history

On a Sunday morning at 08:00 a 36-year-old man was brought to the Accident and Emergency department of a District General Hospital (DGH).

Within the primary survey of his resuscitation, his airway was secure, with no suggestion of cervical spine injury, he was breathing sponta-neously, with no overt ventilatory deficit, he was found to have three stab wounds in his anterior chest: one in the fourth interspace on the left side of the sternum, two others, more lateral on the left side, and three wounds identified on the posterior aspect of his chest. His pulse was 144 bpm, and his systemic blood pressure (BP) was recorded as 90/47. He was diaphoretic and clammy. His abdomen was soft and non-tender, and his limbs were intact. There was a sugges-tion that there had been alcohol consumed and the patient was groaning. He was assessed as having a Glasgow Coma Scale score of 13.

Initial resuscitation involved intravenous access with a 14-G canula to the right external jugular vein, administration of 100% oxygen by a facemask, and insertion of urinary catheter. Two liters of normal (0.9%) saline were administered

Past medical history	None relevant.
Regular medications	None relevant.
Examination	**Primary survey:** Airway intact. Spontaneous respiration. SaO_2 96% on 100% oxygen. Trachea central. Breath sounds equal on left and right. Pulse 144 bpm. BP 90/47. Sweating and clammy with distended neck veins. Stab wounds noted ×3 in anterior and posterior chest wall. Smelling of alcohol. **Secondary survey:** GCS 13. No overt evidence of head injury. No evidence of spinal or limb injury.
Investigations	**CXR:** Left hemothorax, no pneumothorax, no rib fractures seen. AST 26 u l^{-1}, LDH 192 u l^{-1} CK 210 u l^{-1} (NR <175), CK-MB 23 u l^{-1} (NR <21) Hb 13.9 g dl^{-1}, Hct 0.42, WBC 12.4 × 10^9 l^{-1}, platelets 248 × 10^9 l^{-1}

intravenously as first line 'ATLS' resuscitation. An initial chest radiograph showed no pneumothorax but there was a left-sided collection of fluid, which was assumed to be a hemothorax. A size 32-FG chest drain was inserted and an unspecified volume of blood drained. The patient's condition gradually deteriorated and within 15 minutes his systolic blood pressure fell precipitously to 65 mmHg, and he lost consciousness.

A presumptive diagnosis of cardiac tamponade was made and pericardiocentesis by subxiphisternal catheter insertion was performed. Following the aspiration of 100 ml dark blood, there was an immediate improvement in hemodynamics and the blood pressure was rapidly restored to 110/70 mmHg. The pericardiocentesis catheter was secured, and plans made to transfer the patient immediately to the operating theater.

The thoracic surgeon on call for the Regional Thoracic Service was contacted and requested that the patient be prepared and that he would come to the DGH to perform the necessary surgery. The patient arrived in the operating theater at 09:55.

Following a rapid sequence induction with propofol and suxamethonium, tracheal intubation and the institution of mechanical ventilation, anesthesia was maintained with infusions of propofol and remifentanil. Intraoperative monitoring consisted of invasive arterial pressure measurement, SpO2, end-tidal CO_2, central venous pressure (CVP; which was recorded as 12 mmHg) and nasopharyngeal temperature.

Intraoperatively there was a period of hemodynamic instability at the time of median sternotomy, which was treated with a bolus of epinephrine, this being repeated in 50 µg aliquots, to a total of 2 mg during the case. Once the pericardium was opened, a laceration in the right ventricular outflow tract was identified, controlled by digital pressure, and then oversewn. Surgical hemostasis was achieved, and the sternum closed with wires. Minimal inotropic support was required at the end of the surgery. Total fluid administration perioperatively consisted of 2000 ml crystalloid, 6 units packed red cells, 2 units fresh frozen plasma, 6 donor units platelets and 500 ml other colloid. This represented approximately 5 liters fluid administered, and was balanced against an estimated blood loss of 3 liters.

At the end of the procedure mechanical ventilation was continued. The patient was sedated with infusions of remifentanil and propofol, and arrangements were made for his transfer to the Cardiac Surgical Intensive Care Unit (CSICU) in the tertiary referral hospital, approximately 5 miles away, for postoperative intensive care.

On arrival in the CSICU, the patient was hemodynamically stable, with heart rate 110 bpm, blood pressure 125/70 mmHg, CVP 10 mmHg. His arterial blood gases (ABG) on 50% oxygen were: pH 7.39, PaO_2 148 mmHg (19.7 kPa), $PaCO_2$ 40.6 mmHg (5.4 kPa), base excess (BE) –0.8 mmol l^{-1}, standard bicarbonate (SBC) 23.8 mmol l^{-1}. His blood count on admission to CSICU revealed: hemoglobin concentration 14.9 g dl^{-1}, hematocrit 43.7%, leukocytes 10.33 × 10^9 l^{-1} and platelets 120 ×10^9 l^{-1}. His sedation was maintained with a continuous infusion of propofol 100 mg h^{-1}. The infusion of remifentanil was discontinued, and a morphine infusion commenced in its stead. The decision was made to continue mechanical ventilation for a further 24 hours.

This proved to be a very stable period, and the patient was weaned from mechanical ventilation and his trachea extubated early the next morning. ABG analysis (FiO_2 0.5) prior to extubation revealed: pH 7.45, PaO_2 165 mmHg (22 kPa), $PaCO_2$ 38.5 mmHg (5.1 kPa), BE 1.8 mmol l^{-1}, and SBC 26.0 mmol l^{-1}. After extubation (FiO_2 1.0) the first recorded ABG analysis revealed: pH 7.355, PaO_2 98 mmHg (13.1 kPa), SaO_2 98%, $PaCO_2$ 52.0 mmHg (6.9 kPa), BE 1.8 mmol l^{-1} and SBC 26.0 mmol l^{-1}. A chest radiograph immediately following extubation showed signs of right basal collapse and it was felt that his poor gas exchange was explicable on this basis. Auscultation of the precordium revealed a systolic murmur, and a transthoracic echocardiograph (TTE) was requested to visualize the right ventricular outflow tract (RVOT) and main pulmonary artery.

He was treated with a patient-controlled analgesia system (PCAS) device and vigorous physiotherapy over the next few hours saw an improvement in his ABGs with pH 7.32, PaO_2 132.7 mmHg (17.7 kPa), $PaCO_2$ 51.7 mmHg (6.9 kPa), BE 0.5 mmol l^{-1}, SBC 24 mmol l^{-1}. A blood count at this time revealed; hemoglobin 16.4 g dl^{-1}, hematocrit 49%, leukocytes 13.6 × 10^9 l^{-1} and platelets 78 × 10^9 l^{-1}.

At 16:00 a TTE was performed and the suspicion of a connection between the aortic root and main pulmonary artery, consistent with a fistulous connection, was raised. The right ventricular systolic pressure was estimated from the tricuspid regurgitation signal as 40 mmHg. Transesophageal echocardiography (TEE), performed under propofol sedation, subsequently confirmed this suspicion, identifying the site of the fistula as being in the left coronary sinus just above the aortic valve annulus and anterior to the origin of the left coronary artery (Figure 38.1). There was mild mitral valve regurgitation, a hyperdynamic left

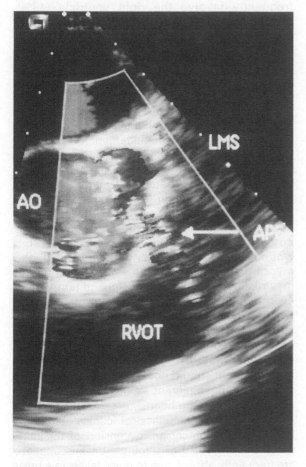

Figure 38.1

Transesophageal echocardiograph demonstrating the fistulous connection from the right ventricular outflow tract to the aorta. APF: aortopulmonary fistula; RVOT: right ventricular outflow tract; AO: aorta; LMS: left main stem coronary artery.

ventricle, and the pulmonary valve was described as normal. It was clear that reparative surgery would be required and the decision made to defer this to an elective operating list the following day.

Subsequently he developed increasing respiratory distress, with respiratory rate increasing to 25 and then to 30 breaths per minute. On auscultion crepitations were audible over all his lung fields. A further chest radiograph confirmed a diagnosis of fulminant pulmonary edema. At this stage it seemed appropriate to reintubate and ventilate the patient as he was becoming increasingly exhausted, and this was achieved without difficulty.

He remained sedated and ventilated overnight, with improvement in ABGs (FiO$_2$ 0.7) from pH 7.35, PaO$_2$ 76 mmHg (10.1 kPa), PaCO$_2$ 54 mmHg (7.2 kPa), BE 2.6 mmol l^{-1} and SBC 20.7 mmol l^{-1} to pH 7.41, PaO$_2$ 139 mmHg (18.5 kPa), PaCO$_2$ 41.2 mmHg (5.5 kPa), BE 1.4 mmol l^{-1} and SBC 25.7 mmol l^{-1}. The radiographic appearances of pulmonary edema remained unchanged.

By the following morning gas exchange had improved: pH 7.52, PaO$_2$ 227.2 mmHg (30.3 kPa), PaCO$_2$ 33.5 mmHg (4.5 kPa), and FiO$_2$ was reduced to 0.5. He was taken to the operating theater, the previous sternotomy was reopened and the patient placed on cardiopulmonary bypass. In addition to confirming the TEE diagnoses, it was also discovered that both pulmonary valve leaflets were partly detached from the commisure, but that the uppermost suspensory ligaments of the cusps were intact. No attempt was made to repair the pulmonary valve leaflets, but all the other defects were repaired appropriately. At the end of the procedure the patient was easily weaned from cardiopulmonary bypass. The pulmonary artery pressure at this time was noted to be significantly lower than it had been at the outset, 34/15 and 50/23 mmHg respectively. He was returned to the CSICU.

On the morning after his second operation he was weaned from mechanical ventilation without incident, and was subsequently discharged from the CSICU the next day. His postoperative recovery was complicated by a chest infection involving the lingular portion of the left lung. This responded to antibiotic therapy and vigorous physiotherapy. He was discharged from hospital 9 days after his original admission to the primary admitting DGH.

Discussion

The incidence of penetrating injuries to the heart is increasing. Penetrating injuries to the heart may be caused by stabbing, which may include anything from a long knife to a fence post, or gunshot or blast injury. The stab wound injury tends to be associated with a better prognosis, as there is less extensive disruption to the myocardium than is associated with the diffuse injury of a high velocity missile, due to the higher kinetic energy of the bullet compared to the blade.[2]

The skills available have resulted in improved prospects of survival particularly in relation to stabbing injuries as compared to gunshot injuries. Some series show a survival of 78% from stabbing compared with 40% from a gunshot injury.[3] Fewer than 3% of these injuries require cardiopulmonary bypass, and therefore are amenable to treatment by a primary trauma team. This case highlights a number of current topics in the management of these patients, including the role of the trauma team, the place of emergency room thoracotomy and the specifics of fluid replacement in thoracic, and specifically, cardiac trauma. All of these will be considered.

In the current climate of hospital closures and superspecialization within surgery, where are these patients best cared for? The policy of 'scoop and run', which has been applied in the management of major trauma in our region, involves the transfer of the injured patient to the Regional Trauma Centre. The journey may take the 'pick up' team past the door of the nearest hospital, but has proven beneficial to many patients. The patient in the case presented was delivered to the local DGH, and thus received his primary resuscitation there.

The primary survey raised the alarm, with stab wounds in the 'danger area', the area including the epigastrium, and the precordium within 3 cm of the sternum.[4] There was an obvious risk of having sustained a cardiac injury.

Stab wounds to the heart present in a number of ways: (1) death; (2) some signs of life but no detectable vital signs; (3) shock; or (4) a stable patient. Eighty per cent of stab wounds present with cardiac tamponade.[5] By comparison, gunshot injury to the heart is associated with tamponade in only 20% of cases, and generally there is significant hypotension present.[6, 7] One published series of gunshot injuries to the heart describes survival in 20/27 (74%) cases with associated tamponade, and no survivors without tamponade.[7] The author concluded that the presence of cardiac tamponade was a good prognostic indicator in patients with gunshot injuries to the heart.

Patients who arrive alive in the Accident and Emergency department or emergency room with a penetrating cardiac injury are a self-selecting population, the majority of studies suggesting that as many as 80% of such injuries, especially gunshot injuries, are fatal before arrival at hospital.[8, 9] Penetrating injuries to the heart most frequently involve the right ventricle (43%), although the left ventricle (34%), right atrium (16%) and left atrium (7%) may also be involved.[10] This is understandable on the basis of the configuration of the structures of the heart within the thoracic cavity. However it is essential to remember that as many as a third of penetrating cardiac injuries involve multiple structures. A high index of suspicion that this is likely is therefore essential in the management of a patient with a penetrating cardiac injury.

The penetrating wound to the pericardium and to the heart is associated with early sealing of the pericardial puncture site. Right ventricular puncture is usually associated with tamponade because the thin (3 mm) myocardial wall does not seal spontaneously. Left ventricular stab wounds tend to seal spontaneously if the myocardial rent is less than 1 cm in length, and may result in the absence of signs of tamponade even though the heart has been lacerated. Stab wounds to the heart bear a close resemblance to surgical incisions, in that there may be little destruction of cardiac tissue. The absence of significant signs of hemodynamic instability in such a patient should not lead to complacency in relation to management as there may still be a serious injury to the heart.

Unfortunately the classical clinical signs of Beck's triad, hypotension, distension of the neck veins and muffled heart sounds on auscultation, are frequently absent, due to noise levels in a busy resuscitation room, loss of circulating blood volume, and resultant hypovolemia.[11, 12] Resuscitation of penetrating cardiac injuries is a contentious area. The ATLS guidelines, which recommend early administration of 2 liters lactated Ringer's solution or normal saline are based on physiological studies in animals and anecdotal clinical evidence.[13, 14] Substantial fluid administration may not be appropriate in all cases. The hemodynamically stable patient with a penetrating cardiac wound is likely to have lost about 500 ml blood, which is contained within the pericardium. A rapid infusion of 2 liters crystalloid will serve to increase CVP without any enhancement of cardiac output. This early fluid load will not help the associated deterioration in left ventricular function. In animal models of crystalloid resuscitation, acute hemodilution is associated with a decrease in tissue oxygen delivery.[15, 16] The patient described in this case study received 5 liters fluid replacement, balanced due to severe pulmonary edema, largely due to his shunt from the fistulous connection between the pulmonary outflow tract and the aorta. The volume load, which he received, no doubt contributed to the degree of heart failure that he suffered.

There have been many publications discussing the options of early surgery in major trauma without fluid resuscitation. The influence of the timing of fluid resuscitation in relation to surgical intervention was assessed in a study performed in Houston.[17] Patients were randomized to have fluid resuscitation either before arriving in the operating room or only in the operating room. The most significant finding in the study was of a greater survival rate in those who were resuscitated in the operating room (70 versus 62%), and also a higher incidence of respiratory and renal complications in those who received fluid resuscitation prior to operative intervention. It would be reasonable to assert that the administration of appropriate volumes, appropriately timed, is an important strand in the management of patients with penetrating cardiac injuries.

Early surgical repair of the causative injury must be the prime objective. Periocardiocentesis may be helpful in buying time to prepare for definitive surgery, but negative periocardiocentesis does not rule out tamponade.[18, 19] The use of echocardiography to identify pericardial fluid is a helpful tool in the patient with stable vital signs, but there is little role for this diagnostic aid in the unstable patient in the emergency room.[20]

The place of emergency thoracotomy in the management of penetrating thoracic injuries has been widely discussed in the literature.[21–23] This maneuver is carried out as a resuscitative exercise, and may be performed at the location of

the injury (e.g. at the roadside in the presence of appropriate personnel), in the emergency room, or in the operating room. The results from this procedure are to a large extent dictated by the preoperative status of the patient. Blunt thoracic trauma has a notoriously bad outcome from this operation,[24] and this reflects the extent of the trauma suffered and the potential for other major organ systems being compromised in the incident. The best results from resuscitative thoracotomy are to be found in patients who have sustained penetrating cardiac injuries: stabbings have a much better prognosis than gun shot wounds, for the reasons described earlier (i.e. the lesser degree of tissue disruption associated with a stab injury as compared with a gun shot).[23]

The factor of greatest prognostic significance in outcome determination for those patients who undergo emergency thoracotomy is the presence or absence of signs of life. Signs of life are taken to be represented by pupillary reaction, agonal respiration and some sort of electrocardiographic rhythm, whether it is an agonal or an idioventricular rhythm. In those patients with no signs of life prior to operation, the survival rate is virtually zero compared to 73% in those with some minimal signs of life who sustained a penetrating cardiac injury.[25] These types of results are well reproduced in a number of studies.[9, 26] It has also been demonstrated that the outcome following emergency thoracotomy is better in those patients who undergo the procedure in the operating room rather than in the emergency room with one series quoting survival rates of 87% and 38% respectively.[23] This again reflects the clinical condition of the patients, indicating the more serious condition of those who undergo the procedure in the emergency room compared to those who were sufficiently stable to be transferred to the operating room instead.[23]

In the case described above, a definitive diagnosis was made in the CSICU 36 hours after the initial injury, by TEE. This diagnostic tool is becoming increasingly useful in trauma management whether it be specific to the heart or not.[27] It is arguable that this man might have been spared the stress of extubation between one operation and the other had TEE been performed earlier in his management. There is no doubt that he required an early surgical intervention for relief of his cardiac tamponade, and that he required to be transferred to the cardiac surgical tertiary referral center, so that there was no other option than a two-stage approach to the repair of his injury.

Conclusions and learning points

- Stab wounds to the heart have the potential to have a high retrieval rate with a heightened awareness in the carers for such patients.
- The potential for more than a single chamber to be involved in a stabbing to the heart should always be borne in mind.
- Fluid resuscitation of the isolated injured heart should be tailored to needs.
- A multidisciplinary approach to the management of penetrating cardiac injuries should allow the well-trained trauma team to liase with the regional cardiac referral center to optimally care for these patients.
- All available diagnostic modalities for management should be brought into play at the first available moment.

References

1. Kim FJ, Moore EE, Moore FA *et al*. Trauma surgeons can render definitive surgical care for major thoracic injuries. *J Trauma* 1994;**36**:871–5.

2. Karrel R, Shaffer MA, Franaszek JB. Emergency diagnosis, resuscitation, and treatment of acute penetrating cardiac trauma. *Ann Emerg Med* 1982;**11**:504–17.

3. Cooley DA, Dunn RJ, Brockman ML *et al*. Treatment of pericardial wounds of the heart. Experimental and clinical observations. *Surgery* 1955;**37**:504–17.

4. Sauer PE, Murdock CE Jr. Immediate surgery for cardiac and great vessel wounds. *Arch Surg* 1967;**95**:7–11.

5. Borja AR, Lansing AM, Ransdell HT Jr. Immediate operative treatment for stab wounds of the heart. Experience with fifty-four consecutive cases. *J Thorac Cardiovasc Surg* 1970;**59**:662–7.

6. Carrasquilla C, Wilson RF, Walt AJ, Arbulu A. Gunshot wounds of the heart. *Ann Thorac Surg* 1972;**13**:208–13.

7. Maynard AD, Brooks HA, Froix CJ. Penetrating wounds to the heart. *Ann Thorac Surg* 1965;**13**:208–13.

8. Asfaw I, Arbulu A. Penetrating wounds of the pericardium and heart. *Surg Clin North Am* 1977;**57**:37–48.

9. Baker CC, Thomas AN, Trunkey DD. The role of emergency room thoracotomy in trauma. *J Trauma* 1980;**20**:848–55.

10. Symbas PN. Cardiothoracic trauma. *Curr Probl Surg* 1991;**28**:741–97.

11. Shoemaker WC, Carey JS, Yao ST *et al*. Hemodynamic alterations in acute cardiac tamponade after penetrating injuries of the heart. *Surgery* 1970;**67**:754–64.

12. Beall AC, Ochsner JL, Morris GC et al. Penetrating wounds to the heart. *J Trauma* 1961;**1**:195.

13. Shires T, Carrico CJ. Current status of the shock problem. *Curr Probl Surg* 1966;3–67.

14. Dillon J, Lynch LJ Jr, Myers R *et al*. A bioassay of treatment of hemorrhagic shock. I. The roles of blood, Ringer's solution with lactate, and macromolecules (dextran and hydroxyethyl starch) in the treatment of hemorrhagic shock in the anesthetized dog. *Arch Surg* 1966;**93**:537–55.

15. Bickell WH, Bruttig SP, Millnamow GA *et al*. The detrimental effects of intravenous crystalloid after aortotomy in swine. *Surgery* 1991;**110**:529–36.

16. Craig RL, Poole GV. Resuscitation in uncontrolled hemorrhage. *Am Surg* 1994;**60**:59–62.

17. Bickell WH, Wall MJ Jr, Pepe PE *et al*. Immediate versus delayed fluid resuscitation for hypotensive patients with penetrating torso injuries. *N Engl J Med* 1994;**331**:1105–9.

18. Breaux EP, Dupont JB Jr, Albert HM *et al*. Cardiac tamponade following penetrating mediastinal injuries: improved survival with early pericardiocentesis. *J Trauma* 1979;**19**:461–6.

19. Steichen FM, Dargan EL, Efron G *et al*. A graded approach to the management of penetrating wounds of the heart. *Arch Surg* 1971;**103**:574–80.

20. Jimenez E, Martin M, Krukenkamp I, Barrett J. Subxiphoid pericardiotomy versus echocardiography: a prospective evaluation of the diagnosis of occult penetrating cardiac injury. *Surgery* 1990;**108**:676–9.

21. Ivatury RR, Shah PM, Ito K *et al.* Emergency room thoracotomy for the resuscitation of patients with 'fatal' penetrating injuries of the heart. *Ann Thorac Surg* 1981;**32**:377–85.

22. Ivatury RR, Rohman M. Emergency department thoracotomy for trauma: a collective review. *Resuscitation* 1987;**15**:23–35.

23. Attar S, Suter CM, Hankins JR *et al.* Penetrating cardiac injuries. *Ann Thorac Surg* 1991;**51**:711–5.

24. Lorenz HP, Steinmetz B, Lieberman J *et al.* Emergency thoracotomy: survival correlates with physiologic status. *J Trauma* 1992;**32**:780–5.

25. Mattox KL, Allen MK. Emergency department treatment of chest injuries. *Emerg Med Clin North Am* 1984;**2**:783–97.

26. Sherman MM, Saini VK, Yarnoz MD *et al.* Management of penetrating heart wounds. *Am J Surg* 1978;**135**:553–8.

27. Porembka DT. Transesophageal echocardiography in the trauma patient. *Curr Opin Anesthesiol* 1997;**10**:130–44.

39
Anesthetic management of the patient with carcinoid heart disease

M Krishna Prasad, Christopher J Rozario and Joseph E Arrowsmith

Introduction

Carcinoid heart disease presents a challenge for the anesthetist involving endocrine, metabolic and cardiac problems.

Case history

A 47-year-old Caucasian female was admitted to hospital for replacement of her tricuspid and pulmonary valves. Three years earlier she had presented with diarrhea, flushing and panic attacks. Investigation at that time revealed a malignant midgut carcinoid tumor with liver metastases. Treatment with long-acting octreotide and interferon produced a significant improvement in her symptoms and she remained well until the development of exertional dyspnea.

Transthoracic echocardiography revealed pulmonary stenosis and torrential tricuspid regurgitation, with enlargement of the right heart chambers. Based on symptom progression and right ventricular dysfunction, pulmonary and tricuspid valve replacement was advised.

On the morning of surgery the patient was premedicated with temazepam 20 mg and ranitidine 150 mg by mouth. An intravenous infusion of octreotide 100 µg h^{-1} was commenced at this time and continued into the postoperative period. On arrival in the anesthetic room electrocardiography, pulse oximetry, and non-invasive blood pressure monitoring were established. A peripheral vein and the right radial artery were cannulated under local anesthetic, an infusion of Hartmann's solution started and arterial blood pressure monitoring established. Anesthesia was induced with midazolam 10 mg, fentanyl 1 mg, propofol 900 mg h^{-1} (15 mg kg^{-1} h^{-1}) and pancuronium 10 mg. Following tracheal intubation the lungs were ventilated with oxygen in air (FiO$_2$ 0.3, F$_{ET}$CO$_2$ 34 mmHg/4.5 kPa) and the propofol infusion rate reduced to 300 mg h^{-1} (5 mg kg^{-1} h^{-1}). A triple-lumen catheter was placed in the right internal jugular vein for central venous pressure monitoring and drug administration.

The patient remained hemodynamically stable during and immediately after the induction of anesthesia. At the time of skin incision, however, there was an increase in heart rate to 115 beats min^{-1} accompanied by cutaneous flushing, which rapidly responded to an intravenous bolus of octreotide 100 µg.

Following the administration of heparin 18 000 u (300 u kg^{-1}; ACT >450 s), hypothermic (30°C) cardiopulmonary bypass (CPB) was established with aortic and bicaval cannulation. A vent was placed in the pulmonary artery, the aorta cross-clamped and cold crystalloid antegrade cardioplegia (St Thomas' I) solution infused through an aortic root cannula.

At operation the right atrium and right ventricle were found to be dilated and hypertrophied. The tricuspid valve leaflets were thickened and shortened, and did not coapt. The pulmonary valve cusps were thickened and there was a central deficit. The tricuspid valve was replaced with a 33-mm Carpentier–Edwards tissue valve and the pulmonary trunk was replaced with an aortic homograft with the coronary ostia oversewn. After closure of the atriotomy suture line, the heart was deaired. Although electrical and mechanical cardiac activity resumed spontaneously after removal of the aortic cross-clamp, epicardial atrioventricular pacing was required to produce an acceptable heart rate. The patient was weaned from CPB without inotropic support.

Past medical history	History of flushes, diarrhea, associated with malignant carcinoid tumor, and liver metastases. Hypothyroidism.
Regular medications	Octreotide (long acting) 30 mg IM every 3 weeks, InotronA (interferon) 5 million units SC five times weekly. Levothyroxin 0.15 mg and 0.10 mg alternate days. Ranitidine 150 mg OD.
Examination	Weight 60 kg, Height 1.72 m, BSA 1.65 m². Good nutrition status, well informed about her condition but anxious. Obvious episodes of flushing during clinical examination. No pedal edema or ascitis. Heart rate 95 min⁻¹, BP 98/62 mmHg, JVP showed features of TR, cardiac apex not displaced. Pansystolic murmur audible at the right sternal edge. Enlarged pulsatile liver, left hypochondrial mass and a mass in the right iliac fossa.
Investigations	Hb 12.8 g dl⁻¹, WBC 4.2 × 10⁹ l⁻¹, platelets 117 × 10⁹ l⁻¹, total bilirubin 1.46 mg dl⁻¹ (25 µmol l⁻¹), alkaline phosphatase 480 u l⁻¹ (8.0 µkat l⁻¹), alanine transaminase (SGPT) 36 u l⁻¹ (0.6 µkat l⁻¹), aspartate transaminase (SGOT) 26 u l⁻¹ (0.44 µkat l⁻¹), creatinine 1.1 mg dl⁻¹ (98 µmol l⁻¹), TSH 0.007 mU (0.39 µmol l⁻¹), total T₃ 85 ng dl⁻¹ (1.3 nmol l⁻¹), P-Chromogranin A 46 nmol l⁻¹ (NR <4), Urinary 5'HIAA 135 and 120 mg day⁻¹ (706 and 629 µmol day⁻¹). **CT scan:** Multiple liver metastases, abdominal lymph node metastases, and rib metastases. **TTE:** Severe TR, moderate PR and PS. PV gradient 14 mmHg. Good left ventricular function.

Anticoagulation was reversed with an infusion of protamine sulfate. The CPB and ischemic times were 96 and 79 minutes respectively.

The patient was transferred to the intensive care unit (ICU) in a stable condition. She was weaned from mechanical ventilation within 24 hours. The octreotide infusion continued for a further 7 days. The postoperative course was complicated by intermittent atrioventricular block and, ultimately, a junctional tachycardia, which responded to oral verapamil. When reviewed in the outpatient clinic 1 month after surgery, her exertional dyspnea had resolved and she was noted to be in sinus rhythm.

Discussion

Carcinoid tumors were first described by Lubarsch over a century ago.[1] The term *karzi-noide* was coined by Oberndorfer in 1907,[2] who described a tumor that, while resembling adeno-carcinoma in appearance, behaved in a more benign and indolent fashion. Since this description, it has become apparent that carcinoid tumors are far from benign in nature.

Carcinoid refers to a neoplastic process of amine- and peptide-producing cells arising from primitive gut neuroectoderm. These tumors stain with silver stains (i.e. argentophilic) and contain granules that contain amines and hormones (Table 39.1).

Table 39.1 Peptides and amines secreted by carcinoid tumours

5-hydroxytryptamine	Prostaglandins	ACTH
Histamine	Neurotensin	Gastrin
Tachykinin	Glycentin	

ACTH: adrenocorticotrophic hormone.

Table 39.2 Distribution of carcinoid tumours[3]

Gastrointestinal tract 73.7%		Liver	0.25%
		Gall bladder	0.3%
		Stomach	3.7%
		Pancreas	0.84%
		Esophagus	0.05%
		Colon	9.6%
		Appendix	9.4%
		Rectum	11.4%
Respiratory tract		Trachea, bronchi and lung	32.1%
		Larynx	0.05%
Other		Ovary	0.73%

Although the primary site of these tumors usually lies within the gastrointestinal tract (predominantly the small bowel) they may also be found in the bronchi and lungs (Table 39.2).

The tumors may be present as a component of the multiple endocrine neoplasia (MEN) type 1 syndrome in association with parathyroid adenoma, pancreatic endocrine tumors, anterior pituitary adenoma, and adrenal adenoma. In the absence of metastases, carcinoid disease is largely asymptomatic whereas classical symptoms of carcinoid syndrome (Table 39.3) develop when the tumor metastasizes to lung or liver and secretes vasoactive amines.

The incidence of carcinoid tumors has been studied in two large series.[3, 5] Godwin analyzed 2837 cases diagnosed between 1959 and 1971 where carcinoid tumors were identified in ovary, lung, the biliary system, and throughout the

Table 39.3 Symptoms and signs of the carcinoid syndrome

Cardiovascular	Angina, hypertension, hypotension, episodic tachycardia, bradycardia, premature atrial ectopics, tricuspid regurgitation, pulmonary stenosis, right heart failure
Respiratory	Bronchospasm, asthma (19%)[4]
Gastrointestinal	Diarrhea (78%),[4] nausea, vomiting, hyperacidosis, abdominal pain, hepatomegaly, liver dysfunction
Metabolic	Hyperglycemia
Integumental	Flushing (94%),[5] telengiectasia, scleroderma, pellagra (diarrhea, dementia and dermatitis)

gastrointestinal tract (Table 39.2). The age-adjusted incidence was highest in the African-American population. Five-year survival rates ranged from 33%, for tumors located in the sigmoid colon, to 99% for those located in the vermiform appendix. More recently, Modlin and Sandor studied 8305 cases of carcinoid diagnosed between 1973 and 1991. They reported a rise in incidence and an overall 5-year survival rate, regardless of tumor site, of 50.4 ±6.4%. It is likely that the true incidence of these tumors is higher as only malignant tumors are reported to cancer registries, the source of these data.

Carcinoid syndrome refers to a constellation of symptoms and signs caused when vasoactive substances bypass hepatic and pulmonary inactivation and enter the systemic circulation. A typical presentation is characterized by cutaneous flushing, wheezing, diarrhea and dyspnea that are induced by alcohol- and tyramine-containing foods. Over time, pellagra and cardiac fibrosis may also arise. Atypical carcinoid syndrome manifests as prolonged episodes of flushing, lachrymation, and bronchoconstriction. Carcinoid crisis is characterized by hemodynamic instability, coronary vasospasm,[6] bronchospasm and metabolic acidosis. Crises may arise spontaneously, or because of stress, the ingestion of certain foodstuffs (e.g. tomatoes), anesthesia and therapeutic embolization of the liver metastases.

The cutaneous manifestations of carcinoid syndrome consist of patches of plethora and cyanosis accompanied by flushing. Over time telengiectasia, enlargement of dermal veins, hypertrophy and non-pitting edema develop. The release of histamine in to the systemic circulation causes facial swelling and lachrymation, which may occur during anesthesia.[7] Gastro-intestinal hypersecretion and excessive gut motility result in malabsorption of bile salts leading to osmotic diarrhea and steatorrhea. In extreme cases, patients may present with protein malnutrition and pellagra-like symptoms (i.e. dementia, diarrhea and dermatitis) secondary to niacin deficiency as dietary tryptophan is preferentially converted into serotonin (5-hydroxytrypt-amine; 5-HT).

Carcinoid heart disease occurs in two-thirds of patients with carcinoid syndrome and appears to be related to the high plasma levels of serotonin and tachykinins.[8] The lesions are characterized by plaque-like endocardial thickening and fibrosis predominantly in the right side of the heart. Lesions similar to carcinoid heart disease have been described associated with use of the anorectic drugs fenfluramine and dexfenflu-ramine, which interfere with serotonin metabo-lism.[9] Tricuspid regurgitation is a universal finding, tricuspid stenosis, pulmonary stenosis and pulmonary regurgitation may also occur. An echocardiographic analysis of patients with carcinoid heart disease demonstrated tricuspid regurgitation in 100% of patients, and pulmonary valve abnormalities in 88% with pulmonary regurgitation (81%) being more common than stenosis (53%).[10] Sclerosis and partial fusion of valve cusps also occurs and may affect bioprosthetic valves as well.[11] Constrictive pericarditis may also occur and may contribute to cardiac dysfunction.[12] Although the left side of the heart is usually spared, a bronchial carcinoid — draining vasoactive amines directly into the heart thus circumventing lung inactivation — may cause left heart involvement. In the series reported by Pellikka et al[10] left-sided valvular involvement was present in 5/74 (7%) of patients. The carcinoid tumor involved the lung in one patient and three patients had a patent foramen ovale, with a right to left shunt. Typically, the mitral and aortic valves showed regurgitant lesions.

The development of right-sided heart failure is an indication for investigation of the tricuspid and pulmonary valves and if necessary, replacement of either or both valves is advisable. Right ventricular failure is a major cause of death in carcinoid disease and is underdiagnosed in clinical practice.[13] Valve replacement in older patients has significant morbidity and mortal-ity.[14] The Minnesota group correlated low limb-lead voltage (i.e. 5 mm) on the preoperative electrocardiogram (ECG) as a predictor of operative mortality. The predictors of late survival included a lower preoperative somatostatin requirement and a lower preoperative level of urinary 5-hydoxy indoleacetic acid (5-HIAA),[14] the principal metabolite of serotonin. Hemodynamic instability may occur because of heart failure or treatment with somatostatin, which has negative inotropic properties.[15] Data from the Duke Carcinoid Database suggests that 30-day mortality following tricuspid valve replacement was 21%. The predictors for mortality were advanced age (>60 years) and the presence of comorbidity.[16] The authors concluded that, although valve replacement can provide prolonged palliation from carcinoid heart disease, it is associated with significant mortality risk. The so-called hepatopulmonary syndrome has been described in carcinoid disease and is believed to be due to intrapulmonary shunting secondary to an imbalance of vasoconstrictor and vasodilator amines.[17]

Treatment

Symptomatic control of the diarrhea associated with carcinoid disease can usually be achieved with loperamide and codeine phosphate. The use of cyproheptadine, a histamine (H_1) and serotonin receptor antagonist, to reduce cutaneous flushing has been superseded by more specific agents, such as ketanserin,[18] a 5-HT_2 receptor antagonist. Ondasetron, a 5-HT_3 receptor antagonist, may be used to control nausea and vomiting.[19]

The introduction of octreotide, a long-acting synthetic somatostatin analog that acts by inhibiting the release of vasoactive substances rather than block their effects, has revolutionized the medical treatment of carcinoid disease. Somatostatin analogs play an important role both in treatment and diagnosis of carcinoid tumors. Somatostatin binds to somatostatin receptors, which belong to the family of G-protein receptors and their activation results in inhibition of adenyl cyclase, decreased conductance of calcium channels, activation of potassium channels and stimulation of tyrosine phosphatase activity.[20] Five subtypes of somatostatin receptors have been identified and octreotide binds to three of them. Although its exact mechanism is unknown, somatostatin and its analogs octreotide and lanreotide act upon somatostatin receptors inhibiting the release of pituitary and gastrointestinal hormones such as serotonin, gastrin, vasoactive intestinal protein, secretin, motilin, insulin, growth hormone, and thyrotropin. In carcinoid syndrome, the use of octreotide and lanreotide results in decreased flushing, diarrhea, wheezing, and urinary 5-HIAA excretion. Radiolabelled somatostatin analogs can be used as a tool for the diagnosis and location of small carcinoid tumors. Antagonist drugs are used when octreotide fails to control symptoms. Octreotide can be administered as subcutaneous injections or as a constant infusion at the rate of 100 µg h^{-1} during surgery with additional boluses of 100 µg to treat a crisis.

Aprotonin, an inhibitor of kallikrein in vitro, has been advocated in the management of patients undergoing carcinoid tumor surgery.[13] The additional benefit of reduced bleeding during cardiac surgery suggests that aprotinin may be a useful adjunct in the management of carcinoid heart disease. Suggested dosing regimens include bolus doses ranging from 20 000 to 400 000 Kiu, and infusions of 50 000 and 100 000 Kiu h^{-1}. Recently published data, however, suggest that much larger doses of aprotinin are required to achieve plasma levels (i.e. $\geq$200 Kiu ml^{-1}) necessary to inhibit kallikrein.[21] When used in combination with octreotide, the antineoplastic agent interferon has been shown to prolong survival in patients with metastatic gastroenteropancreatic tumors.[22] The addition of interferon alpha to somatostatin analog therapy frequently results in an improvement in symptoms that are resistant to somatostatin analogs alone.[23]

Anesthetic management

Anesthesia for patients with carcinoid syndrome is best performed as a planned procedure. The goal of anesthesia is to prevent a carcinoid crisis that may be provoked by anxiety, surgical stimulation and manipulation of the tumor itself. The anesthetist should be familiar with the features of carcinoid crisis: flushing, diaphoresis, tachycardia, hypertension or hypotension, dysrhythmia, confusion and coma. Acute anaphylaxis should be considered as a differential diagnosis.[24]

As previously mentioned, patients may be malnourished, and have fluid and electrolyte disturbances secondary to chronic diarrhea and pellagra.[4] Electrolyte and fluid deficits have to be meticulously replaced before surgery. Concurrent anticarcinoid therapy should be continued. Benzodiazepine premedication is advocated while the use of opiates (e.g. morphine) is discouraged because of the histamine release that accompanies their administration. Histamine (H$_1$ and H$_2$) antagonists may also be useful in reducing the effects of systemic histamine release. An infusion of octreotide 100 µg h^{-1} should be started at the time of premedication and continued into the perioperative period.

Invasive monitoring is mandatory in all cases, although insertion of a pulmonary artery catheter may be difficult, or indeed impossible, in the presence of severe tricuspid regurgitation and/or pulmonary stenosis. If used, a pulmonary artery catheter should be withdrawn during valve replacement. Surgery on the right side precludes use of a transvenous pacing lead hence external transcutaneous pacing should be considered as an option for rate control before skin incision. Transesophageal echocardiography can be used to monitor ventricular function, assist deairing and confirm adequate prosthetic valve function. Etomidate, thiopentone and propofol[25] have been used successfully to induce anesthesia without undue hemodynamic instability. Anesthesia may be maintained with either an infusion of propofol or inhaled isoflurane. Fentanyl provides good analgesia during surgery and lacks the histamine releasing properties of morphine. Virtually any non-depolarizing muscle relaxant may be used. Both tubocurarine and atracurium may cause histamine release. Nevertheless, atracurium may be of use in the presence of significant hepatic dysfunction.

Inotropic agents have traditionally been considered contraindicated in carcinoid disease as their use may cause release of tumor kallikrein, which in turn activates bradykinins resulting in hypotension. For this reason, it has been suggested that catecholamines should be avoided in carcinoid syndrome.[26] The advice to exclude epinephrine from therapeutic options extends to advisory sites on the World Wide Web.[27] More recently, however, epinephrine has been used successfully, and without incident, to treat hypotension following CPB in a patient with carcinoid disease.[25] It should be borne in mind that the recommendation to avoid catecholamines comes from the presomatostatin era.[29] The observation that somatostatin decreases epinephrine-induced kallikrein release, indicates that epinephrine is relatively safe in this setting and should be used if necessary. Evidence that somatostatin may have negative inotropic properties support this suggestion.[15] Alternatives to epinephrine include angiotensin and the phosphodiesterase inhibitor, enoximone.

An infusion of either fentanyl or pethidine may be used for postoperative analgesia. Continuing octreotide in the postoperative period is of paramount importance for successful outcome.

Conclusions and learning points

- Carcinoid syndrome is a distressing disease occurring in some patients with carcinoid tumors.
- Right ventricular failure carries a bad prognosis.
- Continuous administration of octreotide by infusion should reduce the incidence of carcinoid crises and leads to a smooth perioperative course.

References

1. Lubrarsch O. Uber den primaren des ileum, nebst bemerkungen uber das gleichzeitige vorkommen von kerbs und tuberkolose. *Virchows Arch* 1888;**111**:280–317.

2. Oberndorfer S. Karzinoide tumoren des dunndarms. *Frankf Z Pathol* 1907;**1**:425–429.

3. Modlin IM, Sandor A. An analysis of 8305 cases of carcinoid tumors. *Cancer* 1997;**79**:813–29.

4. Veall GR, Peacock JE, Bax ND, Reilly CS. Review of the anaesthetic management of 21 patients undergoing laparotomy for carcinoid syndrome. *Br J Anaesth* 1994;**72**:335–41.

5. Godwin JD. Carcinoid tumors. An analysis of 2 837 cases. *Cancer* 1975;**36**:560–9.

6. Mehta AC, Rafanan AL, Bulkley R et al. Coronary spasm and cardiac arrest from carcinoid crisis during laser bronchoscopy. *Chest* 1999;**115**:598–600.

7. Lippmann M, Cleveland RJ. Anesthetic management of a carcinoid patient undergoing tricuspid valve replacement. *Anesth Analg* 1973;**52**:768–71.

8. Lundin L, Norheim I, Landelius J et al. Carcinoid heart disease: relationship of circulating vasoactive substances to ultrasound-detectable cardiac abnormalities. *Circulation* 1988;**77**:264–9.

9. Connolly HM, Crary JL, McGoon MD et al. Valvular heart disease associated with fenfluramine-phentermine. *N Engl J Med* 1997;**337**:581–8.

10. Pellikka PA, Tajik AJ, Khandheria BK et al. Carcinoid heart disease. Clinical and echocardiographic spectrum in 74 patients. *Circulation* 1993;**87**:1188–96.

11. Ridker PM, Chertow GM, Karlson EW et al. Bioprosthetic tricuspid valve stenosis associated with extensive plaque deposition in carcinoid heart disease. *Am Heart J* 1991;**121**:1835–8.

12. Johnston SD, Johnston PW, O'Rourke D. Carcinoid constrictive pericarditis. *Heart* 1999;**82**:641–3.

13. Holdcroft A. Hormones and the gut. *Br J Anaesth* 2000;**85**:58–68.

14. Connolly HM, Nishimura RA, Smith HC et al. Outcome of cardiac surgery for carcinoid heart disease. *J Am Coll Cardiol* 1995;**25**:410–6.

15. Zonta F, Dondi G, Barbieri A, Grana E. Study of the negative inotropic action of somatostatin. *Arch Int Pharmacodyn Ther* 1989;**300**:149–58.

16. Robiolio PA, Rigolin VH, Harrison JK et al. Predictors of outcome of tricuspid valve replacement in carcinoid heart disease. *Am J Cardiol* 1995;**75**:485–8.

17. Lee DF, Lepler LS. Severe intrapulmonary shunting associated with metastatic carcinoid. *Chest* 1999;**115**:1203–7.

18. Houghton K, Carter JA. Peri-operative management of carcinoid syndrome using ketanserin. *Anaesthesia* 1986;**41**:596–9.

19. Wilde MI, Markham A. Ondansetron. A review of its pharmacology and preliminary clinical findings in novel applications. *Drugs* 1996;**52**:773–94.

20. Reisine T, Bell GI. Molecular biology of somato-statin receptors. *Endocr Rev* 1995;**16**:427–42.

21. Levy JH, Bailey JM, Salmenpera M. Pharmacokinetics of aprotinin in preoperative cardiac surgical patients. *Anesthesiology* 1994;**80**:1013–8.

22. Frank M, Klose KJ, Wied M *et al.* Combination therapy with octreotide and alpha-interferon: effect on tumor growth in metastatic endocrine gastroenteropan-creatic tumors. *Am J Gastroenterol* 1999;**94**:1381–7.

23. Öberg K, Funa K, Alm G. Effects of leukocyte inter-feron on clinical symptoms and hormone levels in patients with mid-gut carcinoid tumors and carci-noid syndrome. *N Engl J Med* 1983;**309**:129–33.

24. Batchelor AM, Conacher ID. Anaphylactoid or carci-noid? *Br J Anaesth* 1992;**69**:325–7.

25. Pratila MG, Pratilas V. Propofol infusion in carcinoid syndrome. *Can J Anaesth* 1991;**38**:943–4.

26. Levine J, Sjoerdsma A. Pressor amines and the carcinoid flush. *Ann Intern Med* 1963;**58**:818–28.

27. Warner RR. Diagnosis, treatment, and management of carcinoid cancer. http://www.carcinoid.org.

28. Hamid SK, Harris DN. Hypotension following valve replacement surgery in carcinoid heart disease. *Anaesthesia* 1992;**47**:490–2.

29. Cross MH. Catecholamines and the carcinoid syndrome. *Anaesthesia* 1993;**48**:81–2.

30. Creutzfeldt W, Stockmann F. Carcinoids and carci-noid syndrome. *Am J Med* 1987;**82**:4–16.

Suggested further reading

Kulke MH, Mayer RJ. Carcinoid tumors. *N Engl J Med* 1999;**340**:858–68.

Index

T - #0326 - 101024 - C0 - 246/189/17 [19] - CB - 9781841841380 - Gloss Lamination